Mind-Body Medicine in Children and Adolescents

Special Issue Editor
Hilary McClafferty

MDPI • Basel • Beijing • Wuhan • Barcelona • Belgrade

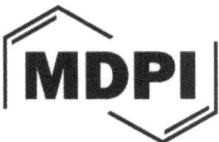

MDPI

Special Issue Editor
Hilary McClafferty
University of Arizona College of Medicine
USA

Editorial Office
MDPI AG
St. Alban-Anlage 66
Basel, Switzerland

This edition is a reprint of the Special Issue published online in the open access journal *Children* (ISSN 2227-9067) in 2017 (available at: http://www.mdpi.com/journal/children/special_issues/mind_body_medicine).

For citation purposes, cite each article independently as indicated on the article page online and as indicated below:

Author 1; Author 2. Article title. *Journal Name* **Year**, *Article number*, page range.

First Edition 2017

ISBN 978-3-03842-528-1 (Pbk)
ISBN 978-3-03842-529-8 (PDF)

Table of Contents

About the Special Issue Editor

Hilary McClafferty, MD, FAAP is an Associate Professor in the Department of Medicine and is Board certified in pediatrics, pediatric emergency medicine, and integrative medicine. Dr. McClafferty received her medical degree from the University of Michigan, Ann Arbor, Michigan, and completed pediatric residency training at Northwestern Children's Memorial Hospital in Chicago, Illinois, and at the University of Arizona in Tucson, Arizona. She is fellowship trained in pediatric emergency medicine through The Children's Hospital, Denver, Colorado, certified in clinical hypnosis through the American Society of Clinical Hypnosis, and trained in medical acupuncture through the University of California, Los Angeles/Helm's Medical Institute. She completed her fellowship training in integrative medicine through University of Arizona Center for Integrative Medicine in 2005 and returned to join the Center's faculty in 2011. She is a leader of the fellowship and Director of the Pediatric Integrative Medicine in Residency program, an international program designed to embed pediatric integrative medicine into residency training, a program that now serves more than 500 residents and faculty. She is immediate past chair of the American Academy of Pediatrics Section on Integrative Medicine and chair of the initiative for Physician Health and Wellness in the Academy. Dr. McClafferty is a founding member of the American Board of Integrative Medicine and serves as Secretary of the Executive Board. She is the author of the textbook: Integrative Pediatrics, Art, Science, and Clinical Application, CRC Press/Taylor Francis Group.

children

MDPI

Editorial

Mind-Body Medicine in Pediatrics

Hilary McClafferty [1,2]

[1] Pediatric Integrative Medicine in Residency, University of Arizona Center for Integrative Medicine, Tucson, AZ 85724, USA; hmcclafferty@email.arizona.edu

[2] Department of Medicine, University of Arizona College of Medicine, Tucson, AZ 85724, USA

Academic Editor: Sari A. Acra

Received: 22 August 2017; Accepted: 24 August 2017; Published: 25 August 2017

Abstract: The primary goals of this Special Issue are to encourage readers to become more familiar with the range of mind-body therapies and to explore their application in the pediatric clinical setting. The Special Issue includes a deliberate mix of case studies and practical clinical guidance, with the dual goals of piquing curiosity and providing resources for clinicians interested in pursuing further training.

Keywords: mind-body medicine; new therapies; self-efficacy

The field of mind-body medicine holds significant promise for children and adolescents. Growing recognition of the intricate connections between thought, emotion, and physiology highlights the need for new therapies that leverage inner resources and offer non-invasive treatment options. Modern imaging techniques such as functional magnetic resonance imaging (fMRI) have advanced our understanding and appreciation of how the mind-body therapies can benefit health, increasing confidence in their use and propelling them into the mainstream of medicine. Mind-body therapies have special value in addressing pain, fear, and stress that accompanies many pediatric medical encounters. Some of the mind-body therapies such as mindfulness, have their roots in ancient traditions and are now being used routinely in the practice of pediatric integrative medicine, an emerging field focused on preventive health that blends conventional and evidence-based complementary therapies [1,2].

The primary goals of this Special Issue are to encourage readers to become more familiar with the range of mind-body therapies and to explore their application in the pediatric clinical setting. The Issue builds on the recent American Academy of Pediatrics Clinical Report: Mind-body Therapies in Children and Adolescents, which provides background and literature updates on several of the most commonly used mind-body therapies including biofeedback, clinical hypnosis, guided imagery, meditation, and yoga [3]. The Special Issue includes a deliberate mix of case studies and practical clinical guidance, with the dual goals of piquing curiosity and providing resources for clinicians interested in pursuing further training.

A central theme of the Special Issue is the importance of enhancing self-efficacy in pediatric patients. The mind-body therapies are unique in that mastery can occur even in the very young, for example the use of relaxation exercises and self-hypnosis techniques in preschoolers. They are also highly versatile and are used in a range of clinical settings, from outpatient clinic to intensive care unit. A child who can acquire even an incremental sense of self-efficacy in a stressful environment will build resilience and ideally gain age-appropriate perspective that can build coping skills. The use of mind-body therapies may also facilitate emotional resilience in other venues, for example in school, sports, or performance arts.

A corollary benefit of use of the mind-body therapies is the potential for stress reduction in the child's caretakers, who can experience extraordinary stress while supporting a child through a medical experience. A third beneficiary are clinicians. The ability to provide options for treatment that are less invasive, cost-effective, and non-pharmacologic has potential to decrease clinician stress and hopefully contribute to reduction of burnout prevalence.

The Issue's contributing authors come from an impressive array of leading academic and private practice centers and are experts in their respective fields. They include specialists in research, infectious disease, psychology, adolescent medicine, neonatology, developmental-behavioral pediatrics, anesthesiology, pediatric intensive care, and general pediatrics. Topics covered touch on some of the most pressing concerns of clinicians and parents, including: childhood stress and trauma—especially related to adverse childhood events; acute, chronic, and perioperative pain; mental health; behavioral and developmental issues; and autoimmune illness such as inflammatory bowel disease.

The mind-body therapies discussed here can be used alone or blended with conventional therapies and include: mindfulness; medical yoga; technology assisted relaxation approaches such as biofeedback; cognitive-behavioral treatment; clinical hypnosis theory and application; neonatal massage; mind-body interventions in pediatric inflammatory bowel disease; mind-body therapies for children with attention deficit-hyperactivity disorder; and the emerging field of immersive virtual reality in pediatric pain patients.

For some clinicians, considering the use of mind-body therapies stretches their definition of 'real medicine'. This may be a result of training bias, personal experience, or insufficient familiarity with the accruing body of research in the field. I encourage readers to peruse this Special Issue with an open mind and, ideally, to entertain the question of not whether, but how the introduction of mind-body therapies into practice could benefit their patients and families.

Conflicts of Interest: The author declares no conflict of interest.

References

1. McClafferty, H.; Dodds, S.; Brooks, A.J.; Brenner, M.G.; Brown, M.L.; Frazer, P.; Mark, J.D.; Weydert, J.A.; Wilcox, G.M.G.; Lebensohn, P.; et al. Pediatric Integrative Medicine in Residency (PIMR): Description of a New Online Educational Curriculum. *Children* **2015**, *2*, 98–107. [CrossRef] [PubMed]
2. Vohra, S.; Surette, S.; Mittra, D.; Rosen, L.D.; Gardiner, P.; Kemper, K.J. Pediatric integrative medicine: Pediatrics' newest subspecialty? *BMC Pediatr.* **2012**, *12*, 123. [CrossRef] [PubMed]
3. AAP SOIM. Mind-Body Therapies in Children and Youth. *Pediatrics* **2016**, *138*, e20161896. [CrossRef]

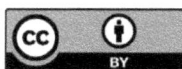

Review

The Role of Mindfulness in Reducing the Adverse Effects of Childhood Stress and Trauma

Robin Ortiz [1] and Erica M. Sibinga [2,*]

[1]   Departments of Internal Medicine and Pediatrics Johns Hopkins Hospital, 1800 Orleans Street,
      Baltimore, MD 21231, USA, Robin.Ortiz@jhmi.edu
[2]   Johns Hopkins School of Medicine, 733 North Broadway, Baltimore, MD 21205, USA
*   Correspondence: esibinga@jhmi.edu

Academic Editor: Hilary McClafferty
Received: 26 January 2016; Accepted: 21 February 2017; Published: 28 February 2017

Abstract: Research suggests that many children are exposed to adverse experiences in childhood. Such adverse childhood exposures may result in stress and trauma, which are associated with increased morbidity and mortality into adulthood. In general populations and trauma-exposed adults, mindfulness interventions have demonstrated reduced depression and anxiety, reduced trauma-related symptoms, enhanced coping and mood, and improved quality of life. Studies in children and youth also demonstrate that mindfulness interventions improve mental, behavioral, and physical outcomes. Taken together, this research suggests that high-quality, structured mindfulness instruction may mitigate the negative effects of stress and trauma related to adverse childhood exposures, improving short- and long-term outcomes, and potentially reducing poor health outcomes in adulthood. Future work is needed to optimize implementation of youth-based mindfulness programs and to study long-term outcomes into adulthood.

Keywords: trauma; mindfulness; adverse childhood events; resilience; MBSR; mind-body; ACEs; at-risk youth; childhood adversity; toxic stress; allostatic load

1. Introduction

The evidence continues to mount that exposure to adverse experiences during childhood has the potential to increase morbidity and mortality both during childhood and across the lifespan into adulthood [1]. Adverse childhood experiences (ACEs) are stressful for children, and include neglect; physical, sexual or emotional abuse; exposure to violence, mental illness, incarceration, or substance abuse in the family; parental absence due to divorce or separation; and low socioeconomic status. Further, significant, traumatic, recurrent, and/or prolonged stress may have a cumulative toxic effect on the child [2,3]. In addition to the psychological toll, stress and toxic stress effect the body through increased allostatic load, the physiologic burden of such stress that may manifest as neuroanatomical changes, increased levels of inflammation, and dysfunction of the hypothalamic-pituitary-adrenal axis [4]. More recent findings are emerging suggesting that resilience, i.e., successful management of and coping with stress, can mitigate the negative consequences of such trauma [5,6]. Findings such as these have sparked a call to action for pediatricians to both recognize that, "many adult diseases should be viewed as developmental disorders that begin early in life and that persistent health disparities associated with poverty, discrimination, or maltreatment could be reduced by the alleviation of toxic stress in childhood" and "to serve as both front-line guardians of healthy child development and strategically positioned, community leaders to inform new science-based strategies that build strong foundations for educational achievement, economic productivity, responsible citizenship, and lifelong health" [2]. This is an emphatic call to work together to enhance the prevention of ACEs, provide early and accessible interventions, and broadly expand the delivery of trauma-informed care. Mindfulness is an evidence-based intervention that supports these important responses to ACEs, fundamentally enhancing self-regulation and resilience in everyday life and in the face of stress and trauma.

This review aims to identify the benefits of mindfulness-based interventions as an approach to mitigating the negative sequelae of childhood trauma by summarizing relevant research in adult and pediatric populations. Additionally, the adaptations for introducing and teaching mindfulness for children and youth will be reviewed. Finally, future directions in the research and clinical realms related to trauma-informed mindfulness interventions will be suggested.

2. ACEs and Trauma

Research suggests that children are often exposed to significant environmental stressors and situational adversities [7]. A Centers for Disease Control and Prevention (CDC) report from five states in 2009 showed that 69% of respondents (n = 26,229) report at least one adverse childhood event (ACE) with 9% experiencing up to five adversities [7]. A smaller study of children found 34% of those screened in school report exposure to at least one trauma and evidence of post-traumatic stress even without a current diagnosis [8]. One of the first studies of ACEs (including traumas such as abuse, neglect, witnessing violence against mother, substance use in the home, household mental illness, parental separation or divorce, or household member incarcerated) showed that not only do ACEs cluster together, but there is a dose response relationship with overall health, such that larger numbers of ACEs are associated with poorer health [1]. Other adversities associated with a risk for exposure to trauma include low socioeconomic status and the associated lower education [9] and risky family environments [10,11]. Such negative experiences in the absence of a protective buffer may manifest as toxic stress, yielding an increased allostatic load to the body causing prolonged activation of physiologic stress responses, which over time may yield poor health outcomes and future illness [3,4,12]. For example, ACEs have been associated with biological markers of disease risk including inflammatory cytokines, metabolic abnormalities, and epigenetic modifications [4,13,14] (Figure 1). Remarkably, such epigenetic modifications may carry across generations, as identified in the glucocorticoid receptor related gene *FKBP5* of holocaust survivors also found in their offspring [15]. Toxic stress can result from different situations, including single stressors that are prolonged in exposure (such as recurrent emotional abuse), multiple stressors that become toxic when aggregated (such as low socioeconomic status), living below the poverty line and having limited educational opportunity, and/or traumatic experiences of greater emotional intensity or severity (such as sexual abuse).

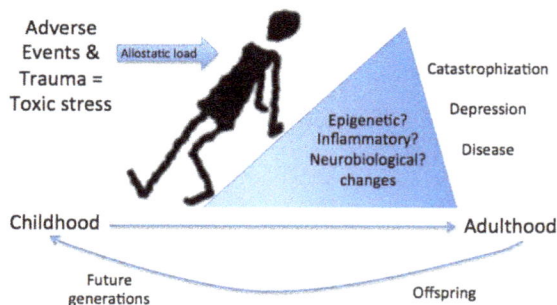

Figure 1. The impact of stress and trauma in childhood. Adverse childhood events, stress, and trauma contribute to toxic stress. Toxic stress that results from prolonged exposure to stress, aggregated trauma experiences, or incidents of significant emotional impact yields an increased allostatic load on the body. Allostatic load, measured by biological markers of disease risk including inflammatory cytokines, neurobiological changes, metabolic abnormalities, and epigenetic modifications, may carry over into future generations.

Specific ACEs, such as those associated with an adverse living environment limited in support and opportunity, have been shown to be associated with negative health outcomes. Such an adverse environment encompasses socioeconomic factors (such as household income, education of parents, and occupational prestige of parents), and risky family environment (such as living with a household member with a substance use disorder, mental illness or history of incarceration, living in a chaotic or disorganized environment, or experiencing violence and lack of parental warmth) [10]. Low socioeconomic status (SES) is associated with reduced access to educational support, or parental involvement in education [16]. Similarly, household chaos is associated with sensitive and harsh parenting, both of which predict childhood misconduct [17]. Low SES also seems to be associated with developmental delay (specifically, a delay in cognitive development of executive functioning including working memory, inhibitory control, and cognitive flexibility), poor conduct, and callous behaviors [17–19]. These lead to consequences of transition to adulthood such that lower SES and early life stress influence both cognitive and associated neurobiological development, which are also associated with poor health outcomes in adulthood and comorbid metabolic and cardiovascular dysfunction [20,21]. Further, adverse living environment, may predispose to the development of characteristics and behaviors that are risk factors for multiple comorbidities, including obesity, smoking, and increased blood pressure trajectory, throughout adolescence into adulthood, and are further specifically associated with metabolic dysfunction and cardiovascular disease in adulthood [10,22–24]. Risky family environments have also been associated with dysfunctional emotional processing, mood disorders, and hypothalamic-pituitary-adrenal (HPA) axis dysfunction [25].

There is diversity in both the types of traumatic experiences that may exist in childhood and the broad systems that may be affected. ACEs are associated with increased poor and risky health behaviors including substance use, smoking, risky sexual activity, and sedentary lifestyle in adulthood. ACEs also show a graded relationship with the presence of mental health disorders, adult ischemic heart disease, cancer, chronic lung disease, skeletal fractures, and liver disease in a study of 9508 Americans in 1998 [1]. In addition, ACEs have also been associated with alcoholism [26], chronic obstructive pulmonary disease [27], autoimmune disease [28], quality of life [29], drug use [23], risk for intimate partner violence [30], sexually transmitted diseases [31], suicide attempts [32], maladjustment and misconduct in and outside of school, as well as risk for incarceration [33,34]. Importantly, many of these conditions begin early in childhood and are reversible or preventable by mitigating risk factors.

Studies have also identified associations between childhood adversity and trauma and specific adult diagnoses including fibromyalgia [35], migraine [36], irritable bowel syndrome [37], insomnia and insufficient sleep [38], cancer [39], cognitive function in mental health disorders [40], as well as learning and behavior problems and obesity in youth [41] and adolescent pregnancy and fetal death [42]. Collectively, this research suggests the significant and pervasive negative impact of childhood ACEs and trauma on short- and long-term health outcomes, and therefore, the necessity and opportunity to prevent and intervene on ACEs, and to provide trauma-informed services broadly to offset the negative consequences in children, the adults they will become, and possibly even future generations.

3. Mindfulness

Mindfulness has origins as a Buddhist concept increased through meditation that has been cultivated into a Western practice of present-focused, non-judgmental awareness [43]. Mindfulness instruction has also been offered through structured training programs such as that developed by Jon Kabat-Zinn in 1979 to enhance non-judgmental attention to the experience of the present moment, entitled Mindfulness Based Stress Reduction (MBSR) [43]. The MBSR program has been shown to increase self-reported mindfulness among participants [44,45]. However, all individuals have the capacity for mindfulness, i.e., non-reactivity, awareness, focus, attention, and nonjudgment [45], though there is variability in the amount and quality of mindfulness among individuals. Therefore, both structured MBSR and unstructured mindfulness practices outside of the MBSR model, may enhance the beneficial characteristics associated with mindfulness.

Structured mindfulness training is available through Kabat-Zinn's MBSR, which typically consists of eight weekly two-and-a-half-hour classes and a full-day retreat, in which participants learn a variety of formal and informal mindfulness practices, learn and discuss the mind-body connection, and have group discussions regarding the challenges to integrating mindfulness into one's life. For particular populations, other programs have been adapted from MBSR, such as Mindfulness-Based Cognitive Therapy (MBCT), shown to be effective in reducing depression recurrences, and one focused on addiction triggers, Mindfulness Based Relapse Prevention (MBRP) [46, 47]. Unstandardized mindfulness may also be offered in other formats such as aspects of educational sessions, art therapy, group therapy, yoga, or other mind-body interventions. Though this review will focus on standardized MBSR and MBSR-related programs to highlight evidence for their practice, there will be brief discussion of the practice and implications of other mindfulness delivery methods.

3.1. Mindfulness in Trauma

Mindfulness instruction has been shown to benefit individuals with a known trauma or ACE. Mindfulness may do this by both an indirect effect of negating the acute response to trauma and stress, but also by inhibiting underlying consequences of chronic exposure to stress and trauma such as psychiatric, metabolic and cardiovascular disease through the influence on lifestyle choices, underlying biochemistry and neurobiology (Figure 2). In 50 women exposed to trauma including witnessing family violence, experiencing childhood physical or sexual abuse, or sudden loss of a loved one, an 8-week MBSR program was associated with decreased symptoms of stress and trauma exposure including perceived stress, depression, trait and state anxiety, emotion dysregulation, and posttraumatic stress symptoms [48]. Additionally, 27 female survivors of sexual abuse in childhood, experienced significantly reduced symptoms of depression, posttraumatic stress disorder (PTSD), and anxiety after an 8-week MBSR intervention [49]. This beneficial effect continued at follow-up 2.5 years later [50], which highlights that mindfulness may have an effect on the formation of related psychiatric comorbidities. This was demonstrated in two populations at risk for high rates of trauma and/or ACEs and related psychiatric disease. In a group of incarcerated women (n = 33) improvements in perceived stress, anxiety and depression were seen with a 12-week mindfulness intervention [51]. In a small qualitative study of a population of survivors (n = 12) of political violence, when mindfulness was combined with art therapy in a unique 4-day intensive program, themes of resilience emerged [52].

Research also suggests a role for mindfulness to mitigate consequences of toxic stress, by identifying benefit in individuals exposed to high stress environments by both enhancing long-term coping, and influencing the related physiologic effects of stress on the HPA axis. Klatt et al. studied intensive care unit workers finding that a mindfulness intervention was linked to increased resilience [53]. In active duty military personnel preparing for deployment, mindfulness was shown to mitigate the response to stressful experience [54], which suggests that it may both reduce current stress experience and predispose to enhanced coping prior to stress exposure. However, mindfulness, additionally, has lasting effects beyond exposure to prolonged stress as demonstrated by numerous studies in veteran populations and those exposed to war and bereavement. Veterans (n = 58) who participated in an 8-week long mindfulness intervention including a day long retreat, saw clinically significant improvements in their Post Traumatic Stress Disorder (PTSD) symptoms up to 17 weeks afterward, and another study suggests a shorter duration (n = 62, 4-session program) intervention may also decrease PTSD symptoms though only studied up to 8-weeks post [55,56]. The same group found that mindfulness also decreased cortisol levels in the veterans [57]. To suggest that this may be a global effect, other studies have supported these similar findings. A study that used mindfulness through mantra based meditation also showed decreased PTSD symptoms in veterans [58]. In one of the largest mindfulness studies of the veteran population, a mediation program that elicited mindfulness as an outcome, also reduced PTSD symptoms in 391 veterans in a uniquely implemented Department of Veteran Affairs meditation program through six medical centers [59]. In veterans with mental health comorbidities mindfulness improved sleep quality [60].

These underlying influences of mindfulness may mitigate mental health outcomes, enhance quality of life, and reduce somatic symptoms. A short 4-session intervention incorporating mindfulness in the mind-body approach, modestly increased resilience and also decreased depressive and anxiety symptoms and perceived stress in veterans though only assessed post-intervention [61]. These effects translate to improvements in quality of life [62] with a reduction in somatic symptoms including dizziness, fatigue and tension in addition to depressive symptoms as shown in veterans with PTSD [63]. Undergraduates ages 18–36, who participated in a mindfulness activity interrelated with expressive writing exercises about a past stress or trauma demonstrated decreased physical symptoms, poor sleep, and negative affect; with beneficial findings apparently linked to the mindfulness component, given expressive writing alone was not predictive of improvement [64]. Mindfulness is also inversely associated with functional disability in Iraq and Afghanistan war veterans (n = 115) [65], and with PTSD in a trauma exposed Iranian population (n = 1708) [66]. It may also offer protection in burn-out and compassion fatigue, such as in a study of traumatic bereavement workers [67].

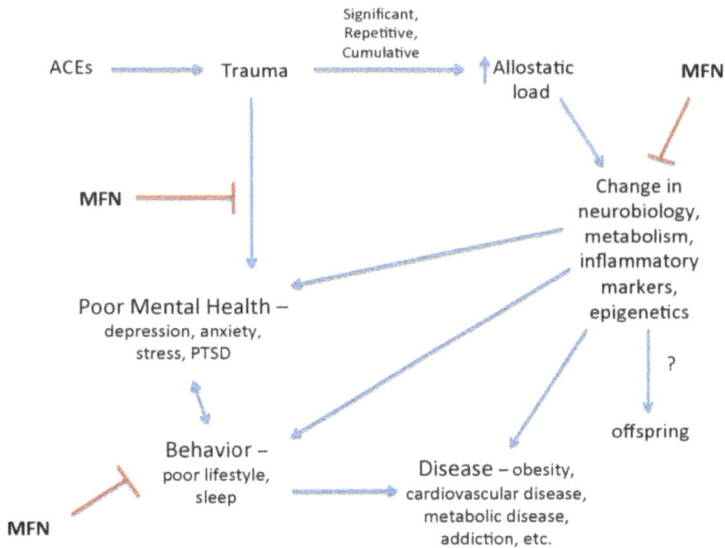

Figure 2. The negative impact of adverse childhood events (ACEs) and trauma in childhood is reduced by mindfulness (MFN). Mindfulness has been shown to mitigate the psychological, behavioral, and physiological changes associated with ACEs and trauma and increased allostatic load. MFN, specifically, reduces symptoms of depression and posttraumatic stress disorder (PTSD) associated with stress and trauma, and is inversely associated with poor health behavior and biological makers of metabolic, neurologic, and inflammatory dysfunction and disease. Stress has been demonstrated to be associated with epigenetic modifications that may persist in offspring; therefore, mindfulness interventions may reduce these negative influences.

Further, research has shown that these beneficial effects of mindfulness may be generalizable to healthy populations, regardless of known exposure to stress and trauma. In large meta-analyses, mindfulness was shown to reduce stress in healthy adult individuals [68] and to reduce anxiety, depression, and pain in diverse clinical populations [69]. Mindfulness is inversely related to anxiety, experiential avoidance, distress and uncertainty, external stimulus reactivity (poorer executive control), and persistence of negative affect [70,71]. Mindfulness programs can improve coping and resiliency in specific conditions including quality of life in patients with multiple sclerosis [72], depression and anxiety in patients with cancer [73], and specifically in trauma-exposed individuals with human immunodeficiency virus (HIV), can reduce PTSD symptoms [74].

Importantly, the beneficial effects of mindfulness on psychological and somatic symptoms and foundations for disease extend beyond negating the psychological impact of stress and may influence physiologic dysfunction (Figure 2). In general, mindfulness has been modestly associated with alterations in markers of inflammation, cell-mediated immunity, and biological aging [75]. Specifically, in women with interpersonal trauma ($n = 50$), not only were their psychological symptoms improved, as discussed above, but their inflammatory cytokine, interleukin-6 (IL-6) levels decreased [48]. Mindfulness has neurobiological modification potential as demonstrated by enhanced resting state functional connectivity as well as executive control via the dorsolateral prefrontal cortex, both coinciding with decreased levels of peripheral IL-6 levels [76]. Such biomarkers may be modulated by epigenetic changes through, histone-modifying enzymes also found to be associated with mindfulness interventions [77]. These neurobiological changes may represent modifications that can influence behavior and disease risk factors in adults and possibly the predisposition to disease in children, especially those at higher risk when exposed to stress, trauma, and/or toxic stress.

Though children may be exposed to different types of trauma then adults, these studies collectively suggest that mindfulness may serve to buffer the effects of stress and trauma in children and into adulthood.

3.2. Mindfulness in Youth

Recent mindfulness studies in youth, specifically in populations with known trauma exposure or populations at high risk for ACEs suggest promise in improving a variety of outcomes, including mental health symptoms, behavior and quality of life, and coping (Table 1). In one randomized control trial (RCT) of a population of urban youth in a low-income environment, middle-school age male children ($n = 41$) underwent a 12-week school-based mindfulness intervention that resulted in decreased negative coping [78]. The group additionally yielded decreases in anxiety and rumination and possibly school related stress response as suggested by a flatter cortisol curve over the course of the study (three months) and school term compared to the attention, social experience and time matched control, health education group. A larger RCT in two urban public middle schools ($n = 300$) showed that the 12-week, school-based MBSR program led to reduced depression, self-hostility, negative affect, negative coping, rumination, somatization, and post-trauma stress symptoms [79]. Additionally, one study of mindfulness in youth in foster care, ages 14–21 ($n = 42$), showed a trend toward post-intervention changes in state anxiety, qualitative gains in-group effectiveness in social gains, and coping with stress was observed [80].

These studies with foster care youth and in urban low-resourced areas likely represent children affected by or at risk for on-going stresses, and/or trauma [78–82], especially illustrated by the reduction in post-stress trauma symptoms in the MBSR arm. Other studies also support the promising hypothesis that mindfulness may offer coping skills, emotional processing and resilience. Many of these studies are done in the school environment. In a RCT of 522 children ages 12–16, the mindfulness arm post-intervention outcomes included lower stress, greater well-being, and fewer depressive symptoms [83]. It is important to note that the control group in this study was a usual school curriculum and did not control for peer experience, attention, or time. In a study of 101 sixth grade children, a 6-week mindfulness curriculum decreased suicidal ideation and self-harm [84] compared to a matched experiential activity control group. Though this study did not show an effect on internalizing or externalizing problems, others have demonstrated it to improve classroom behavior, and attention [85,86] (Table 1). Mindfulness may also offset the psychiatric comorbidities accompanied by traumatic experiences that impact the lives of youth in and outside of the classroom. Biegel and colleagues showed that 104 adolescents ages 14–18 benefited with improved state anxiety, sleep, stress, self-esteem, psychiatric symptoms (such as somatization and hostility) and global assessment functioning [87].

Though mindfulness has been demonstrated to be beneficial across a variety of domains when taught directly to youth, it may also influence youth outcomes when those surround them learn mindfulness, such as teachers and parents [88]. A study by Singh and colleagues demonstrated that an intervention administered to preschool teachers resulted in decreases in difficult behaviors, decreases in negative interactions, and an increase in compliance among students [89]. Similarly, Jennings and colleagues observed that mindfulness training improved teacher well-being and characteristics of impactful teaching including improved efficacy, and reduced stress ($n = 35$) [90].

Resilience in children may also arise through mindful parenting. Less parenting stress, increased parental warmth, and increased parental attention to their children may also contribute to buffering against the poor health outcomes associated with ACEs [10,91]. Given the number of studies that suggest mindfulness may reduce parental dismissal of their children, mindful parenting may also contribute to resilience against trauma [92]. Mindfulness in parents was associated with each individual's positive perspective on quality of the relationship in black families of stepparents and their child [93]. Mindfulness in parents also may be protective against poor psychobehavioral outcomes in children as has been demonstrated by an inverse association between internalizing and externalizing problems in youth across multiple age groups (young childhood, middle childhood, and adolescence, $n = 215$) [94]. Mindful parenting interventions may improve parent-child relationship qualities [94], but there is mixed evidence regarding the effectiveness of mindful parenting in general depending on the outcomes of interest [92]. However, one study specifically showed benefit that may be extrapolated to relate to parenting children exposed to ACEs. Parents in inner-city methadone programs demonstrated reduced ratings on the Child Abuse Potential Inventory indicating lower potential for physical abuse [95], and therefore show promise to reducing the sequelae of ACEs.

Table 1. Beneficial outcomes seen in research of mindfulness programs for children and youth.

Outcome	Reference
Decreased anxiety	Sibinga et al., 2013 [78] / Jee et al., 2015 [80]
Decreased rumination	Sibinga et al., 2013 [78]
Decreased school related stress, coping with stress	Sibinga et al., 2013 [78] / Jee et al., 2015 [80]
Flatter cortisol curve	Sibinga et al., 2013 [78]
Lower levels of somatization	Sibinga et al., 2016 [79] / Biegel et al., 2009 [87]
Decreased depressive symptoms	Sibinga et al., 2016 [79] / Kuyken et al., 2013 [83]
Effectiveness in social gains	Jee et al., 2015 [80]
Classroom behavior	Black et al., 2015 [86] / van de Weijer-Bergsma et al., 2012 [85]
Decreased hostility	Biegel et al., 2009 [87] / Sibinga et al., 2016 [79]
Decreased suicidal ideation	Britton et al., 2014 [84]
Decreased self-harm	Britton et al., 2014 [84]
Reduced child abuse potential by parents	Dawe and Harnett, 2007 [95]
Conflict avoidance	Sibinga et al., 2014 [81]
Improved attention	van de Weijer-Bergsma et al., 2012 [85]
Greater well-being	Kuyken et al., 2013 [83]
Decreased post traumatic symptoms severity	Sibinga et al., 2016 [79]

In summary, high-quality structured mindfulness programs for youth show promise by reducing mood and emotion dysregulation (decrease depressive, self-hostility, PTSD, anxiety and negative affect symptoms), negative-coping with stress, and improved school adaptation (classroom behavior and discipline, social and academic competence), and attention, mitigating negative effects and potential exacerbations of ACEs. Mindfulness has also been shown to benefit those important to youth, including parents and teachers.

3.3. Resilience and Mindfulness

In order to understand how the practice of mindfulness might be offered as an intervention mitigating the relationship between childhood trauma and health outcomes, one must appreciate the contribution of mindfulness to enhancing resiliency [6]. Resilience is buffering, through successful coping, against adverse outcomes after exposure to traumatic experiences. Conceptually, the lack of resilience may predispose to conditions like PTSD and further unfavorable health consequences as seen in those who experience trauma. In an adult urban inner-city population resilience was found to be inversely associated with symptoms of PTSD [5] and depression, but childhood trauma was positively associated with the presence of PTSD and depression symptoms [96]. Further, there may be neurobiological underpinnings to the buffering effect of resilience on ACEs. Though ACEs have been associated with neurocognitive impairment, trait resilience is associated with better neurocognitive skills such as non-verbal memory [20,21,97]. Importantly, a limitation to exploring this concept is the assessment of resilience, which in research investigations is done by collecting data on related concepts such as perseverance and self-confidence as assessed by the Connor-Davidson-Resilience Scale (CD-RISC) questionnaire, or other concepts measures like coping, social support, emotional and behavioral reactivity, and compassion [98,99]. Nonetheless, enhancing these important domains through mindfulness may serve collectively or independently as buffers against trauma.

Mindfulness may increase resilience in those who have experienced trauma, because it offers an alternative to the common psychological dissociation that occurs after trauma, which can prevent healthy processing or coping [100]. The mindfulness characteristics of accepting without judgment, and acting with awareness are inversely associated with PTSD symptoms [101]. This is likely due to the mindfulness teaching of non-judgmental acceptance of painful and unpleasant thoughts, as well as feelings and practice of decreased reactivity to them [102]. In a cross-sectional study of 125 individuals with substance dependence and a history of trauma, the characteristic of mindfulness was inversely associated with thought suppression, which may represent a form of dissociation and which was strongly associated with PTSD symptoms [103]. Accordingly, trait mindfulness was also associated with decreased cravings.

4. Mindfulness Program Considerations

4.1. Mindfulness Practice and Instructor Training

Mindfulness instruction as a practice has taken on many forms, but MBSR is structured as a 26-h (eight 2.5 h sessions with 1 full day) involving mindful exercises, such as body-scans, mindful breathing, and yoga with meditation instruction, group discussions and encouragement of home practice [43,104]. However, some programs have found effect with as few as 12-h of instruction, with no clear association between hours of instruction and effect size of post-MBSR effects, but studies are varied and limited in their duration of effect [105]. Britton et al. implemented a 15-min daily 6-week course in children, and Kalmanowitz et al. demonstrated that even a 4-day long intensive program in adults demonstrated benefit [52,84].

There is no centralized credentialing required for teaching mindfulness. While there are certificate programs to become an MBSR instructor [106], many programs have branched off from Jon Kabat-Zinn's original model and even studies of mindfulness interventions vary in the qualifications of those implementing instruction to subjects. It is a further challenge to find practitioners that have completed both MBSR and trauma-informed training, and still further, rarely so with specific qualifications to work with youth. Importantly, even trauma therapists who offer mindfulness in practice, have varying degrees of self-practice that may impact their level of involvement [107].

There have been attempts at unique modifications to programming for children or those with special focused needs (Tables 2 and 3). Some studies have specifically involved instructors who have had years of experience specifically with children [78–82]. One study partnered a mental health therapist with adolescents in the community to co-facilitate a mindfulness meditation practice, though the study does not comment on the level of experience of the mental health therapist with mindfulness [108]. For mindfulness training implementation in schools, many programs have branched from the classic MBSR program as described by Meiklejohn et al., 2012 [109]. For example, The Mindfulness in Schools Project (UK based), based on MBSR, is one that has been studied with successful outcomes including fewer depressive symptoms in adolescents, and the Mindful Schools (US based) improved teacher-based perceptions of classroom behavior in a 6th grade public elementary school children [110,111]. Many similar programs to The Mindfulness in Schools Project and Mindful Schools, as seen in Table 3, share in their methodology that mindfulness trained individuals lead practices in the school environment and also educate teachers to lead students [109].

Though many studies have administered mindfulness interventions to teachers, showing benefits for teaching work-environment and temperament [88], none have assessed associated student outcomes directly as a result of the teachers training in isolation. However, the training of teachers is a promising approach to improved classroom outcomes. One study cited by Gouda et al., 2016, showed that schoolteachers (n = 82) had self-reported improvements in mood as well as measures of improved emotional regulation (decreased reactivity, increased compassion) as compared to controls, though the subjects were all female [112], and another showing decreased distress [113]. A smaller study (n = 15) with similar outcome measures also suggested reduction in burnout [114]. Based on such studies, programs have launched to improve classroom learning environments such as the "Cultivating Awareness and Resilience in Education" Program [90]. Since, a larger combined RCT recently showed improvements in schoolteacher sleep and work satisfaction and decreased bad mood, but this was of a workplace mindfulness training not specific to educational environments [115]. Though only one small case study in preschool students showed decrease in negative social interactions [89], taken with the teacher trials, these studies suggest that it may be worth considering that future studies assess the effects and consider if training teachers alone may impact resiliency against ACEs. Therefore, perhaps implementation of programming for both students and teachers is ideal, as found by Gouda et al., 2016 in that both students and teachers showed improvement in interpersonal problems, and affect, whereas students also showed improved school-specific self-efficacy by specific developed self-assessment questionnaires [88]. It is important to keep in mind that lack of benefit of mindfulness in schools programs can be due to lack of teacher experience [116].

Even outside of the school, teacher-led environment, children are never cared for in isolation. It may be beneficial to consider methodology of mindfulness implementation that addresses their caretakers. Given that mindful parenting yields reduced parental stress, with increased parental warmth toward their children [10,91], suggests that mindful parenting training should also be included in interventions for youth. However, many caretakers are involved in influencing children. As examples, one intervention partnered therapists with peer instructors, and another allowed time for individualized intervention for youth (average age 11.5 years) and their parents, then partnered them for family intervention [88,108,117]. The intervention to strengthen families (n = 9) involved seven 2-h sessions with the first hour individualized between youth and their parents and the second hour for family training. It also allowed time for mindful parenting training with teaching and practice exercises on being mindful (attentive, reducing emotional reactivity, being less judgmental) [117], demonstrating how a holistic approach including caretakers, parents and children may be implemented.

Table 2. Variations in mindfulness programs and implementation.

Population	Program	Instruction	Setting	Duration	Reference
Public urban middle school (5th–8th grade; avg. 12 years), $n = 300$	Adapted MBSR	Trained MBSR instructors and personal practice 10+ years	School	12 weekly 50-min sessions	Sibinga et al., 2016 [79]
Foster care youth ages 14–21, $n = 42$	Adapted MBSR	Psychologist with expertise in mindfulness, two pediatrician lead group activities	Conference room of a joint family visitation and clinic space	10 weekly 2-h sessions	Jee et al., 2015 [80]
Kindergarten through 6th grade, low-income and ethnic minority students, $n = 409$	Mindful Schools (MS) Program or MS Plus	MS instructor with 3–20 years mindful meditation experience and classroom teacher facilitated	School	5-week (MS) or 7-week (MS Plus), 15-min sessions running three times per week	Black and Fernando, 2014 [118]
Ages 13–21, underserved youth, $n = 43$	Adapted MBSR	Instructors trained in MBSR, 10+ years' experience	Primary care pediatric clinic	8 weekly 2-h sessions	Sibinga et al., 2014 [81]
Middle-school, urban youth, $n = 41$	Adapted MBSR	Trained MBSR instructor, 10+ years' experience	School	12 weekly 50-min sessions	Sibinga et al., 2013 [78]
Adolescents ages 12–16 years, multiple schools, $n = 522$	School teacher facilitated adapted MBSR (Mindfulness in Schools Project – UK)	Teachers trained by instructors with MBSR training	School	9-week	Kuyken et al., 2013 [83]
6th grade students, $n = 101$	Meditation instruction and student writing exercises	One teacher with meditation training and 5+ years' experience, one teacher who completed MBSR course, no experience	School	Daily for 6 weeks	Britton et al., 2014 [84]
Adolescents ages 14–18, $n = 104$	Adapted MBSR	Instructors MBSR trained	Outpatient psychiatric facility	8-week, 2 h/week, home 20–25 min homework daily	Biegel et al., 2009 [87]
Age 11–15 years, with ADHD, parents, and tutors; $n = 38$	Adapted MBSR combining Mindfulness in Schools Project, and methods for children with ADHD	Instructors trained in MBSR	Group program at an academic treatment center	8-week	van de Weijer-Bergsma et al., 2012 [85]
Ages 13–21, HIV infected, $n = 11$	Adapted MBSR	Instructor trained in MBSR, prior experience	Group at specialty HIV clinic	Eight 2-h sessions and a 3-h retreat	Sibinga et al., 2008 [82]

MBSR, Mindfulness Based Stress Reduction; ADHD, attention-deficit/hyperactivity disorder; HIV, human immunodeficiency virus.

Table 3. Examples of structured mindfulness programs for children.

Program Title	Website
Inner Resilience Program	http://www.innerresilience-tidescenter.org/
Wellness and Resilience Program	http://sbsd.schoolfusion.us/modules/cms/pages.phtml?pageid=195404&SID
Mindful Schools	www.mindfulschools.org
Learning to Breathe	www.learning2breathe.org
Mindfulness in Schools Project (".b", or "Stop and Be!" curriculum)	www.mindfulnessinschools.org
Still Quiet Place	www.stillquietplace.com
Stressed Teens	www.stressedteens.com
Wellness Works in Schools	www.wellnessworksinschools.com
Center for Mindful Awareness	www.centerformindfulawareness.org

The type and location of intervention taught varies tremendously in the literature. As discussed and seen in Table 2, many interventions are integrated directly into school curriculum [88], but also have been offered as extracurricular, in the clinic setting (primary care and specialty), during incarceration, and to parents [81,82,85,87,95,108,119]. Some offer mindfulness only as an addition to a structured and detailed training program with other included skillsets including cognitive therapy, behavioral therapy, resilience training for healthy behaviors, and meditation [6,108,119,120]. There is no study to date that has compared settings, but variation may be dependent on population and outcome of interest. For example, if targeting improvements in mood dysfunction, this has been seen across settings by various different outcome measures for PTSD, depression and anxiety. Attention and behavior outcomes are more commonly measures in studies of school-based interventions, though importantly, there is no evidence that interventions outside of school would not produce effects in the school environment. Given the broad exposure to traumas and ACEs, and the generalizable benefits of mindfulness, mindfulness programs offered through school and/or primary care sites may be most suited to reaching the broadest population of children.

The methods of mindfulness implementation may vary given the diversity of existing academic curricula and environments for youth. Generally, schools offer the most appropriate environment to reach a broad spectrum of children across developmental stages, diagnoses, and socioeconomic circumstances, as well as stressor exposure [116]. Incorporation of mindfulness practice directly into the school curriculum addresses the suggestion of the school environment as a means to reach broad categories of children [78,79,81,86,88]. Examples of broad reaching implementations were postulated by Britton et al. who allotted half a semester on a course to mindfulness with the second half preserved for other curriculum and a mid-year switch of groups, or by Johnstone et al., who proposes to complete a study with a 2-semester health class incorporating eight weeks of mindfulness into the class [84,121]. Kuyken et al. replaced studies in either religious studies or personal, social and health education, offering the idea that perhaps mindfulness could be offered as an elective course in the curriculum [83].

Though the school environment offers a promising delivery format for teaching mindfulness, other methods have been suggested. Home practice is one such model and may offer shorter study formats requiring as little as 5 min [122]. Some formats have even bridged home study with one-on-one in home training [95]. Clinic groups if advertised as a 'social' group rather than a 'stress management' group may pose another potential format [80]. To enhance participation regardless of the format studies have implemented facilitating transportation to class, reminder phone calls, and providing snacks, for example [123]. Other organizations are implementing mindfulness into women and children's shelters and community centers [124].

In school, home and clinic environments, a generalized training in mindfulness allows for broad population applicability, but individualized programs also may be helpful in certain specified populations. An example of individualization of mindfulness intervention methodology for a unique trauma exposed population was accomplished by a program that identified reactivity as a problem in incarcerated individuals and tailored the program "S.T.I.C". S.T.I.C. involves the following steps: stop, take a breath, imagine, and choose, allowing the mindfulness and attention to be directed at consequences and redirection of choices [119]. Though S.T.I.C. was individualized by targeting a specific population, personalization can also be accomplished in school or clinic settings by narrowing the target population such as by diagnosis or age. For example, one study clustered female students with any eating disorder history into a mindfulness program finding improved psychosocial outcomes relative to control by six months post-intervention [120]. Grouping by diagnosis has also been beneficial in the diagnoses of attention-deficit/hyperactivity disorder (ADHD), HIV, or psychiatric conditions [82,85,87], with incorporation of mindfulness into existing therapeutic interventions like cognitive or rehabilitation therapy, MBCT or MBRP, specifically. The RAP Club was offered exclusively to 7th and 8th grade students and catered to adolescent specific life challenges in the program design [108], whereas others incorporated simplistic terminology that can be applied to younger and older students such as, "FOFBOC: Feet on the floor and bum on chair", and "Beditation" referring to a body scan done while lying down [116]. Finally, mindfulness technique has been applied in combination with other therapies including sound and music, touch, walking, daily routines, and even "mindful texting" to allow for the inclusion of mindfulness in regular activities with the idea of "checking in" with the self as much as possible throughout the day [125]. For translating concepts of mindfulness to children, metaphors can be helpful and many children's books are available including those authored by Thich Nhat Hahn, a Buddhist monk who has helped bring the practice of mindfulness to western society with John Kabat-Zinn [126].

4.2. Trauma-Informed Care

Per the Substance Abuse and Mental Health Services Administration (SAMHSA) a program that is trauma-informed realizes trauma prevalence and its common adverse effects, recognizes signs and symptoms of trauma, responds with standard operating procedures, and seeks to resist re-traumatization. SAMHSA provides various examples of well-known trauma-informed intervention programs and they all include general principals of safety, connection and trustworthiness, collaboration, empowerment, and current and historical societal and cultural competency [127]. Formal mindfulness instructor training incorporates a number of these elements and lays the foundation for mindfulness as a trauma-informed care (TIC) practice.

In trauma-informed care, an intervention may be primary (preventive), secondary (reduction of severity and acuity of consequences), or tertiary (treatment of long-term sequelae) [128]. Though it is important for clinicians involved in intervention administration to be cognizant of the above principals of TIC, this does not necessarily mean that the specific stressors or traumas need to be identified for mindfulness to have a beneficial effect, though this has not specifically studied. There is a high prevalence of stress and trauma, with up to 34% of children in school reporting exposure to at least one trauma and evidence of post-traumatic stress even without a current diagnosis [8]. Further, it is known that abuse and trauma is underreported [129] and poorly recalled [130]. Even when reported, child memory of trauma can include intrusions or inaccurate recall [131], and symptoms of PTSD are often poorly recognized by parents [132]. In studies assessing previous trauma, methods of quantification vary widely from general indication of trauma domain to specifics of traumatic event(s). Further, PTSD may mask itself through generalized somatic complaints in children including trouble sleeping, low energy, stomach pain, dizziness, and headaches [133]. Taken together, these studies suggest that one cannot rely on always and accurately identifying the presence of traumatic experience in children. Yet, mindfulness may have an impact in children whether they report a trauma exposure, or not. Trait mindfulness is associated with resilience in face of adverse events, and is associated with strong cognitive abilities, and mindfulness interventions can reduce somatic manifestations of psychiatric undertones [6,70,71,87,134,135]. In populations with high likelihood of ACEs, such as low-income urban areas, school-based mindfulness instruction provided to all students (primary prevention) has been shown to improve psychological symptoms and coping and to reduce post-trauma stress symptoms [79]. Therefore, mindfulness interventions that lead to enhanced coping and resilience can be beneficial when offered to all children regardless of specific identification of trauma exposure.

5. Conclusions and Future Directions

In conclusion, research has demonstrated that high-quality, structured mindfulness interventions improve mental, behavioral, and physical outcomes in youth. Further, these results in combination with the well-studied interventions in adults suggest promise in preventing the poor health outcomes associated with trauma exposure in childhood. Future work should aim to optimize the implementation of high-quality mindfulness programs in youth populations. Further research should explore the mechanisms of mindfulness and the long-term outcomes of mindfulness interventions in childhood into adulthood, as well as outcomes in offspring.

Conflicts of Interest: The authors declare no conflict of interest.

References

1. Felitti, V.J.; Anda, R.F.; Nordenberg, D.; Williamson, D.F.; Spitz, A.M.; Edwards, V.; Koss, M.P.; Marks, J.S. Relationship of childhood abuse and household dysfunction to many of the leading causes of death in adults. The adverse childhood experiences (ACE) study. *Am. J. Prev. Med.* **1998**, *14*, 245–258. [CrossRef]
2. Shonkoff, J.P.; Garner, A.S.; Committee on Psychosocial Aspects of Child and Family Healty; Committee on Early Childhood Adoption, and Dependent Care; Section on Developmental and Behavioral Pediatrics. The lifelong effects of early childhood adversity and toxic stress. *Pediatrics* **2012**, *129*, e232–e246. [CrossRef] [PubMed]
3. Johnson, S.B.; Riley, A.W.; Granger, D.A.; Riis, J. The science of early life toxic stress for pediatric practice and advocacy. *Pediatrics* **2013**, *131*, 319–327. [CrossRef] [PubMed]
4. Danese, A.; McEwen, B.S. Adverse childhood experiences, allostasis, allostatic load, and age-related disease. *Physiol. Behav.* **2012**, *106*, 29–39. [CrossRef] [PubMed]
5. Wrenn, G.L.; Wingo, A.P.; Moore, R.; Pelletier, T.; Gutman, A.R.; Bradley, B.; Ressler, K.J. The effect of resilience on posttraumatic stress disorder in trauma-exposed inner-city primary care patients. *J. Natl. Med. Assoc.* **2011**, *103*, 560–566. [CrossRef]
6. Chandler, G.E.; Roberts, S.J.; Chiodo, L. Resilience intervention for young adults with adverse childhood experiences. *J. Am. Psychiatr. Nurses Assoc.* **2015**, *21*, 406–416. [CrossRef] [PubMed]
7. *Adverse Childhood Experiences Reported by Adults—Five States, 2009*; CDC: Atlanta, GA, USA, 2010; pp. 1609–1613.
8. Gonzalez, A.; Monzon, N.; Solis, D.; Jaycox, L.; Langley, A.K. Trauma exposure in elementary school children: Description of screening procedures, level of exposure, and posttraumatic stress symptoms. *Sch. Ment. Health* **2016**, *8*, 77–88. [CrossRef] [PubMed]
9. Umeda, M.; Oshio, T.; Fujii, M. The impact of the experience of childhood poverty on adult health-risk behaviors in japan: A mediation analysis. *Int. J. Equity Health* **2015**, *14*, 145. [CrossRef] [PubMed]
10. Carroll, J.E.; Gruenewald, T.L.; Taylor, S.E.; Janicki-Deverts, D.; Matthews, K.A.; Seeman, T.E. Childhood abuse, parental warmth, and adult multisystem biological risk in the coronary artery risk development in young adults study. *Proc. Natl. Acad. Sci. USA* **2013**, *110*, 17149–17153. [CrossRef] [PubMed]
11. Harter, S.L. Psychosocial adjustment of adult children of alcoholics: A review of the recent empirical literature. *Clin. Psychol. Rev.* **2000**, *20*, 311–337. [CrossRef]
12. Garner, A.S.; Shonkoff, J.P.; Committee on Psychosocial Aspects of Child and Family Health; Committee on Early Childhood, Adoption, and Dependent Care; Section on Developmental and Behavioral Pediatrics. Early childhood adversity, toxic stress, and the role of the pediatrician: Translating developmental science into lifelong health. *Pediatrics* **2012**, *129*, e224–e231. [PubMed]
13. Danese, A.; Moffitt, T.E.; Harrington, H.; Milne, B.J.; Polanczyk, G.; Pariante, C.M.; Poulton, R.; Caspi, A. Adverse childhood experiences and adult risk factors for age-related disease: Depression, inflammation, and clustering of metabolic risk markers. *Arch. Pediatr. Adolesc. Med.* **2009**, *163*, 1135–1143. [CrossRef] [PubMed]

14. Demetriou, C.A.; van Veldhoven, K.; Relton, C.; Stringhini, S.; Kyriacou, K.; Vineis, P. Biological embedding of early-life exposures and disease risk in humans: A role for DNA methylation. *Eur. J. Clin. Investig.* **2015**, *45*, 303–332. [CrossRef] [PubMed]

15. Yehuda, R.; Daskalakis, N.P.; Bierer, L.M.; Bader, H.N.; Klengel, T.; Holsboer, F.; Binder, E.B. Holocaust exposure induced intergenerational effects on *FKBP5* methylation. *Biol. Psychiatry* **2016**, *80*, 372–380. [CrossRef] [PubMed]

16. Benner, A.D.; Boyle, A.E.; Sadler, S Parental involvement and adolescents' educational success: The roles of prior achievement and socioeconomic status. *J. Youth Adolesc.* **2016**, *45*, 1053–1064. [CrossRef] [PubMed]

17. Mills-Koonce, W.R.; Willoughby, M.T.; Garrett-Peters, P.; Wagner, N.; Vernon-Feagans, L.; Family Life Project Key Investigators. The interplay among socioeconomic status, household chaos, and parenting in the prediction of child conduct problems and callous-unemotional behaviors. *Dev. Psychopathol.* **2016**, *28*, 757–771. [CrossRef] [PubMed]

18. Potijk, M.R.; Kerstjens, J.M.; Bos, A.F.; Reijneveld, S.A.; de Winter, A.F. Developmental delay in moderately preterm-born children with low socioeconomic status: Risks multiply. *J. Pediatr.* **2013**, *163*, 1289–1295. [CrossRef] [PubMed]

19. Ursache, A.; Noble, K.G.; Pediatric Imaging, Neurocognition and Genetics Study. Socioeconomic status, white matter, and executive function in children. *Brain Behav.* **2016**, *6*, e00531. [CrossRef] [PubMed]

20. Ursache, A.; Noble, K.G. Neurocognitive development in socioeconomic context: Multiple mechanisms and implications for measuring socioeconomic status. *Psychophysiology* **2016**, *53*, 71–82. [CrossRef] [PubMed]

21. Saleh, A.; Potter, G.G.; McQuoid, D.R.; Boyd, B.; Turner, R.; MacFall, J.R.; Taylor, W.D. Effects of early life stress on depression, cognitive performance and brain morphology. *Psychol. Med.* **2017**, *47*, 171–181. [CrossRef] [PubMed]

22. Scharoun-Lee, M.; Adair, L.S.; Kaufman, J.S.; Gordon-Larsen, P. Obesity, race/ethnicity and the multiple dimensions of socioeconomic status during the transition to adulthood: A factor analysis approach. *Soc. Sci. Med.* **2009**, *68*, 708–716. [CrossRef] [PubMed]

23. Anda, R.F.; Croft, J.B.; Felitti, V.J.; Nordenberg, D.; Giles, W.H.; Williamson, D.F.; Giovino, G.A. Adverse childhood experiences and smoking during adolescence and adulthood. *JAMA* **1999**, *282*, 1652–1658. [CrossRef] [PubMed]

24. Su, S.; Wang, X.; Pollock, J.S.; Treiber, F.A.; Xu, X.; Snieder, H.; McCall, W.V.; Stefanek, M.; Harshfield, G.A. Adverse childhood experiences and blood pressure trajectories from childhood to young adulthood: The Georgia stress and heart study. *Circulation* **2015**, *131*, 1674–1681. [CrossRef] [PubMed]

25. Taylor, S.E.; Lerner, J.S.; Sage, R.M.; Lehman, B.J.; Seeman, T.E. Early environment, emotions, responses to stress, and health. *J. Personal.* **2004**, *72*, 1365–1393. [CrossRef] [PubMed]

26. Rothman, E.F.; Edwards, E.M.; Heeren, T.; Hingson, R.W. Adverse childhood experiences predict earlier age of drinking onset: Results from a representative us sample of current or former drinkers. *Pediatrics* **2008**, *122*, e298–e304. [CrossRef] [PubMed]

27. Yao, H.; Rahman, I. Current concepts on the role of inflammation in COPD and lung cancer. *Curr. Opin. Pharmacol.* **2009**, *9*, 375–383. [CrossRef] [PubMed]

28. Li, M.; Zhou, Y.; Feng, G.; Su, S.B. The critical role of toll-like receptor signaling pathways in the induction and progression of autoimmune diseases. *Curr. Mol. Med.* **2009**, *9*, 365–374. [CrossRef] [PubMed]

29. Salinas-Miranda, A.A.; Salemi, J.L.; King, L.M.; Baldwin, J.A.; Berry, E.L.; Austin, D.A.; Scarborough, K.; Spooner, K.K.; Zoorob, R.J.; Salihu, H.M. Adverse childhood experiences and health-related quality of life in adulthood: Revelations from a community needs assessment. *Health Qual. Life Outcomes* **2015**, *13*, 123. [CrossRef] [PubMed]

30. Mair, C.; Cunradi, C.B.; Todd, M. Adverse childhood experiences and intimate partner violence: Testing psychosocial mediational pathways among couples. *Ann. Epidemiol.* **2012**, *22*, 832–839. [CrossRef] [PubMed]

31. Hillis, S.D.; Anda, R.F.; Felitti, V.J.; Nordenberg, D.; Marchbanks, P.A. Adverse childhood experiences and sexually transmitted diseases in men and women: A retrospective study. *Pediatrics* **2000**, *106*, E11. [CrossRef] [PubMed]

32. Fuller-Thomson, E.; Baird, S.L.; Dhrodia, R.; Brennenstuhl, S. The association between adverse childhood experiences (ACES) and suicide attempts in a population-based study. *Child Care Health Dev.* **2016**, *42*, 725–734. [CrossRef] [PubMed]

33. Duke, N.N.; Pettingell, S.L.; McMorris, B.J.; Borowsky, I.W. Adolescent violence perpetration: Associations with multiple types of adverse childhood experiences. *Pediatrics* **2010**, *125*, e778–e786. [CrossRef] [PubMed]

34. Skarupski, K.A.; Parisi, J.M.; Thorpe, R.; Tanner, E.; Gross, D. The association of adverse childhood experiences with mid-life depressive symptoms and quality of life among incarcerated males: Exploring multiple mediation. *Aging Ment. Health* **2016**, *20*, 655–666. [CrossRef] [PubMed]

35. Ortiz, R.; Ballard, E.D.; Machado-Vieira, R.; Saligan, L.N.; Walitt, B. Quantifying the influence of child abuse history on the cardinal symptoms of fibromyalgia. *Clin. Exp. Rheumatol.* **2016**, *34*, S59–S66. [PubMed]

36. Tietjen, G.E.; Khubchandani, J.; Herial, N.A.; Shah, K. Adverse childhood experiences are associated with migraine and vascular biomarkers. *Headache* **2012**, *52*, 920–929. [CrossRef] [PubMed]

37. Park, S.H.; Videlock, E.J.; Shih, W.; Presson, A.P.; Mayer, E.A.; Chang, L. Adverse childhood experiences are associated with irritable bowel syndrome and gastrointestinal symptom severity. *Neurogastroenterol. Motil.* **2016**, *28*, 1252–1260. [CrossRef] [PubMed]

38. Bader, K.; Schafer, V.; Schenkel, M.; Nissen, L.; Schwander, J. Adverse childhood experiences associated with sleep in primary insomnia. *J. Sleep Res.* **2007**, *16*, 285–296. [CrossRef] [PubMed]

39. Brown, M.J.; Thacker, L.R.; Cohen, S.A. Association between adverse childhood experiences and diagnosis of cancer. *PLoS ONE* **2013**, *8*, e65524. [CrossRef] [PubMed]

40. Poletti, S.; Colombo, C.; Benedetti, F. Adverse childhood experiences worsen cognitive distortion during adult bipolar depression. *Compr. Psychiatry* **2014**, *55*, 1803–1808. [CrossRef] [PubMed]

41. Burke, N.J.; Hellman, J.L.; Scott, B.G.; Weems, C.F.; Carrion, V.G. The impact of adverse childhood experiences on an urban pediatric population. *Child Abus. Negl.* **2011**, *35*, 408–413. [CrossRef] [PubMed]

42. Hillis, S.D.; Anda, R.F.; Dube, S.R.; Felitti, V.J.; Marchbanks, P.A.; Marks, J.S. The association between adverse childhood experiences and adolescent pregnancy, long-term psychosocial consequences, and fetal death. *Pediatrics* **2004**, *113*, 320–327. [CrossRef] [PubMed]

43. Kabat-Zinn, J. *Full Catastrophe Living: Using the Wisdom of Your Body and Mind to Face Stress, Pain, and Illness*; Dell Publishing: New York, NY, USA, 1990.

44. Carmody, J.; Baer, R.A. Relationships between mindfulness practice and levels of mindfulness, medical and psychological symptoms and well-being in a mindfulness-based stress reduction program. *J. Behav. Med.* **2008**, *31*, 23–33. [CrossRef] [PubMed]

45. Baer, R.A.; Smith, G.T.; Hopkins, J.; Krietemeyer, J.; Toney, L. Using self-report assessment methods to explore facets of mindfulness. *Assessment* **2006**, *13*, 27–45. [CrossRef] [PubMed]

46. Batink, T.; Peeters, F.; Geschwind, N.; van Os, J.; Wichers, M. How does MBCT for depression work? Studying cognitive and affective mediation pathways. *PLoS ONE* **2013**, *8*, e72778. [CrossRef] [PubMed]

47. Bowen, S.; Chawla, N.; Collins, S.E.; Witkiewitz, K.; Hsu, S.; Grow, J.; Clifasefi, S.; Garner, M.; Douglass, A.; Larimer, M.E.; et al. Mindfulness-based relapse prevention for substance use disorders: A pilot efficacy trial. *Subst. Abus.* **2009**, *30*, 295–305. [CrossRef] [PubMed]

48. Gallegos, A.M.; Lytle, M.C.; Moynihan, J.A.; Talbot, N.L. Mindfulness-based stress reduction to enhance psychological functioning and improve inflammatory biomarkers in trauma-exposed women: A pilot study. *Psychol Trauma* **2015**, *7*, 525–532. [CrossRef]

49. Kimbrough, E.; Magyari, T.; Langenberg, P.; Chesney, M.; Berman, B. Mindfulness intervention for child abuse survivors. *J. Clin. Psychol.* **2010**, *66*, 17–33. [PubMed]

50. Earley, M.D.; Chesney, M.A.; Frye, J.; Greene, P.A.; Berman, B.; Kimbrough, E. Mindfulness intervention for child abuse survivors: A 2.5-year follow-up. *J. Clin. Psychol.* **2014**, *70*, 933–941. [CrossRef] [PubMed]

51. Ferszt, G.G.; Miller, R.J.; Hickey, J.E.; Maull, F.; Crisp, K. The impact of a mindfulness based program on perceived stress, anxiety, depression and sleep of incarcerated women. *Int. J. Environ. Res. Public Health* **2015**, *12*, 11594–11607. [CrossRef] [PubMed]

52. Kalmanowitz, D.L.; Ho, R.T. Art therapy and mindfulness with survivors of political violence: A qualitative study. *Psychol. Trauma* **2016**. [CrossRef] [PubMed]

53. Klatt, M.; Steinberg, B.; Duchemin, A.M. Mindfulness in motion (MIM): An onsite mindfulness based intervention (MBI) for chronically high stress work environments to increase resiliency and work engagement. *J. Vis. Exp.* **2015**, e52359. [CrossRef] [PubMed]

54. Johnson, D.C.; Thom, N.J.; Stanley, E.A.; Haase, L.; Simmons, A.N.; Shih, P.A.; Thompson, W.K.; Potterat, E.G.; Minor, T.R.; Paulus, M.P. Modifying resilience mechanisms in at-risk individuals: A controlled study of mindfulness training in marines preparing for deployment. *Am. J. Psychiatry* **2014**, *171*, 844–853. [CrossRef] [PubMed]

55. Polusny, M.A.; Erbes, C.R.; Thuras, P.; Moran, A.; Lamberty, G.J.; Collins, R.C.; Rodman, J.L.; Lim, K.O. Mindfulness-based stress reduction for posttraumatic stress disorder among veterans: A randomized clinical trial. *JAMA* **2015**, *314*, 456–465. [CrossRef] [PubMed]

56. Possemato, K.; Bergen-Cico, D.; Treatman, S.; Allen, C.; Wade, M.; Pigeon, W. A randomized clinical trial of primary care brief mindfulness training for veterans with PTSD. *J. Clin. Psychol.* **2016**, *72*, 179–193. [CrossRef]

57. Bergen-Cico, D.; Possemato, K.; Pigeon, W. Reductions in cortisol associated with primary care brief mindfulness program for veterans with PTSD. *Med. Care* **2014**, *52*, S25–S31. [CrossRef] [PubMed]

58. Bormann, J.E.; Oman, D.; Walter, K.H.; Johnson, B.D. Mindful attention increases and mediates psychological outcomes following mantram repetition practice in veterans with posttraumatic stress disorder. *Med. Care* **2014**, *52*, S13–S18. [CrossRef] [PubMed]

59. Heffner, K.L.; Crean, H.F.; Kemp, J.E. Meditation programs for veterans with posttraumatic stress disorder: Aggregate findings from a multi-site evaluation. *Psychol. Trauma* **2016**, *8*, 365–374. [CrossRef] [PubMed]

60. Kluepfel, L.; Ward, T.; Yehuda, R.; Dimoulas, E.; Smith, A.; Daly, K. The evaluation of mindfulness-based stress reduction for veterans with mental health conditions. *J. Holist Nurs.* **2013**, *31*, 248–255. [CrossRef]

61. Sylvia, L.G.; Bui, E.; Baier, A.L.; Mehta, D.H.; Denninger, J.W.; Fricchione, G.L.; Casey, A.; Kagan, L.; Park, E.R.; Simon, N.M. Resilient warrior: A stress management group to improve psychological health in service members. *Glob. Adv. Health Med.* **2015**, *4*, 38–42. [CrossRef] [PubMed]

62. Azad Marzabadi, E.; Hashemi Zadeh, S.M. The effectiveness of mindfulness training in improving the quality of life of the war victims with post traumatic stress disorder (PTSD). *Iran. J. Psychiatry* **2014**, *9*, 228–236. [PubMed]

63. Omidi, A.; Mohammadi, A.; Zargar, F.; Akbari, H. Efficacy of mindfulness-based stress reduction on mood states of veterans with post-traumatic stress disorder. *Arch. Trauma Res.* **2013**, *1*, 151–154. [CrossRef] [PubMed]

64. Poon, A.; Danoff-Burg, S. Mindfulness as a moderator in expressive writing. *J. Clin. Psychol.* **2011**, *67*, 881–895. [CrossRef] [PubMed]

65. Dahm, K.A.; Meyer, E.C.; Neff, K.D.; Kimbrel, N.A.; Gulliver, S.B.; Morissette, S.B. Mindfulness, self-compassion, posttraumatic stress disorder symptoms, and functional disability in U.S. Iraq and Afghanistan war veterans. *J. Trauma. Stress* **2015**, *28*, 460–464. [CrossRef] [PubMed]

66. Basharpoor, S.; Shafiei, M.; Daneshvar, S. The comparison of experiential avoidance, [corrected] mindfulness and rumination in trauma-exposed individuals with and without posttraumatic stress disorder (PTSD) in an Iranian sample. *Arch. Psychiatr. Nurs.* **2015**, *29*, 279–283. [CrossRef]

67. Thieleman, K.; Cacciatore, J. Witness to suffering: Mindfulness and compassion fatigue among traumatic bereavement volunteers and professionals. *Soc. Work* **2014**, *59*, 34–41. [CrossRef]

68. Chiesa, A.; Serretti, A. Mindfulness-based stress reduction for stress management in healthy people: A review and meta-analysis. *J. Altern. Complement. Med.* **2009**, *15*, 593–600. [CrossRef]

69. Goyal, M.; Singh, S.; Sibinga, E.M.; Gould, N.F.; Rowland-Seymour, A.; Sharma, R.; Berger, Z.; Sleicher, D.; Maron, D.D.; Shihab, H.M.; et al. Meditation programs for psychological stress and well-being: A systematic review and meta-analysis. *JAMA Intern. Med.* **2014**, *174*, 357–368. [CrossRef] [PubMed]

70. Mahoney, C.T.; Segal, D.L.; Coolidge, F.L. Anxiety sensitivity, experiential avoidance, and mindfulness among younger and older adults: Age differences in risk factors for anxiety symptoms. *Int. J. Aging Hum. Dev.* **2015**, *81*, 217–240. [CrossRef] [PubMed]

71. Patterson, P.; McDonald, F.E. "Being mindful": Does it help adolescents and young adults who have completed cancer treatment? *J. Pediatr. Oncol. Nurs.* **2015**, *32*, 189–194. [CrossRef] [PubMed]

72. Senders, A.; Bourdette, D.; Hanes, D.; Yadav, V.; Shinto, L. Perceived stress in multiple sclerosis: The potential role of mindfulness in health and well-being. *J. Evid. Based Complemen. Altern. Med.* **2014**, *19*, 104–111. [CrossRef] [PubMed]

73. Sharplin, G.R.; Jones, S.B.; Hancock, B.; Knott, V.E.; Bowden, J.A.; Whitford, H.S. Mindfulness-based cognitive therapy: An efficacious community-based group intervention for depression and anxiety in a sample of cancer patients. *Med. J. Aust.* **2010**, *193*, S79–S82. [PubMed]

74. Gonzalez, A.; Locicero, B.; Mahaffey, B.; Fleming, C.; Harris, J.; Vujanovic, A.A. Internalized Hiv stigma and mindfulness: Associations with PTSD symptom severity in trauma-exposed adults with HIV/AIDS. *Behav. Modif.* **2016**, *40*, 144–163. [CrossRef] [PubMed]
75. Black, D.S.; Slavich, G.M. Mindfulness meditation and the immune system: A systematic review of randomized controlled trials. *Ann. N. Y. Acad. Sci.* **2016**, *1373*, 13–24. [CrossRef] [PubMed]
76. Creswell, J.D.; Taren, A.A.; Lindsay, E.K.; Greco, C.M.; Gianaros, P.J.; Fairgrieve, A.; Marsland, A.L.; Brown, K.W.; Way, B.M.; Rosen, R.K.; et al. Alterations in resting-state functional connectivity link mindfulness meditation with reduced interleukin-6: A randomized controlled trial. *Biol. Psychiatry* **2016**, *80*, 53–61. [CrossRef] [PubMed]
77. Kaliman, P.; Alvarez-Lopez, M.J.; Cosin-Tomas, M.; Rosenkranz, M.A.; Lutz, A.; Davidson, R.J. Rapid changes in histone deacetylases and inflammatory gene expression in expert meditators. *Psychoneuroendocrinology* **2014**, *40*, 96–107. [CrossRef] [PubMed]
78. Sibinga, E.M.; Perry-Parrish, C.; Chung, S.E.; Johnson, S.B.; Smith, M.; Ellen, J.M. School-based mindfulness instruction for urban male youth: A small randomized controlled trial. *Prev. Med.* **2013**, *57*, 799–801. [CrossRef] [PubMed]
79. Sibinga, E.M.; Webb, L.; Ghazarian, S.R.; Ellen, J.M. School-based mindfulness instruction: An RCT. *Pediatrics* **2016**, *137*. [CrossRef] [PubMed]
80. Jee, S.H.; Couderc, J.P.; Swanson, D.; Gallegos, A.; Hilliard, C.; Blumkin, A.; Cunningham, K.; Heinert, S. A pilot randomized trial teaching mindfulness-based stress reduction to traumatized youth in foster care. *Complement. Ther. Clin. Pract.* **2015**, *21*, 201–209. [CrossRef]
81. Sibinga, E.M.; Perry-Parrish, C.; Thorpe, K.; Mika, M.; Ellen, J.M. A small mixed-method RCT of mindfulness instruction for urban youth. *Explore* **2014**, *10*, 180–186. [CrossRef] [PubMed]
82. Sibinga, E.M.; Stewart, M.; Magyari, T.; Welsh, C.K.; Hutton, N.; Ellen, J.M. Mindfulness-based stress reduction for hiv-infected youth: A pilot study. *Explore* **2008**, *4*, 36–37. [CrossRef] [PubMed]
83. Kuyken, W.; Weare, K.; Ukoumunne, O.C.; Vicary, R.; Motton, N.; Burnett, R.; Cullen, C.; Hennelly, S.; Huppert, F. Effectiveness of the mindfulness in schools programme: Non-randomised controlled feasibility study. *Br. J. Psychiatry* **2013**, *203*, 126–131. [CrossRef] [PubMed]
84. Britton, W.B.; Lepp, N.E.; Niles, H.F.; Rocha, T.; Fisher, N.E.; Gold, J.S. A randomized controlled pilot trial of classroom-based mindfulness meditation compared to an active control condition in sixth-grade children. *J. Sch. Psychol.* **2014**, *52*, 263–278. [CrossRef] [PubMed]
85. Van de Weijer-Bergsma, E.; Formsma, A.R.; de Bruin, E.I.; Bogels, S.M. The effectiveness of mindfulness training on behavioral problems and attentional functioning in adolescents with adhd. *J. Child Fam. Stud.* **2012**, *21*, 775–787. [CrossRef] [PubMed]
86. Black, D.S.; O'Reilly, G.A.; Olmstead, R.; Breen, E.C.; Irwin, M.R. Mindfulness meditation and improvement in sleep quality and daytime impairment among older adults with sleep disturbances: A randomized clinical trial. *JAMA Intern. Med.* **2015**, *175*, 494–501. [CrossRef] [PubMed]
87. Biegel, G.M.; Brown, K.W.; Shapiro, S.L.; Schubert, C.M. Mindfulness-based stress reduction for the treatment of adolescent psychiatric outpatients: A randomized clinical trial. *J. Consult. Clin. Psychol.* **2009**, *77*, 855–866. [CrossRef] [PubMed]
88. Gouda, S.; Luong, M.T.; Schmidt, S.; Bauer, J. Students and teachers benefit from mindfulness-based stress reduction in a school-embedded pilot study. *Front. Psychol.* **2016**, *7*, 590. [CrossRef] [PubMed]
89. Singh, N.N.; Lancioni, G.E.; Winton, A.S.W.; Karazsia, B.T.; Singh, J. Mindfulness training for teachers changes the behavior of their preschool students. *Res. Human Dev.* **2013**, *10*, 211–233. [CrossRef]
90. Jennings, P.A.; Frank, J.L.; Snowberg, K.E.; Coccia, M.A.; Greenberg, M.T. Improving classroom learning environments by cultivating awareness and resilience in education (care): Results of a randomized controlled trial. *Sch. Psychol. Q.* **2013**, *28*, 374–390. [CrossRef]
91. Bethell, C.; Gombojav, N.; Solloway, M.; Wissow, L. Adverse childhood experiences, resilience and mindfulness-based approaches: Common denominator issues for children with emotional, mental, or behavioral problems. *Child Adolesc. Psychiatr. Clin. N. Am.* **2016**, *25*, 139–156. [CrossRef] [PubMed]
92. Townshend, K.; Jordan, Z.; Stephenson, M.; Tsey, K. The effectiveness of mindful parenting programs in promoting parents' and children's wellbeing: A systematic review. *JBI Database Syst. Rev. Implement. Rep.* **2016**, *14*, 139–180. [CrossRef] [PubMed]

93. Parent, J.; Clifton, J.; Forehand, R.; Golub, A.; Reid, M.; Pichler, E.R. Parental mindfulness and dyadic relationship quality in low-income cohabiting black stepfamilies: Associations with parenting experienced by adolescents. *Couple Fam. Psychol.* **2014**, *3*, 67–82. [CrossRef] [PubMed]

94. Parent, J.; McKee, L.G.; J, N.R.; Forehand, R. The association of parent mindfulness with parenting and youth psychopathology across three developmental stages. *J. Abnorm Child Psychol.* **2016**, *44*, 191–202. [CrossRef] [PubMed]

95. Dawe, S.; Harnett, P. Reducing potential for child abuse among methadone-maintained parents: Results from a randomized controlled trial. *J. Subst. Abus. Treat.* **2007**, *32*, 381–390. [CrossRef] [PubMed]

96. Wingo, A.P.; Wrenn, G.; Pelletier, T.; Gutman, A.R.; Bradley, B.; Ressler, K.J. Moderating effects of resilience on depression in individuals with a history of childhood abuse or trauma exposure. *J. Affect. Disord.* **2010**, *126*, 411–414. [CrossRef] [PubMed]

97. Wingo, A.P.; Fani, N.; Bradley, B.; Ressler, K.J. Psychological resilience and neurocognitive performance in a traumatized community sample. *Depress Anxiety* **2010**, *27*, 768–774. [CrossRef] [PubMed]

98. Connor, K.M.; Davidson, J.R. Development of a new resilience scale: The Connor-Davidson Resilience Scale (CD-RISC). *Depress Anxiety* **2003**, *18*, 76–82. [CrossRef] [PubMed]

99. Sinclair, V.G.; Wallston, K.A. The development and psychometric evaluation of the brief resilient coping scale. *Assessment* **2004**, *11*, 94–101. [CrossRef] [PubMed]

100. Thompson, R.W.; Arnkoff, D.B.; Glass, C.R. Conceptualizing mindfulness and acceptance as components of psychological resilience to trauma. *Trauma Violence Abus.* **2011**, *12*, 220–235. [CrossRef] [PubMed]

101. Vujanovic, A.A.; Youngwirth, N.E.; Johnson, K.A.; Zvolensky, M.J. Mindfulness-based acceptance and posttraumatic stress symptoms among trauma-exposed adults without axis i psychopathology. *J. Anxiety Disord.* **2009**, *23*, 297–303. [CrossRef] [PubMed]

102. Perry-Parrish, C.; Copeland-Linder, N.; Webb, L.; Sibinga, E.M. Mindfulness-based approaches for children and youth. *Curr. Probl. Pediatr. Adolesc. Health Care* **2016**, *46*, 172–178. [CrossRef] [PubMed]

103. Garland, E.L.; Roberts-Lewis, A. Differential roles of thought suppression and dispositional mindfulness in posttraumatic stress symptoms and craving. *Addict. Behav.* **2013**, *38*, 1555–1562. [CrossRef] [PubMed]

104. Kabat-Zinn, J. An outpatient program in behavioral medicine for chronic pain patients based on the practice of mindfulness meditation: Theoretical considerations and preliminary results. *Gen. Hosp. Psychiatry* **1982**, *4*, 33–47. [CrossRef]

105. Carmody, J.; Baer, R.A. How long does a mindfulness-based stress reduction program need to be? A review of class contact hours and effect sizes for psychological distress. *J. Clin. Psychol.* **2009**, *65*, 627–638. [CrossRef] [PubMed]

106. Mindfulness-Based Professional Education. Available online: http://www.umassmed.edu/cfm/training/ (accesses on 20 December 2016).

107. Waelde, L.C.; Thompson, J.M.; Robinson, A.; Iwanicki, S. Trauma therapists' clinical applications, training, and personal practice of mindfulness and meditation. *Mindfulness* **2016**, *7*, 622–629. [CrossRef] [PubMed]

108. Mendelson, T.; Tandon, S.D.; O'Brennan, L.; Leaf, P.J.; Ialongo, N.S. Brief report: Moving prevention into schools: The impact of a trauma-informed school-based intervention. *J. Adolesc.* **2015**, *43*, 142–147. [CrossRef] [PubMed]

109. Meiklejohn, J.; Phillips, C.; Freedman, M.L.; Griffin, M.L.; Biegel, G.; Roach, A.; Frank, J.; Burke, C.; Pinger, L.; Soloway, G.; et al. Integrating mindfulness training into k-12 education: Fostering the resilience of teachers and students. *Mindfulness* **2012**, *3*, 291–307. [CrossRef]

110. Mindful in Schools Project. Available online: https://mindfulnessinschools.org (accesses on 20 December 2016).

111. Mindful Schools. Available online: http://www.mindfulschools.org/ (accesses on 20 December 2016).

112. Kemeny, M.E.; Foltz, C.; Cavanagh, J.F.; Cullen, M.; Giese-Davis, J.; Jennings, P.; Rosenberg, E.L.; Gillath, O.; Shaver, P.R.; Wallace, B.A.; et al. Contemplative/emotion training reduces negative emotional behavior and promotes prosocial responses. *Emotion* **2012**, *12*, 338–350. [CrossRef] [PubMed]

113. Franco, C.; Manas, I.; Cangas, A.J.; Moreno, E.; Gallego, J. Reducing teachers' psychological distress through a mindfulness training program. *Span. J. Psychol.* **2010**, *13*, 655–666. [CrossRef] [PubMed]

114. Flook, L.; Goldberg, S.B.; Pinger, L.; Bonus, K.; Davidson, R.J. Mindfulness for teachers: A pilot study to assess effects on stress, burnout and teaching efficacy. *Mind Brain Educ.* **2013**, *7*. [CrossRef] [PubMed]

115. Crain, T.L.; Schonert-Reichl, K.A.; Roeser, R.W. Cultivating teacher mindfulness: Effects of a randomized controlled trial on work, home, and sleep outcomes. *J. Occup. Health Psychol.* **2016**. [CrossRef] [PubMed]

116. Johnson, C.; Burke, C.; Brinkman, S.; Wade, T. Effectiveness of a school-based mindfulness program for transdiagnostic prevention in young adolescents. *Behav. Res. Ther.* **2016**, *81*, 1–11. [CrossRef] [PubMed]
117. Duncan, L.G.; Coatsworth, J.D.; Greenberg, M.T. Pilot study to gauge acceptability of a mindfulness-based, family-focused preventive intervention. *J. Prim. Prev.* **2009**, *30*, 605–618. [CrossRef] [PubMed]
118. Black, D.S.; Fernando, R. Mindfulness Training and Classroom Behavior Among Lower-Income and Ethnic Minority Elementary School Children. *J. Child. Fam. Stud.* **2014**, *23*, 1242–1246. [CrossRef] [PubMed]
119. Himelstein, S.; Saul, S.; Garcia-Romeu, A.; Pinedo, D. Mindfulness training as an intervention for substance user incarcerated adolescents: A pilot grounded theory study. *Subst. Use Misuse* **2014**, *49*, 560–570. [CrossRef] [PubMed]
120. Atkinson, M.J.; Wade, T.D. Mindfulness-based prevention for eating disorders: A school-based cluster randomized controlled study. *Int. J. Eat. Disord.* **2015**, *48*, 1024–1037. [CrossRef] [PubMed]
121. Johnstone, J.M.; Roake, C.; Sheikh, I.; Mole, A.; Nigg, J.T.; Oken, B. School-based mindfulness intervention for stress reduction in adolescents: Design and methodology of an open-label, parallel group, randomized controlled trial. *Contemp. Clin. Trials Commun.* **2016**, *4*, 99–104. [CrossRef] [PubMed]
122. Lee, L.; Semple, R.J.; Rosa, D.; Miller, L. Mindfulness-based cognitive therapy for children: Results of a pilot study. *J. Cogn. Psychother.* **2008**, *22*, 15–28. [CrossRef]
123. Kerrigan, D.; Johnson, K.; Stewart, M.; Magyari, T.; Hutton, N.; Ellen, J.M.; Sibinga, E.M. Perceptions, experiences, and shifts in perspective occurring among urban youth participating in a mindfulness-based stress reduction program. *Complement. Ther. Clin. Pract.* **2011**, *17*, 96–101. [CrossRef] [PubMed]
124. Connolly, A. Center for mindful awareness. Available online: http://centerformindfulawareness.org/ (accessed on 20 December 2016).
125. Thompson, M.; Gauntlett-Gilbert, J. Mindfulness with children and adolescents: Effective clinical application. *Clin. Child Psychol. Psychiatry* **2008**, *13*, 395–407. [CrossRef] [PubMed]
126. Hanh, T.N. *Planting Seeds: Practicing Mindfulness with Children*; Parallax Press: Berkeley, CA, USA, 2007.
127. Trauma-informed approach and trauma-specific interventions. Available online: https://www.samhsa.gov/nctic/trauma-interventions (accessed on 20 December 2016).
128. Oral, R.; Ramirez, M.; Coohey, C.; Nakada, S.; Walz, A.; Kuntz, A.; Benoit, J.; Peek-Asa, C. Adverse childhood experiences and trauma informed care: The future of health care. *Pediatr. Res.* **2016**, *79*, 227–233. [CrossRef] [PubMed]
129. Luce, H.; Schrager, S.; Gilchrist, V. Sexual assault of women. *Am. Fam. Physician* **2010**, *81*, 489–495. [PubMed]
130. Williams, L.M. Recall of childhood trauma: A prospective study of women's memories of child sexual abuse. *J. Consult. Clin. Psychol.* **1994**, *62*, 1167–1176. [CrossRef] [PubMed]
131. Howe, M.L.; Courage, M.L.; Peterson, C. Intrusions in preschoolers' recall of traumatic childhood events. *Psychon. Bull. Rev.* **1995**, *2*, 130–134. [CrossRef] [PubMed]
132. Meiser-Stedman, R.; Smith, P.; Yule, W.; Glucksman, E.; Dalgleish, T. Posttraumatic stress disorder in young children 3 years posttrauma: Prevalence and longitudinal predictors. *J. Clin. Psychiatry* **2016**. [CrossRef] [PubMed]
133. Zhang, Y.; Zhang, J.; Zhu, S.; Du, C.; Zhang, W. Prevalence and predictors of somatic symptoms among child and adolescents with probable posttraumatic stress disorder: A cross-sectional study conducted in 21 primary and secondary schools after an earthquake. *PLoS ONE* **2015**, *10*, e0137101. [CrossRef] [PubMed]
134. Keng, S.L.; Tong, E.M. Riding the tide of emotions with mindfulness: Mindfulness, affect dynamics, and the mediating role of coping. *Emotion* **2016**, *16*, 706–718. [CrossRef] [PubMed]
135. Teper, R.; Inzlicht, M. Meditation, mindfulness and executive control: The importance of emotional acceptance and brain-based performance monitoring. *Soc. Cogn. Affect. Neurosci.* **2013**, *8*, 85–92. [CrossRef] [PubMed]

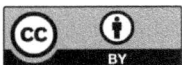

![children logo] **children**

MDPI

Essay

Incorporating Hypnosis into Pediatric Clinical Encounters

Robert A. Pendergrast Jr.

Department of Pediatrics, Medical College of Georgia, Augusta University, 1120 15th Street, Augusta, GA 30912, USA; rpenderg@augusta.edu; Tel.: +1-706-721-2457; Fax: +1-706-721-3912

Academic Editor: Hilary McClafferty
Received: 31 December 2016; Accepted: 7 March 2017; Published: 16 March 2017

Abstract: Increasing numbers of licensed health professionals who care for children have been trained in clinical hypnosis. The evidence base for the safety and efficacy of this therapeutic approach in a wide variety of conditions is also growing. Pediatricians and other health professionals who have received training may wish to apply these skills in appropriate clinical scenarios but still may be unsure of the practical matters of how to incorporate this skill-set into day to day practice. Moreover, the practical application of such skills will take very different forms depending on the practice setting, types of acute or chronic conditions, patient and family preferences, and the developmental stages of the child or teen. This article reviews the application of pediatric clinical hypnosis skills by describing the use of hypnotic language outside of formal trance induction, by describing natural trance states that occur in children and teens in healthcare settings, and by describing the process of planning a clinical hypnosis encounter. It is assumed that this article does not constitute training in hypnosis or qualify its readers for the application of such skills; rather, it may serve as a practical guide for those professionals who have been so trained, and may serve to inform other professionals what to expect when referring a patient for hypnotherapy. The reader is referred to specific training opportunities and organizations.

Keywords: hypnosis; pediatric hypnosis; pediatric skills development; self-hypnosis; primary care; therapeutic use of language; hypnosis consult; practice style

1. Introduction

Though called by different names, there has been interest in the concept of clinical hypnosis by health professionals caring for children at least as far into Western history as the 18th century. This has been reviewed briefly by Kohen and Kaiser [1] and in more detail in Kohen and Olness' Hypnosis and Hypnotherapy in Children [2]. Since the 1960s, there has been a rapid expansion of dissemination of knowledge in the field, numbers of professionals receiving training and certification, and the development of a specifically pediatric curriculum. Since 1987, annual pediatric training workshops have been offered, initially under the auspices of the Society for Developmental and Behavioral Pediatrics, and since 2010 by the National Pediatric Hypnosis Training Institute, both American organizations. In Germany, the Kindertagung (the largest child hypnosis congress in the world) has been held periodically since 1990, with thousands of participants and an international faculty. There are excellent textbooks in the field, including Hypnosis and Hypnotherapy in Children [2], and Therapeutic Hypnosis with Children and Adolescents [3]. The American Journal of Clinical Hypnosis has published special issues on pediatric specific themes [4]. However, despite increasingly rich training and education resources, the number of licensed health professionals regularly utilizing hypnosis in practice is relatively small compared, say, to other similar skill sets such as active listening, motivational interviewing, or mindfulness training for example. Even after training, a practitioner may face the difficulty of local access to mentoring or modeling of the practical matters of incorporating hypnosis into pediatric clinical encounters. While not a substitute for training, this article will review some of those matters of practical application, the use of language, and may demystify the hypnosis referral process for other professionals.

2. Utilizing and Planning

A clinician who wishes to be purposeful in utilizing hypnosis in clinical encounters can begin by simply noticing the number of ways that children demonstrate spontaneous trance, or display behaviors that may be interpreted or understood as spontaneous self-hypnosis skills. While these are not quite conscious or intentional, they are nonetheless common in the context of everyday clinical encounters [5]. These quite natural states may take the form of imaginative language or play during a clinical encounter, intense focus or concentration on an activity, game, book, or puzzle, intense (and even fearful) focus on a physical sensation or injury, or distracted daydreaming that serves the purpose of adaptive dissociation for the child in an otherwise unpleasant situation. The fact that natural trance states occur so frequently in children in healthcare settings leads to the inescapable conclusion that *all* clinicians, whether trained in hypnosis or not, must be very careful with word choices around children. During any trance state, a person is much more likely to accept a suggestion as true (and act upon it); even unintentional suggestions or developmentally misinterpreted statements may have a larger than expected impact on a child [6]. For example, a clinician attempting humor with a 5-year-old with a wrist fracture may say something like "it's OK, you won't miss using that arm for a while . . . ." While an adult would be able to process such language as jest, a child in the trance of pain and injury may hear those words as suggestions for disuse or loss of the arm. Both children and adults interpret suggestions made during a trance state very literally and concretely. The concept of "trance logic" implies that during trance, a person may have very limited reality testing and would likely accept and act upon whatever suggestion is offered [7]. A natural trance state may be generated by a variety of healthcare encounters, such as an illness visit, awaiting an immunization, pre-operative preparation, or hearing an interpretation of lab tests or radiology results. Clinicians in these settings must think carefully about their choice of words and the effect of unintentional suggestions.

Conversely, natural trance states give clinicians the opportunity to decide when and how to utilize the child's demonstrated strengths by the purposeful use of language to build positive expectancy and positive outcomes. Thoughtful use of hypnotic language includes choice of words, tone of voice, and reflective listening. The decision to utilize the child's own natural self-hypnosis may be implemented immediately (e.g. "I'm impressed by how you are helping yourself right now" for a child with Tourette's who is not having tics in the office), or implemented later when appropriate in the conversation (e.g., "remember a few minutes ago when you were enjoying your new book? Did you know *you can do that* while the nurse is giving you medicine in your arm so it doesn't have to *bother you so much?*").

Natural trance states in children can be understood as the child's spontaneous and subconscious attempt to organize their experiences (especially novel and perhaps frightening experiences) and make new connections in four areas of self-regulation: cognitive, affective/emotional, physiologic, and behavioral. When clinicians are attentive and prepared, they can notice and then facilitate the child's nascent self-regulatory capacity by "being hypnotic" in a clinical conversation. For example, an observant clinician dealing with a child with a delayed sleep onset disorder may be watching for a child's attempts at emotional self-regulation and learning about how the child might self-soothe from anxiety symptoms. Based on moment-to-moment observation of the child, the clinical interview might include something like "I notice you took a nice deep breath just now . . . I wonder why/how your brain chose *right now* to do that?" Or to access the child's ability for physiologic self-regulation, a clinician could ask "what have you done in the past to help that tummy feel better when stress or worry had made it uncomfortable?" This approach is quite different from one that would take a clinical history, view all of that as devoid of trance or hypnotic phenomena, and then verbally move into a new section of the appointment understood or even labeled as "doing hypnosis." The concept of utilizing children's trance as a way of enhancing self-regulatory skills has been expertly reviewed by Kaiser [8].

This approach to enhancing children's self-regulatory capacity by utilizing hypnotic language without "doing hypnosis" can be characterized as noticing and cultivating the natural hypnotic state, or "using the hypnosis" in the encounter. It usually occurs in the context of taking a clinical history. But the history taking process can and should be more of a conversation than a question and answer checklist, in which clinical questions and open-ended reflection are designed to help the child begin to reframe their experiences, expand their cognitive capacity by attaching new labels to experience, and expand their emotional fluency and self-awareness. The clinician can be extremely helpful to children and teens by simply using reflective listening skills to enhance self-awareness, knowing that self-awareness is a foundational first step to self-regulation. For example, a child may present to the medical office with both chronic abdominal pain and separation anxiety, but has never comprehended the connection between the two. The clinical conversation helps the child to make sense of his or her disconnected experiences and understand that they are not separate phenomena. Because of curiosity and novelty, this conversation is often hypnotic, but is not "doing hypnosis" in the sense that there is a formal sequence of invitation, induction or any script. It is important in this type of clinical conversation for the clinician to provide observations of the co-incidence of phenomena in the child's life, but in the end each patient must make the connections for themselves by responding to questions like "tell me what you make of that . . . ."

Complementary to the concept of utilizing natural trance states, it is equally important for clinicians to be deliberate in planning or designing hypnotic encounters, especially before entering a consult in which the reason for the appointment is already known. This implies intentional planning, a carefully crafted encounter with a patient that is more likely to have been thought out ahead of time, reviewing a clinical history that is (mostly) known and planning the structure and content of an appointment, including the type of induction and the metaphors/suggestions that would be most appropriate based on the clinical history. It may be helpful for the clinician to outline in writing some expected steps of the appointment, following a predicted sequence: interim history, today's therapeutic goals, induction technique, intensification strategy, suggestions/metaphors, post-hypnotic suggestions, alerting and ratification, and follow-up plan. It involves giving therapeutic, specific suggestions related to specific goals for that particular clinical encounter. (Induction and intensification techniques and the specific use of hypnotic suggestion and therapeutic metaphor are beyond the scope of this article.) Thoughtful planning of each of the expected steps of the appointment can make a positive outcome more likely. Still, even when carefully planned and conceived ahead of time, in any given appointment a clinician must be prepared to flexibly follow cues from the child, adapting strategies based on how the child demonstrates readiness for help in cultivating these skills.

Whether "doing hypnosis" or "noticing and utilizing and being hypnotic", clinicians must recognize in this model that patients, especially children, bring trance with them into the setting without being aware of it. Trance is what the brain does naturally when it encounters something for the first time, giving attention to novelty: "I never saw that before," "I never thought of it that way before," "I never met anyone quite like you before," or even "I never had a pain quite like this before." Trance can be elevating and activating (like a 6-month old reaching for a cardboard picture book), or it can be terrible like the fight or flight response of someone who encounters a phobic object. Within that trance, there is often an openness to change, a readiness to see and experience the world differently, that is, to learn. That may occur with or without the patient having any cultivated self-hypnosis skills, but the attentive clinician will often find that children and teens arrive at appointments with some skills they have already discovered for themselves in this area.

Thus, whether the encounter is spontaneous or planned, clinicians bring their own skill sets and attentiveness to the encounter, ready to cultivate change for the patient, but only when and if the child or teen allows that to happen. In any encounter where the clinician is doing something formally or informally planned to be hypnotic or to evoke hypnosis in the patient, nothing happens at all unless the patient is willing and open to this. In this model, one may see hypnosis as an interpersonal interaction by which the clinician cultivates a trance that the patient makes accessible, for the purpose of a specific health related outcome.

3. Primary Care Pediatrics

In the primary care pediatric setting, there are four areas in which a clinician's choice of words can intersect with a child's curiosity and become a spontaneously hypnotic encounter that facilitates positive outcomes. They are: developmental mastery, positive expectation, behavior change/motivation, and discovering self-regulation.

Developmental mastery: Even during well-child checkups for infants and toddlers, a clinician can reinforce the child's own growing sense of competence or the maternal-infant dyad's resilience by making the screening history conversational. For example, pointing out to a new mother how alert and attentive a nursing infant is, talking with parents about how their newborn is constantly learning, commenting on how focused is the 6-month old reaching for a cardboard picture book (demonstrating trance, encountering novelty). In these settings, the mother is often also in trance focusing on her child, so these are opportune moments for positive comments and suggestions regarding the multitude of opportunities that parents and caregivers have to interact with the child in ways that build resilience and developmental mastery.

Pediatric practitioners have daily opportunities to reinforce the child's growing developmental competence. The verbal content of the well-child history changes with age and developmental stages, but at each age, the words that a clinician chooses can be powerfully reinforcing. The child's natural trance state in the healthcare encounter creates an opportunity for purposeful suggestions that are specific to the developmental stage of the child or teen. Any pediatric health provider wishing to apply clinical hypnosis must first become fluent in the normal stages of child development and learn how to connect with children in a developmentally appropriate way [9]. For example, a 3-year-old (in Erikson's stage of autonomy versus shame and doubt) would have his/her developmental mastery reinforced by a comment like, "look how well you climbed onto the exam table *by yourself*! When you were a baby you couldn't do that!," or during a checkup saying to a 10-year-old (stage of industry versus inferiority, where competence is the key strength to be developed) "You're good at lots of things! I wonder how many things you'll learn to be good at by this time next year?."

Positive expectation: Setting positive expectations for children in pediatric healthcare settings is an important and often neglected challenge. Immunizations, phlebotomy, or the uncertainty and anxiety regarding the physical examination all create strongly negative expectations for children and teens in medical offices. Using distraction and other hypnotic approaches to reduce children's discomfort in medical offices is a very important subject in its own right and will not be covered in detail in this paper [10]. A growing body of literature supports the idea that measures to reduce pain of immunizations and procedures in children are both important and achievable [11]. Even without structured office interventions to reduce discomfort, each clinician can help children and teens feel more comfortable, physically and emotionally, by careful choice of words. Because children and teens are often in a natural trance state (albeit a negative one full of intense focus on a feared event) in the medical office, a carefully crafted statement that reframes the experience and opens the child to new expectations can be powerful. For example, "I don't really know just what it will feel like for you, but I do know that you may be surprised at how little it will have to bother you, and how easy it may be for you just to pay attention to something else while the nurse takes good care of that arm over there … ." On the other hand, suggestions such as "it's not going to *hurt*," can be pro-nociceptive. A child's thoughts will invariably focus on the word "hurt" and ignore the word "not." Finding ways to use words to substitute for "pain" and "hurt" is important. Use "bother" in place of "hurt," and "discomfort" instead of "pain".

Behavior change/motivation: Any primary care office caring for adolescents will present daily opportunities to use hypnotic language to promote behavior change. In this context, there is a large overlap between the use of hypnotic language and the principles of motivational interviewing [12,13]. One of the core concepts of motivational interviewing is Developing Discrepancy. This is the process in which the clinician facilitates the patient's awareness of his/her current state versus a desired future state. A respectful and empathetic conversation that provokes the teen to think deeply about this discrepancy can often lead to spontaneous trance experiences in the patient. For example, asking a teen, "I wonder what sort of things you picture or think about when you think about yourself one year from now ... " can be followed by an expectant silence, in which trance phenomena may be observed. This can be a very useful way to gauge readiness to change. Another key concept of motivational interviewing is that of Exploring Ambivalence. A question such as "will you miss the extra weight when it is gone?" is an implied hypnotic suggestion that the weight will in fact be gone at some future time. Second, it implies that the patient may be ambivalent about it and can (perhaps in spontaneous trance induced by such a novel question) explore the pros and cons of continuing current behaviors versus changing. One can also explore other motivational interviewing domains while the patient is in trance, either from a formal hypnotic induction or spontaneous. A suggestion for future visualization of the self (either with the positive health behavior change or not) can assist the patient in exploring his/her readiness to change, and in affirming his/her own goals. For example, "while these thoughts are on your mind, take a moment to picture yourself, as if on a 'future TV screen' and get a sense of what you like about that picture, what you don't like about that picture, and what choices you can make now that affect that future." This clinical encounter may be in the mental health office or in the primary care office around issues of health behavior.

Self-regulation: Another important way in which purposeful language in outpatient settings can be hypnotic is in facilitating discovery of psychophysiological self-regulation (e.g., breath awareness). Many opportunities for this in clinical care. For example, a brief intervention in the office for a child with anxiety can start with a question like, "Can you put your hand on the place where that worry shows up most in your body?" Most children will readily identify the site of the most troubling somatic symptoms related to stress. A follow-up question can immediately follow: "Would it be OK to learn how to help yourself feel better there?" Teaching the child or teen simple techniques of abdominal breathing and then noticing how they feel differently can be a powerful first step in enhanced self-regulation. It is also important during the clinical encounter to encourage the child or teen to reflect on how they may have already discovered their own methods of physiologic self-regulation. It is not uncommon for a patient to disclose their own techniques to the clinician, such as "I already use my imagination and breathing when I am nervous at bedtime." The clinician's task then is to reinforce and ratify the child's own strengths with statements like "helping you learn to help yourself is going to be easier than I thought, since you are *already good at changing things*".

4. Hospital and Acute Care Settings

Hypnotic language can often be utilized in hospital settings or in preparation for medical procedures [14]. This can be very informal, without a formal induction, and may occur in the routine course of daily work for a pediatric hospitalist or a Child Life professional. A clinician may also set a longer appointment time for more formal hypnotherapy to prepare for an anticipated procedure. Fundamentally, this involves rehearsing the procedure in trance and creating positive expectations. However, any such intervention must be developmentally appropriate, and expecting a preschooler to sit quietly and visualize is not developmentally on target. Such a child could be encouraged to bring a doll or favorite toy with them, and a playful conversation about how well the doll can experience the upcoming procedure may be sufficient, as long as the child is engaged in the imaginative experience. More formal trance induction in an older child could be followed by imaginal desensitization (the "future TV of me") using imagery and suggestions that reframe and change the child or teen's expectations. In urgent care and emergency settings, clinicians have opportunities to help children in crisis. The negative trance that children and teens bring with them into that circumstance in fact makes the use of hypnotic language easier, and is also a reminder of the critical importance of choice of words in acute care settings. Our language in such settings is important, because the children are already in a highly suggestible state. During evaluation of an acute injury, it is possible to embed hypnotic suggestions such as "I can tell it hurts, and you know it may keep on keep on hurting until it feels better, or until it doesn't need to any more . . . ." The likelihood is that the words that "stick" in the child's consciousness are the words "it feels better," which is, after all, the desired outcome. Reframing is possible as well, such as "isn't it nice that your body knows how to use all that good healthy blood to clean out the cut?"

5. The Hypnotherapy Consult

Clinicians who are trained and develop their clinical hypnosis practice will invariably be consulted by other clinicians, usually regarding patients who remain symptomatic despite all the usual diagnostic and therapeutic approaches of more conventional pediatric medicine. For such appointments, it is wise to block a longer extended appointment time, at least 45 min, in order to establish rapport, gather the clinical history, explain hypnosis and self-hypnosis to the child and parent(s), clarify the rationale for using hypnotherapy for the troubling symptoms, reassure the parents (more than the child) that a referral for hypnotherapy does not imply that anyone believes the symptoms are not "real," and then (perhaps) to begin self-hypnosis coaching for the child or teen. Often there is not sufficient time in a first appointment to give adequate attention to the actual use of hypnotherapy, and a quick return appointment is expected.

There are a number of ways that hypnotic language shows up in these appointments even well before anything that looks like hypnosis, and should start during the process of gathering the medical history. The clinician should be alert to signs of trance in the child, and then reflecting their own trance state back to them in several ways. First, find out what they do well, and what resources they have already discovered for wellness and self-regulation. Short phrases that can be useful include:

Tell me about something you do so well, and is so much fun, that you often or usually forget most everything else . . .

What was going on the last time you felt really good?

Can we talk about that time when you felt really worried but didn't (throw-up, have a headache, etc.)?

This process always involves the clinician noticing what the patient is saying, how s/he is saying it, the moments which appear to be moments of trance in which s/he is attempting to make sense of connections and novel ideas, and then offering new interpretations of what s/he has said, as a way of opening possibilities to change based on what s/he already knows.

Words and phrases that can help as therapeutic reflection of child's own trance, specifically planned to cultivate and nurture the child's own curiosity include:

How do YOU think is the best way to learn that?

You have lots of skills (in whatever areas already discussed), are you ready to learn some new things or new ways to help yourself solve that problem with . . . ?

How does your bladder know to keep the gate shut while you are sitting in school during the day?

Is there a time when pain can be useful?

Do you know about the pain switches?

I wonder how soon you will be able to turn off the pain switch when it's not needed . . .

How did you do that?

Preparation is critical for these consult appointments. The prepared clinician will review prior medical records, referral documents, and his/her own notes for return appointments. This implies that one should keep very detailed notes of appointments. Write down in the medical record the child's own words that describe their situation; record the history from the parents' perspective; record observations of the child's demeanor during the appointment and how that may have changed over the course of the appointment; record their likes and dislikes, things they do well, who they live with, how they are doing in school, and any special circumstances of the family, such as military deployments for example. When the child returns for the second appointment, the prepared clinician has already reviewed these notes in order to build on that rapport and to remember what worked well and what did not work well.

During the appointment, it is advisable to direct most of the conversation to the child, not to the parent. One can explicitly say to the child at the outset that s/he is important, what s/he thinks is important, what s/he says is important, *and* that the parent will also have a turn to talk, because *s/he has some important things to say too*, but that can wait.

This deliberately child-centric posture is, in all likelihood, completely different from any prior experience this child has had with medical professionals, who tend to talk *about* them *to* their parents, but not talking *with* them and acting respectful of what they have to say. This implies to the child that one is confident in them to articulate and express their own wishes and desires. It builds their trust in the clinician, and it most certainly builds their curiosity in what is about to happen because it breaks previously held expectations about conversations with doctors. It creates the space and opportunity to transform old cognitive, emotional, physiologic, or behavioral patterns of self-regulation. It implies a belief that they *themselves* can be an effective change agent for their own issues. This conversation with the child must always be done in a developmentally appropriate way, remembering to talk with a 7-year-old *very* differently than with a 14-year-old.

After planning and preparation is done, the clinician's behavior toward the patient is that of leading with permission. Leading implies that one has a skill set to use in order to show the patient in a collaborative way *how* they can get to their goals. The patient came to the appointment with a need and did not know on their own how to meet that need; it is the clinician's job to lead them there. Equally as important, it is the clinician's job to recognize that all of this happens only if the patient wants it to happen. That is true not just of the hypnotherapy itself, but also of the appointment in general. A useful introductory comment is that "things happen in hypnosis because you want them to happen, not because I want them to happen." This "leading with permission" posture and behavior continues even during hypnosis, so that the language of suggestions is not prescriptive (e.g., "you will have the pain down to zero by the time I count down from 10"), but permissive (e.g., "I wonder how soon you will find that old pain completely gone ... let me know when you get it down to zero ... ").

There are pros and cons of keeping parents in the consult room while working with a child or teen [15]. Many clinicians keep the parent in the room for most if not all of the first appointment, enhancing insights into the parent-child interaction and whether it may be a strength or a liability; it can also help to get two different perspectives on the issues at hand. At subsequent appointments, it may not be advisable to keep a parent in the room during hypnotherapy, as a parent can be distracting and cause the child to "perform" in a way that they believe their parents would expect rather than exercising their own autonomy and mastery. Similar to the child's performance expectations with parents watching, the clinician may also become overly self-conscious with parents watching. A clinician who is personally attached to creating a certain outcome in the clinical encounter or who is consciously or unconsciously trying to please a parent is not likely to give his or her best energy to creating a therapeutic alliance with the child or teen. This can inadvertently sabotage the very clinical outcome the clinician is anxious to demonstrate to the parent. A clinician who is anxious about what a parent is thinking about him or her is not likely to be clinically effective. If a child is very anxious, one may more strongly consider keeping the parent in the room, hoping to gradually wean the child from that anxious attachment to facilitate their mastery of new skills in self-regulation.

Audio recordings of hypnotherapy sessions can be very helpful as a tool to help the child/teen practice at home, and most families now have a smart phone with a voice recorder app, making recording almost effortless. One may want to introduce the idea of using the recording at home with a comment like "you can find this a helpful way to start practicing, until you don't need the audio anymore."

On return appointments, the interim history will reveal if things have gone well or not. If the patient's experience was positive or neutral, they will expect to have a repeat hypnotherapy session with more guidance for self-hypnosis practice at home. It may be advisable on the second visit to use the same hypnotic induction as at the first appointment in order to help reinforce what may still be a fragile practice of self-hypnosis at home. On future appointments with a patient who is making progress, it can be a good idea to teach them a new type of self-induction for themselves at home, to build skills and the opportunity for new types of self-discovery.

If parents or children report that things did not go well after the first appointment, the clinician must gather all the details about what happened in the interim, and re-assess the child/teen's interest and willingness to use such techniques to feel better. All that may be required is a different approach, along with continued optimism that a child who is motivated to feel well will discover (with expert guidance) a way to enhance their own self-regulatory ability in order to resolve an issue.

6. Resources and Training

It is incumbent on all professionals who care for children in healthcare settings to be aware of the power of words in affecting the mental and physical health of children, for better or for worse. Experienced and thoughtful pediatric clinicians are aware of this even without specific training in clinical hypnosis. Over time, most clinicians become more careful in how they speak during clinical encounters, helping children become more comfortable in healthcare settings. However, many of the concepts described in this paper are quite different from widespread practice patterns. A thoughtful clinician wanting to interact with children and teens in such new ways will soon realize that specific and more concentrated training is needed. The annual training workshops conducted by the National Pediatric Hypnosis Training Institute (NPHTI, a United States registered non-profit 501(c)(3) corporation) are directed by experienced clinician educators and achieve consistently high ratings from attendees. More information is available [16]. The American Society of Clinical Hypnosis (ASCH) conducts annual meetings, national and regional workshops, and is the certifying body for health professionals in the United States who have had clinical hypnosis training. There is a small but consistent presence of pediatric offerings the annual workshops by ASCH [17]. Professionals in Europe can avail themselves of the resources and training events from the European Society of Hypnosis [18]. And while one does not become skilled in clinical hypnosis by reading articles or books, there are seminal readings which should form the foundation of basic knowledge of any pediatric clinician. These include Michael Yapko's book, Trancework [19], and the more specific pediatric titles Hypnosis and Hypnotherapy in Children [2], and Therapeutic Hypnosis with Children and Adolescents [3]. ASCH publishes pediatric specific articles frequently to keep professionals abreast with progress in the field [4]. With frequent attendance at hypnosis training workshops and meetings, a commitment to reading core books and articles, a thoughtful pediatric clinician can not only facilitate transformation for his or her patients, but also transform his or her own professional life and satisfaction.

Acknowledgments: I am grateful to my colleagues and mentors in the National Pediatric Hypnosis Training Institute and to the children and families with whom I am privileged to work.

Conflicts of Interest: The author declares no conflict of interest.

References

1. Kohen, D.P.; Kaiser, P. Clinical Hypnosis with Children and Adolescents—What? Why? How? Origins, Applications, and Efficacy. *Children* **2014**, *1*, 74–98. [CrossRef] [PubMed]
2. Kohen, D.P.; Olness, K.N. *Hypnosis and Hypnotherapy with Children*, 4th ed.; Routledge Publications: New York, NY, USA, 2011.

3.   Wester, W.; Sugarman, L.I. *Therapeutic Hypnosis with Children and Adolescents*; Crown House Publishing: Carmarthen, Wales, UK, 2007.
4.   Anbar, R.D. Guest Editorial: Clinical Pearls Gleaned from Pediatric Hypnosis. *Am. J. Clin. Hypn.* **2011**, *54*, 3–4. [CrossRef] [PubMed]
5.   Olness, K.N.; Gardner, G.G. Some Guidelines for uses of hypnotherapy in pediatrics. *Pediatrics* **1978**, *62*, 228. [PubMed]
6.   Kohen, D.P.; Olness, K.N. *Hypnosis and Hypnotherapy with Children*, 4th ed.; Routledge Publications: New York, NY, USA, 2011; pp. 109–112.
7.   Yapko, M. *Trancework*, 4th ed.; Routledge Publications: New York, NY, USA, 2012; pp. 185–186.
8.   Kaiser, P. Childhood anxiety, worry and fear: Individualizing hypnosis goals and suggestions for self-regulation. *Am. J. Clin. Hypn.* **2011**, *54*, 16–31. [CrossRef] [PubMed]
9.   *Growth and crises of the "healthy personality"*; Erikson, E.H.; Senn, M.J.E. (Eds.) Symposium on the healthy personality; Josiah Macy Jr. Foundation: Oxford, England, 1950; pp. 91–146.
10.   Berberich, F.R.; Landman, Z. Reducing immunization discomfort in 4 to 6 year old children: A randomized clinical trial. *Pediatrics* **2009**, *124*, e203–e209. [CrossRef] [PubMed]
11.   Lee, G.Y.; Yamada, J.; Shorkey, A.; Stevens, B. Pediatric Clinical Practice Guidelines for Acute Procedural Pain: A Systematic Review. *Pediatrics* **2014**, *133*, 1–16. [CrossRef] [PubMed]
12.   Miller, W.R.; Rollnick, S. *Motivational Interviewing: Helping People Change*, 3rd ed.; Guilford Press: New York, NY, USA, 2013.
13.   Barnes, A.J.; Gold, M.A. Promoting Healthy Behaviors in Pediatrics. *Pediatr. Rev.* **2012**, *33*, e57–e68. [CrossRef] [PubMed]
14.   Kuttner, L. Management of young children's acute pain and anxiety during invasive medical procedures. *Pediatrician* **1989**, *16*, 39–45. [PubMed]
15.   Linden, J. Hypnosis and Parents: Pattern interruptus. *Am. J. Clin. Hypn.* **2011**, *54*, 70–81. [CrossRef] [PubMed]
16.   National Pediatric Hypnosis Training Institute. Available online: www.nphti.org (accessed on 14 March 2017).
17.   American Society of Clinical Hypnosis. Available online: www.asch.net (accessed on 14 March 2017).
18.   European Society of Hypnosis. Available online: http://esh-hypnosis.eu (accessed on 14 March 2017).
19.   Yapko, M. *Trancework*, 4th ed.; Routledge Publications: New York, NY, USA, 2012.

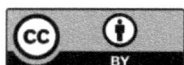

children

MDPI

Review

Mind–Body Interventions for Pediatric Inflammatory Bowel Disease

Ann Ming Yeh [1],*, Anava Wren [1] and Brenda Golianu [2]

[1] Department of Pediatrics, Division of Pediatric Gastroenterology, Hepatology and Nutrition,
   Stanford University, Palo Alto, CA 94304, USA; awren2@stanford.edu
[2] Department of Anesthesia, Perioperative and Pain Medicine, Stanford University, Palo Alto, CA 94304, USA;
   bgolianu@stanford.edu
* Correspondence: annming@stanford.edu; Tel.: +1-650-723-5070

Academic Editor: Hilary McClafferty
Received: 15 February 2017; Accepted: 27 March 2017; Published: 3 April 2017

Abstract: Pediatric inflammatory bowel disease is an autoimmune disease that causes chronic inflammation of the gastrointestinal mucosa. There is emerging evidence that the brain–gut connection affects inflammatory bowel disease (IBD) patients more than previously thought. This is evidenced by comorbid mood disorders, irritable bowel symptoms concurrent with quiescent IBD, and the potential of psychosocial stressors to trigger IBD flares. Mind–body interventions such as psychotherapy, relaxation, mindfulness, biofeedback, yoga, and clinical hypnosis offer an adjunct to standard medical treatment for IBD. We will review the current evidence base for these mind–body interventions in the treatment of pediatric IBD, illustrate a case study, and offer suggestions for future research for this promising field.

Keywords: mind-body; inflammatory bowel disease; pediatric; biofeedback; psychotherapy; hypnosis; yoga; relaxation

1. Introduction

Inflammatory bowel disease (IBD) is a chronic and relapsing inflammatory condition involving all or part of the gastrointestinal (GI) tract. The most common forms of IBD are Crohn's Disease (CD) and Ulcerative Colitis (UC), where CD may involve the entire GI tract and UC involves only the large intestine. The pathophysiology of IBD is thought to be multifactorial, involving a complex interplay between genetic predisposition, the gut microbiota, gut mucosal integrity, the immune system, and environmental triggers such as nutrition and psychosocial stressors [1,2]. Conventional treatments for pediatric IBD include anti-inflammatory pharmacologic therapies (5-aminosalicylic acid derivatives), corticosteroids, immunomodulators (6-mercaptopurine, methotrexate), and biologics [3]. Nutritional therapies such as enteral nutrition can also be effective for small bowel Crohn's disease [4–6].

Patients with IBD commonly seek integrative and complementary medicine treatment due to beliefs that medications are not effective, concern about medication side effects/risks, and interest in adjunct therapies to optimize disease management and help to improve symptoms and quality of life [7]. Integrative medicine is considered a healing-oriented medicine that reaffirms the importance of the relationship between practitioner and patient, focuses on the whole person, and utilizes empirically supported therapeutic approaches. According to the National Institute of Health, integrative medicine is an umbrella term that can include various modalities such as natural products (e.g., herbs and supplements), whole systems medicine (e.g., traditional Chinese medicine, Ayurveda), and mind–body interventions (e.g., relaxation, yoga, clinical hypnosis). The term integrative refers to the coordinated approach of utilizing conventional and complementary therapies together in an integrative way [8].

Over the past decade, mind–body interventions (MBI) have received increased attention. These interventions are categorized as those that 'employ a variety of techniques designed to facilitate the mind's capacity to affect bodily function and symptoms' [9]. Mind–body interventions are thought to be dynamic, and some definitions of MBI include manipulative modalities such as acupuncture, massage, and spinal manipulation. For the purposes of this review, however, we will focus on non-manipulative MBI, including psychotherapy, relaxation techniques, mindfulness-based therapies, biofeedback, yoga, and clinical hypnosis. Mind–body interventions are emerging as popular treatment modalities amongst IBD patients [10] and provide safe, inexpensive, non-pharmacologic ways to target the autonomic nervous system by decreasing the stress response and increasing the relaxation response.

The aim of this paper is to: (1) provide background information and a rationale for the use of mind–body interventions in pediatric IBD populations; (2) provide a brief overview of key mind–body interventions for pediatric IBD; (3) review the safety and efficacy of these mind–body interventions and highlight areas for future research; and (4) present a sample case demonstrating a multidisciplinary approach to mind–body IBD treatment.

Regarding the criteria for considering studies for this review, all controlled clinical trials, quasi-randomized trials, and non-randomized trials including pediatric patients with UC or CD and mind–body interventions were included. The search criteria were expanded to include adult patients with IBD or youth with irritable bowel syndrome (IBS) when no literature was available in pediatric IBD samples. Studies published between 1980 and 2017 were considered in this review. Pubmed was utilized as the primary search engine. The search strategies included terms related to pediatrics, IBD, IBS, mind–body interventions identified for this review, and common synonyms for the aforementioned terms.

2. Background

While the pathophysiology of IBD is thought to be due to interrelated factors, increasing evidence has shown the intimate connection between the brain and the gut and the effect of this bidirectional interaction on gut and psychological health [11]. It is noteworthy to highlight that IBD patients readily identify stress as a contributing factor to disease flares [12,13]. Numerous studies have noted a significant association between perceived stress, negative mood, and major life events and disease relapse, hospitalization, and abdominal surgery risk [12,14]. Prospective studies show that exposure to stressful events as well as perceived stress (i.e., the individual's view of a demand relative to their resources) may contribute to relapse risk [15–17]. One study found that pediatric patients with IBD who had low stress levels and used non-avoidant coping strategies had fewer relapses [15], suggesting the potential benefit of stress management interventions in this population.

The bidirectional brain-gut relationship is especially notable in youth who have IBD with associated IBS-type symptoms. Despite adequate control of their IBD, patients may continue to suffer from refractory IBS symptoms. At times, this situation may present a diagnostic and treatment challenge, as it may be difficult to distinguish between 'true' IBS symptoms versus a subclinical form of IBD. Children with IBD in clinical remission, as defined in the abbreviated-PCDAI (pediatric Crohn's disease activity index) or the PUCAI (pediatric ulcerative colitis activity index), have a 6.4% prevalence of IBS-type symptoms. In patients who have biochemical markers of quiescent or minimal disease, with a calprotectin in <250 µg/g, IBS symptom prevalence is 16.1% (95% confidence interval (CI): 7.6–25.8%; Crohn's disease: 16.7%; ulcerative colitis: 10.8% [18]. A meta-analysis of 1703 patients showed that patients with IBD had a higher prevalence of IBS symptoms, compared to non-IBD controls [19].

Patients in IBD remission may suffer from a variety of somatic complaints, including recurrent abdominal pain, urgency, diarrhea, constipation, bloating, gas, and cramping sensations. Symptoms of pain and discomfort may persist even after inflammation is adequately controlled due to visceral hyperalgesia, somatic-parietal abdominal pain, referred pain, strictures or adhesions, small intestinal bacterial overgrowth (SIBO), dysmotility, and central sensitization [20]. Factors that may increase central sensitization include disordered sleep, social stressors, and the presence of anxiety or depression [20]. IBD and IBS have overlapping and interacting mechanisms of illness. Subsets of IBS patients may have low grade inflammation, and some studies suggest that IBS and IBD exist on a similar disease continuum [21,22]. Furthermore, both IBD and IBS patients may have derangements in the gut microbiota that lead to disease [23–25].

A multidisciplinary approach to the management of IBD and IBS symptoms is essential to successful symptom improvement and disease treatment [26–28]. This approach includes thorough assessment and management by a pediatrician in consultation with a gastroenterology specialist to ensure adequate control of inflammation and gut physiological factors. Additional providers include a dietician to assess nutritional concerns; a pain specialist if pain is a presenting complaint; a physical or occupational therapist if there is significant deconditioning or loss of quality of life; and a clinical psychologist, pediatric pain psychologist, or other mental health therapist if there are psychosocial, adjustment, or symptom management concerns. An effective multidisciplinary team will work in tandem to guide appropriate interventions and disease modifying therapies for patients, optimize their physiologic and psychological wellbeing, and help to improve and sustain their ongoing quality of life [29].

IBD patients, specifically those with persistent IBS symptoms despite quiescent inflammation, may benefit from integrating mind–body interventions into multidisciplinary care. Research has demonstrated that mind–body interventions are commonly utilized by patients with IBS and IBD and may help to decrease anxiety and improve coping abilities [10]. Of note, up to 84% of pediatric patients with IBD already utilize some sort of integrative medicine therapy, according to a single-center survey at a tertiary care center [10]. Among these, 61% of patients used stress management and 35% utilized special exercises (e.g., yoga, swimming). In another survey of 67 adolescents with IBD, 40% used relaxation and 21% used guided imagery once a day to once a week for symptom management [30]. Younger adolescents were more likely to regularly use meditation, and adolescents with more severe disease were more willing to consider using relaxation as an adjunct therapy. Given the high utilization of mind–body interventions among pediatric IBD patients and the potential efficacy of MBI for this population, providers should be knowledgeable and open to discussing common mind–body interventions.

3. Mind–Body Interventions

3.1. Psychotherapy

Patients with IBD endorse elevated levels of emotional distress and poor quality of life compared to the general population [28,31]. Anxiety and depressive disorders have been documented to be higher among patients with IBD compared to non-IBD cohorts [31–33]. In pediatric IBD populations, high rates of anxiety and depression have been documented and there is an increased risk of developing depression compared to youth with other chronic illnesses and healthy controls [33–35]. Symptoms of anxiety and depression have been negatively associated with psychological well-being and disease-related outcomes in IBD populations, including lower quality of life, increased perceived stress, IBD relapse, inflammation, pain, poor medication adherence, and increased risk of surgery [28,33,36–39]. Unfortunately, psychiatric comorbidities are often under-diagnosed and undertreated across the lifespan. Recently, there has been growing support for multidisciplinary IBD treatment in order to treat the whole patient, including psychological interventions for youth and adults with IBD [28]. Psychological interventions have received increasing attention in the mind–body IBD literature [7], given the comorbidity between psychological conditions and IBD and the preliminary efficacy of such treatments on both psychological and physical outcomes.

Psychological interventions aimed at improving emotional distress and disease outcomes among IBD patients have generally focused on psychotherapy, stress management, hypnosis, and psychoeducation [40]. Over the past decade, numerous systematic reviews and meta-analyses have explored the effect of psychological interventions on children, adolescents, and adults with IBD. Overall, the findings have been mixed. A Cochrane review from 2011 [41] concluded that there was no evidence for psychological interventions in adults with IBD; however, the authors noted more empirical evidence for the use of psychotherapy among pediatric populations with IBD. Specifically, such interventions were found to improve depression and quality of life among youth [41]. More recent reviews have found psychological interventions to have some benefit on psychological outcomes and growing potential to reduce physical symptoms such as pain and fatigue, relapse rate, hospitalization, and medication adherence [40,42]. These mixed findings have been partially attributed to the limited body of research, comparing interventions with varying psychological content and methodological limitations.

Cognitive Behavioral Therapy

Cognitive behavioral therapy (CBT) is one type of psychological intervention that has demonstrated particular promise among pediatric populations with IBD. While there are many types of psychotherapy, CBT is the most common and has the greatest evidence base in pediatric IBD populations [35,43]. CBT is based on the premise that emotions, thoughts, and behaviors are interconnected and that psychological functioning can improve by working to understand and change maladaptive thoughts and behaviors. Significant literature supports the use of CBT among children with anxiety and mood disorders [44,45], and growing research has demonstrated the efficacy of CBT protocols among youth with chronic illnesses [46].

Szigethy and colleagues conducted some of the first studies exploring the effectiveness of CBT among youth with IBD [47]. They modified a manual-based CBT protocol to address the impact of physical illness on youth with depression. The intervention focused on physical illness narrative, social skills training, and family education. The protocol consists of nine individual modules focused on behavioral activation, cognitive restructuring, and problem-solving skills and three family sessions focused on psychoeducation and family problem-solving skills. An early pilot study demonstrated promising results among 11 adolescents (12–17 years). Specifically, there were significant reductions in child and parent-reported depression symptoms pre- to post-treatment ($p < 0.001$; 0.65–0.92 effect size), as well as significant improvements in global adjustment ($p < 0.01$) and physical functioning ($p < 0.05$) among youth [47]. Despite these positive results, there were several study limitations, including the small sample size and the lack of a control group and long-term follow-up, limiting assumptions of causality and generalizability.

Later larger randomized controlled groups by Szigethy et al. [48] demonstrated that, among 41 youth with IBD, the protocol could lead to clinically significant improvements in depression symptoms ($p < 0.01$; 1.01 effect size) and functioning ($p < 0.05$, 0.86 effect size), compared to treatment as usual. Of note, these benefits persisted one-year post-treatment. When the protocol was compared to supportive non-directive therapy (SNDT), the results showed that both interventions equally reduced depression symptoms (37.3% for CBT; 31.9% for SNDT) among 217 youth [43]. There were also significant improvements across groups on measures of global functioning, quality of life, and disease activity; however, the CBT intervention showed a significantly greater reduction in IBD activity compared to SNDT ($p = 0.04$). Disease activity was measured by the PCDAI and PUCAI disease activity scoring scales for CD and UC, respectively. Lastly, follow-up analyses on a smaller study sample of youth with CD ($N = 70$) showed that both CBT and SNDT were associated with decreased GI-related health care utilization, specifically GI-hospitalization frequency, inpatient days, ER visits, and endoscopies [49]. Overall, these results support CBT as a beneficial adjunct to the medical management of IBD among pediatric patients.

Recent research supports Szigethy and colleagues' findings over the past decade, demonstrating the benefits of CBT protocols for youth with IBD and emotional distress. Of note, Levy et al. [50] randomized 187 youth (8–17 years) to a brief three session CBT intervention or an education support condition and conducted follow-up assessments up to one year post-treatment. The findings demonstrated that the CBT intervention led to significantly more pre- to post-treatment improvement compared to the control group on measures of pain coping abilities ($p < 0.05$), IBD-related quality of life ($p < 0.05$), parent-reported solicitous behavior ($p < 0.05$), and missed days of school in the six months following treatment ($p < 0.05$). Children reported significant improvement in depression symptoms post-treatment with no significant between group differences ($p = 0.10$). Interestingly, exploratory sub-group analyses demonstrated that children in the CBT intervention with higher levels of flares pre-baseline had significantly fewer flares post-treatment compared to the control (16.7% versus 52.9%; $p < 0.05$). Future studies should further explore the possibility that brief CBT protocols can affect disease activity in a larger sample of youth with IBD using more rigorous methodology, such as PCDAI/PUCAI measures of disease activity, and the concurrent measurement of calprotectin and inflammatory cytokines. The strengths of this study include the large sample size, controlling for time and attention in the educational support condition, and developing a brief intervention to address the accessibility and adherence issues common to psychotherapy protocols.

Currently, a multicenter randomized controlled trial (RCT) is underway to investigate the efficacy of a CBT protocol in reducing symptoms of depression and anxiety and improving quality of life and disease course in youth with IBD [51]. Larger RCTs such as this are greatly needed in order to address past study limitations and further assess the feasibility, efficacy, and generalizability of CBT interventions for youth with IBD and co-occurring emotional distress.

Overall, there is promising preliminary evidence for the feasibility of CBT interventions in tertiary pediatric GI/IBD clinics and the efficacy of such protocols in improving psychological wellbeing and disease-related outcomes. Effective non-pharmacological treatments for emotional distress are especially important given the comorbidity between IBD and depression and anxiety and the potential for antidepressants to exacerbate GI symptoms and complicate medical regimens [47].

3.2. Relaxation and Stress Management

Given the relationship between stress, emotional distress, and negative IBD-related outcomes, researchers have explored the efficacy of relaxation and stress-management protocols for IBD patients. The goal of such interventions is to teach patients skills to relax and reduce daily stress in order to support improved psychological and physical wellbeing. The content of these interventions varies, as well as the format (individual versus group sessions), delivery (nurse, psychiatrist, psychologist), and duration (one session versus eight weekly sessions). Relaxation-based interventions usually focus on teaching patients a subset of relaxation strategies, such diaphragmatic breathing techniques, guided imagery (e.g., focus on imagination and distraction), progressive muscle relaxation (PMR) (e.g., focus on building and releasing muscle tension), and autogenic training (i.e., focus on physical manifestations of relaxation in the body like heaviness in the musculoskeletal system or warmth of the circulatory system) [41]. Stress management protocols tend to include psychoeducation (e.g., related to IBD and treatment; stress and relaxation response) and a variety of relaxation and coping skills (e.g., problem solving, communication, identifying and modifying negative thoughts). Exercise and diet support are also integrated into some stress management treatments [40,41].

The majority of research investigating the use of relaxation and stress management interventions in IBD populations has been conducted in adult samples. Randomized controlled trials investigating the efficacy of PMR and guided imagery-based relaxation protocols have shown significant improvements in psychological functioning, quality of life, and pain variables among adults with IBD [52,53]. Stress management interventions have shown mixed efficacy. Some RCTs have demonstrated that stress management protocols can improve psychological functioning [54–56] and disease-related outcomes [55,57,58], while other studies show no significant changes in IBD outcomes across conditions [59].

Research exploring more integrative CBT interventions (CBT with greater emphasis on relaxation-based coping skills) has shown promise in pediatric patients with IBD. McCormick and colleagues [60] developed a one-day CBT intervention for adolescents and parents focused on disease-related coping skills, pain management, relaxation, communication, and limit setting

(N = 24 parent–child dyads). Treatment was followed by six weeks of web-based skill review that focused on weekly homework, coping skills, and group chat sessions related to treatment modules. Separate adolescent and parent sites were created. Following the integrative CBT treatment, there were significant improvements in child and parent-reports of somatic symptoms ($p < 0.01$) and adaptive coping ($p < 0.05$). While there were no significant differences between the CBT and wait-list control condition, no changes in the above symptoms were found for the control group. Despite preliminary support for the intervention among adolescents with IBD and their parents, there was a lack of random assignment to groups, limiting conclusions about intervention efficacy. Overall, it appears that no studies to date have explored the efficacy of relaxation or stress management interventions in pediatric IBD populations.

Future research exploring the feasibility and efficacy of relaxation-focused interventions among pediatric samples is needed. Brief relaxation protocols could be particularly helpful in pediatric GI clinics, as they could be easily delivered by a variety of providers and integrated into multidisciplinary care.

3.3. Mindfulness

Over the past decade, mindfulness-based interventions have received increasing attention in mind–body research and are emerging as a point of interest among researchers exploring psychotherapeutic interventions for patients with IBD. Mindfulness-based stress reduction (MBSR) and mindfulness-based cognitive therapy (MBCT) are typically the most common mindfulness treatments in clinical and research settings. Across these protocols, the primary treatment aim is to teach patients mindfulness, which is the ability to be aware of the present moment and one's thoughts, emotions, and body sensations in a purposeful, non-judgmental manner [61,62]. Mindfulness is usually practiced via a series of breathing, meditation, and movement exercises, all of which support non-judgmental and compassionate awareness. Bringing one's focus and attention to the present can buffer one from ruminating on negative cognitions (e.g., catastrophizing about IBD flares) or bothersome physical sensations (e.g., abdominal pain).

To date, it appears that mindfulness-based interventions for patients with IBD have been exclusively conducted in adult samples. One of the first randomized controlled studies investigated the feasibility and efficacy of an eight week mindfulness-based stress reduction (MBSR) group among 55 patients with ulcerative colitis compared to an attention control condition with mind–body psychoeducation [63]. MBSR was developed by John Kabat-Zinn and consists of eight weekly 2.5 h sessions, weekly homework, and a seven hour weekend session, all focused on promoting mindfulness in daily life. Results demonstrated that the MBSR intervention was highly feasible and acceptable among IBD patients; however, the protocol did not impact psychological or disease outcomes compared to the control condition. Interestingly, among patients who flared during the study, those randomized to the MBSR condition reported significantly higher quality of life compared to the control condition ($p = 0.001$). Additionally, post-hoc analyses demonstrated that MBSR may be effective in reducing flares among patients with heightened states of stress, supporting the approach of tailoring treatments to patient characteristics as is routinely done with pharmacotherapy [63].

A more recent controlled trial [64] provided preliminary support for the feasibility, acceptability, and efficacy of an eight week modified MBSR protocol for adults with IBD (N = 60). Post-treatment, there were significant improvements in anxiety ($p < 0.05$), depression ($p < 0.05$), quality of life ($p < 0.01$), and mindfulness ($p < 0.01$), compared to a treatment as usual control condition. Of note, significant reductions in depression and improvements in mindfulness were present six months following the intervention ($p < 0.001$). The corresponding effect sizes ranged from medium ($d = 0.56$) to large ($d = 1.27$), providing support for clinically meaningful outcomes. However, additional randomized controlled trials are needed to further support these findings.

Schoultz and colleagues [65] have also explored the efficacy of a MBCT intervention among 44 adults with IBD. MBCT was developed by Zindel Segal and colleagues and is largely based on

MBSR [66]. It is an eight-week group treatment that integrates mindfulness and cognitive therapy techniques to support stress management and self-care. Schoultz et al. [65] found that MBCT led to significant improvements in depression ($p < 0.05$), trait anxiety ($p < 0.05$), and dispositional mindfulness ($p < 0.05$) among patients with IBD, compared to a wait-list control condition. These findings persisted at a six-month follow-up assessment. No changes were noted on disease activity and IBD quality of life. Thomas and colleagues also developed a form of psychotherapy, entitled multi-convergent therapy (MCT), that combines mindfulness with cognitive and behavioral techniques [67]. A randomized controlled pilot study assessed the efficacy of MCT among 66 adults with IBD. The results demonstrated significant pre- to post-treatment improvements in the MCT condition, compared to the control on quality of life among IBD patients with IBS-type symptoms (determined by Rome III criteria at baseline) ($p = 0.021$) [68]. These findings offer further support to the notion that mindfulness protocols could be effective for sub-groups of IBD patients.

While, to our knowledge, there is no published research investigating the use of mindfulness-based interventions among youth with IBD, preliminary support for mindfulness protocols in adult IBD populations and youth with IBS [69] suggest that this could be a promising line of future research. Going forward, investigators should explore the feasibility and efficacy of age appropriate mindfulness treatments among children and adolescents with IBD, particularly in patients with heighted states of stress, concurrent psychological diagnoses, or IBS-IBD symptoms. This research should also address some of the methodological limitations highlighted in the adult literature. Specifically, future studies should include a bigger sample size and multiple control groups and include attention and wait list control, assess treatment adherence and engagement, and collect psychological, physiological, and disease activity-related outcomes.

3.4. Biofeedback

Biofeedback is a process in which the electronic monitoring of normally automatic bodily functions (e.g., heart rate, blood pressure, skin temperature) is used to train a patient to acquire voluntary control of that function. The autonomic nervous system is the primary target of biofeedback, particularly the sympathetic nervous system, or the body's 'fight or flight' system. The autonomic nervous system received its name because it was once believed that this system operated without our control. However, research has shown that a person can, in fact, control this part of the nervous system when provided with appropriate feedback of its functioning [70]. In pediatric gastroenterology, mind–body research suggests that biofeedback may be helpful in treating symptoms of IBS and functional abdominal pain (FAP) such as dyspepsia, bloating, and cramping [71,72].

Heart Rate Variability Biofeedback

Heart rate variability biofeedback (HRVB) is a type of biofeedback that can directly improve autonomic dysfunction and restore vagal tone [70]. Heart rate variability (HRV) is the change in time intervals between adjacent heartbeats. HRV can be measured non-invasively as a physiologic marker of autonomic nervous system function. Optimal HRV reflects a self-regulatory capacity, specifically a person's adaptability and resilience to respond to and recover from stressful stimuli [73]. HRV varies from person to person depending on age, gender, health, and fitness. Lower HRV, or less variability in heart rate in various positions and activities, suggests higher persistent sympathetic tone and less resilience to stressful triggers [73]. Analysis of HRV involves power spectral analysis filtering techniques to separate the heart rate waveform into frequency ranges [74,75]. The high frequency (HF) band reflects parasympathetic activity, whereas the low frequency (LF) band reflects sympathetic activity [76]. The LF/HF ratio is used by some researchers to assess the balance between sympathetic and parasympathetic activity [74,77]. Non-invasive instruments that connect to an earlobe, finger, or to the chest via electrocardiogram leads measure HRV. The user then engages in breathing and relaxation exercises to visualize how this may affect their HRV directly on the screen [73]. HRVB is a novel modality and research on its efficacy and utilization is still emerging.

A study by Sowder et al. [72] investigated the effect of HRVB in children with FAP. Children participated in six sessions of HRVB aimed at normalizing autonomic balance. At baseline, children with FAP in this study had greater autonomic dysregulation than children without FAP, as indicated by a higher LF/HF ratio ($t_{(28)}$ = 2.95; p = 0.006). After the treatment sessions, the FAP group was able to significantly reduce their symptoms which correlated with significant increases in their autonomic balance, as evidenced by a decrease in the LF/HF ratio($t_{(19)}$ = 2.57, p = 0.019). Another prospective open-label study by Stern et al. looked at 27 children with either IBS or FAP who underwent HRVB to treat their presenting symptoms for an average of eight 30-min sessions. They concluded that almost 70% of IBS patients and 63% of FAP patients achieved full remission (defined as having no symptoms for at least two full weeks) [71]. Qualitative data from this study showed that patients with both IBS and FAP expressed satisfaction with the intervention and their clinical outcomes and felt validated in the 'reality' of their symptoms.

Although no studies to date have looked at HRVB in IBD patients, a study by Jelenova et al. found that adolescents with mild IBD had less adaptability to stress compared to healthy controls [78]. The HRV of the IBD patients showed significantly lower levels of spectral activity in low frequency bands of HRV at both supine and standing positions (p < 0.005 and p < 0.01 respectively). This study was limited by the small sample size (25 IBD patients, 35 controls) and the fact that HRV was measured over five min, which may not be as accurate as 24 h measurements. Larger studies investigating normal values of HRV within healthy adolescent populations as compared to IBD populations would help to identify clinically significant HRV abnormalities within a pediatric IBD population. Although the effect of biofeedback on pediatric IBD has not yet been explored in depth, this modality offers a non-invasive way to decrease physiologic reactivity to stress, which may lead to IBD flares, decreased pain threshold, and IBS-IBD symptoms. Further research in this area is clearly warranted.

3.5. Yoga

Yoga is a mind–body technique arising from ancient India that combines physical postures, breath control, and meditation to promote health and relaxation. Yoga is believed to have mood-enhancing properties that inhibit physiologic stress and inflammation [79,80]. A systematic review of 25 randomized controlled trials provides evidence that yoga improves regulation of the sympathetic nervous system and hypothalamic–pituitary–adrenal system, as evidenced by multiple physiologic parameters including blood pressure, heart rate, cortisol, and cytokine expression [81]. Yoga also increases personal empowerment, which is the ability to develop the confidence and strength to set realistic goals and fulfill one's potential [82]. Personal empowerment is a measure vital to one's wellness and emotional health, and increased empowerment leads to improved patient activation. Of note, patient activation towards medical care can improve health outcomes, reduce medical system costs, and improve the patient's overall healthcare experience [83,84]. Yoga is a low cost, high reward form of self-care that has the potential to fill a known health care gap by decreasing stress, promoting wellness, and reducing disease burden.

Yoga protocols have been shown to be a feasible and safe adjunctive therapy for adolescents and young adults with IBS [85]. Nearly half of the participants in a brief yoga intervention for adolescents with IBS reported a significant reduction in pain and global symptom improvement, and young adults in the yoga group were significantly more likely to endorse symptom improvement compared to wait-list controls (χ^2 = 11.13, p = 0.03) [85]. Another randomized trial of yoga for adolescents with IBS found significantly improved gastrointestinal symptoms (p < 0.01), lower levels of functional disability (p = 0.073), less use of emotion-focused avoidance (p = 0.09), and less anxiety (p = 0.09) compared to wait-list controls [86]. A systematic review of six randomized controlled trials studying yoga as a treatment for IBS in adults found significant improvements in quality of life, global improvement, and physical functioning [87]. However, the review was limited by the small overall sample size (total of 273 patients), heterogeneity of control groups, and unclear risk of bias in observed studies (no allocation concealment or adequate random sequence generation described). Despite these studies' positive findings, there are no studies to date evaluating yoga as a potentially effective adjunct therapy for youth with IBD. Given the overlapping and interacting mechanisms between IBD and IBS, these preliminary yoga studies for IBS may also apply to the IBD population. Thus, there is a clear need for studies to investigate the potential benefits of yoga as a mind–body therapy in children and adolescents with IBD.

3.6. Clinical Hypnosis

Clinical hypnosis is a common MBI and refers to the specific ability to focus one's attention narrowly and deepen one's concentration, while simultaneously diminishing awareness of external stimuli. In this state of awareness, it is thought that the individual may be able to modulate some physiological processes not ordinarily under conscious control [88]. In the treatment of abdominal pain, most hypnosis or hypnotherapy studies have focused on the management of symptoms related to IBS, while a few have examined the action of hypnosis on IBD [89]. The strongest evidence for the efficacy of hypnotherapy in IBD is its association with reduced IBD related inflammation and improved quality of life. Mixed results have been obtained regarding its effects on psychological and pain outcomes [90]. The mechanism of action of hypnotherapy is believed to be via the 'brain–gut axis', through the modulation of vagal visceral afferent signals via the pontomedullary nuclei, limbic regions including the amygdala, hippocampus, and insula, and vagal efferent signaling via pathways of descending modulation. These pathways may be dysregulated by cognitive and environmental demands, leading to the overriding of local reflex functions that occur during sleep or in the context of digestion [11].

Hypnotherapy normally begins with an introduction by the practitioner, development of rapport, and receipt of permission to perform the hypnosis exercise. Following, a hypnosis induction is performed, with the aim of allowing the individual to enter an altered consciousness or trance state (e.g., similar to a narrow state of focused attention). This state is readily achieved by children, who naturally are able to enter a state of focus and attention during play or while engaging their imagination. Once in the hypnotic state, gentle suggestions are made for enhancing one's ability to regulate or normalize gastro-intestinal function, including the minimization of pain, nausea, vomiting or other symptomatology. Various metaphors can be employed to facilitate this process; for example, the gut may be likened to a smoothly flowing river, whose flow can be guided by the patient's gentle encouragement. The placing of the patient's hands over the abdomen, or taking specific medicines, can be seen as a way to engender calm and protection against pain, bloating, discomfort, or abnormal bowel habits. Subsequently, patients are encouraged to utilize the technique to calm their symptoms at other times during their daily life. Hypnotherapy has been demonstrated to be safe and effective for use in youth; however, it should only be employed by appropriately trained individuals [91].

In a randomized controlled study of 54 adult patients with ulcerative colitis, clinical remission was prolonged in 26 patients by a mean of 78 days compared to 29 attention controls. The intervention consisted of a seven-session standardized treatment protocol. Patients were also provided with an audio recording to practice outside of sessions five days per week during the study. The control intervention consisted of non-directive discussion about Ulcerative Colitis and the 'mind–body connection'. In addition, analysis of the group maintaining remission at one year showed a significantly higher remission rate among those in the hypnosis condition (68%) compared to control patients (40%) [92]. While mechanisms of action are unknown, stress management and increased self-efficacy have been posited as possible mediators.

In another study, 15 adult patients with severe or very severe IBD on corticosteroids, but not responding to medication, received 12 sessions of 'gut-focused hypnotherapy' and were followed up for a mean duration of 5.4 years. Sixty percent of patients were able to entirely stop corticosteroids and did not require them at follow-up [93]. In a similar study, 15 patients with severe IBD underwent 12 sessions of gut directed hypnosis, which focused on tactile stimuli as well as visualization. In 14 out of the 15 patients, disease severity was reduced from severe to either mild or moderate following treatment, and quality of life was improved from 'very poor' and 'poor' to 'good' and 'excellent' [94]. Of note, one session of 'gut-directed hypnotherapy' has been shown to reduce systemic and rectal mucosal inflammatory responses. Serum interleukin-6 concentration was reduced by 53%, circulating natural killer cell numbers were reduced by 18%, rectal mucosal release of substance P was reduced by 81%, histamine was reduced by 35%, and interleukin-13 was reduced by 53% [95].

In the pediatric population, hypnotherapy was successfully utilized in a case series for six children with IBD. The children received between four and 12 sessions over three months, and treatment resulted in improved symptoms and decreased inflammatory markers, though the exact values are not provided in the report [96]. In a randomized controlled study of 53 pediatric patients (aged eight to 18) with IBS and functional abdominal pain, patients underwent six sessions of hypnotherapy (HT) over a three-month period. The control intervention was standard medical care, with six sessions of supportive therapy. Pain intensity decreased in the HT group from 13.5 to 1.3 and in the control group from 14.1 to 8 ($p < 0.001$). Pain frequency reporting also decreased in the HT group from 13.1 to 1.1 and in the control group from 14.4 to 9.3 ($p = 0.007$). The three-month pain remission rate was 59% in the HT group compared to 12% in the standard care group ($p < 0.001$). Interestingly, there continued to be post-treatment improvement and remission rates at one year (85% and 25% respectively; $p < 0.001$) [97].

While no larger studies have investigated how some of these effects might be mediated in children with IBD, an interesting study in adults with IBS showed that gut-directed hypnotherapy had a normalizing effect on the aberrant central processing of visceral signals. Forty-four female adult patients were randomized to hypnosis or educational therapy. They received seven weekly one hour long sessions of hypnotherapy, including CD recordings for home use. Rectal distention was performed while the patient underwent functional magnetic resonance imaging of the brain to assess the central nervous system response to the distention stimulus. Both groups showed reduction in blood oxygen level dependent signals, including anterior insula, albeit by different centrally acting mechanisms [98]. The normalization of autonomic nervous system functions may also play a role in symptom management, as gut directed hypnotherapy has been shown to reduce heart and respiratory rates independently of emotional content [99]. Hypnotherapy is a promising therapy that may support symptom management in inflammatory bowel disease and potentially decrease the inflammatory response itself. More studies are needed to explore the feasibility, efficacy, and dose-response relationship of hypnotherapy interventions among pediatric patients suffering from IBD.

4. Sample Case

A 14-year-old female with a diagnosis of ileocolonic Crohn's disease for one year presented for a second opinion for IBD evaluation and management. The important findings on initial endoscopy were chronic ileitis of the terminal ileum, moderately active chronic colitis of the ascending colon, and colonic mucosa with rare branching crypt. Magnetic resonance enterography demonstrated a segment of borderline mild circumferential thickening of the small bowel in the ileum. Previous laboratories showed an elevated C-reactive protein (17 mg/L) and erythrocyte sedimentation rate (42 mm/h), fecal calprotectin (839 mcg/g), and low vitamin D (12 ng/mL). Her weight was 48 kg (24%), and her BMI was 21.28 kg/m^2 (50%). She was initially started on sulfasalazine, folic acid, and prednisone taper with the plan to transition to 6-mercaptopurine. However, she was only currently compliant with iron supplementation due to concerns about medication side effects.

The patient's presenting symptoms included watery diarrhea two times daily without hematochezia, frequent abdominal pain limiting her activity, and fatigue requiring a three hour nap every afternoon. She described significant stress related to Crohn's and school and became tearful when discussing her disease and desire to be normal. She also endorsed medical-related anxiety, needle phobia, and increasing frustration about her recurrent abdominal pain. During the evaluation, disease management options were discussed, including biologics, re-induction with steroids, use of immunomodulators, and enteral therapy. The patient was also referred for psychotherapy with a pediatric pain psychologist.

Psychological evaluation suggested significant academic and social anxiety related to IBD. Specifically, the patient endorsed difficulties concentrating in class due to symptoms, embarrassment about bathroom needs at school, body image concerns around peers, pain catastrophizing when out with friends, and anxiety around upcoming required blood draws. Weekly psychotherapy was initiated, and treatment goals included teaching her anxiety and pain management strategies, increasing daily functioning, and supporting her adjustment to life with a chronic illness.

Treatment initially focused on validating her past experiences, supporting increased trust with medical professionals, and empowering her to be more engaged in her health care. The mind–body modalities used in treatment included: (1) biofeedback for stress and pain management (e.g., HRV via emWave—a commonly used biofeedback program by HeartMath LLC, Boulder Creek, CA, USA); (2) hypnosis for needle phobia and pain management (e.g., comfort and relaxation dials in her 'control center', the brain); (3) mindfulness for stress and anxiety management; (4) CBT for needle phobia (e.g., graded exposures to feared stimulus like needles and blood draw); (5) and CBT for general anxiety and pain management (e.g., increasing awareness of negative pain-related thoughts, cognitive restructuring, behavioral activation to increase daily functioning).

During the first month of treatment, each session began with biofeedback and/or hypnosis exercises, such as playing the Garden Game on emWave (HeartMath LLC, Boulder Creek, CA, USA) or utilizing her relaxation dial to release worries and tension. CBT techniques were incorporated into the last 30 min of the session, focusing on graded needle exposures. For example, she practiced looking at pictures of blood draws and preparing her arm for a blood draw, with rubbing alcohol and tourniquet placement, and applying relaxation-based coping skills. Daily homework included practicing mind–body skills using biofeedback applications such as Bellybio [100] and Breathe2Relax [101], listening to a hypnosis recording about her comfort dial, and creating a weekly behavioral activation log. Treatment focused on a top-down and bottom-up approach to anxiety and pain management. After four weekly sessions working with these mind–body interventions, the patient was able to have her blood drawn with minimal difficulty. She also endorsed less anxiety at school and spent more time out of the house with friends.

At the patient's follow-up gastroenterology visit, she agreed to restart disease modifying medications. Of note, her calprotectin values subsequently normalized to 70 mcg/g, and her anemia and inflammatory markers also improved. The patient continued psychotherapy for 12 weeks. This multidisciplinary approach allowed for shared decision making in a case where the patient and family had at first demonstrated medical noncompliance due to medical-related anxiety. This case highlights the benefit of integrating mind–body interventions into IBD treatment.

When considering this case, and the biopsychosocial challenges associated with IBD, it is also important to highlight that ongoing psychotherapy is often recommended by multidisciplinary IBD teams to support mood, IBD symptom management, and health promotion (e.g., medication adherence, transitioning care). As studies have demonstrated, psychotherapy can have long-term positive effects on psychological and IBD-related outcomes. While most empirical evidence supports CBT for youth with IBD, acceptance and mindfulness-based treatment strategies should be considered when working with patients on adjustment and identity concerns related to IBD. Continued research in this area is warranted.

5. Conclusions

Mind–body interventions may be an effective non-invasive adjunctive therapy to standard medical care in pediatric IBD populations. Research shows that psychotherapy, specifically cognitive behavioral therapy, may be helpful in improving depression, functioning, and quality of life in youth with IBD. Relaxation and mindfulness-based interventions appear to improve psychological functioning among adult IBD populations, with particular benefit for subpopulations of patients experiencing heightened states of stress and concurrent IBS symptoms. Heart rate variability biofeedback and yoga may offer a way to help patients decrease pain and IBS-IBD symptoms, as well as improve anxiety and elevated persistent sympathetic tone. Preliminary data also suggests that clinical hypnosis and other mind–body interventions may have the potential to affect IBD activity (e.g., reduced inflammatory response). Further research needs to be conducted in pediatric samples in order to further validate the feasibility, efficacy, and cost effectiveness of these mind–body interventions in pediatric IBD. Manipulative therapies, such as acupuncture and massage, and dietary therapies may also improve overall well-being in IBD patients and be an area worthy of further investigation.

Mind–body interventions can be implemented in the clinical setting by various providers, including GI physicians, nurse practitioners, and physician assistants. Mental health providers such as social workers, pediatric pain psychologists, or clinical psychologists can also be trained in mind–body interventions. For the time being, insurance may not cover specific mind–body treatments. However, providers often can bill for services through evaluation and management codes based on time (for medical providers) or health and behavior codes based on time (for mental health providers). As evidence emerges on the efficacy of mind–body interventions to improve IBD outcomes, hopefully insurance companies will deem these interventions as medically necessary and gradually incorporate them into part of mainstream care.

We encourage pediatric IBD providers to reflect on the importance of the brain–gut connection with patients and families, assess their interest in mind–body interventions, and engage in multidisciplinary treatment with mind–body treatments when appropriate and supported by empirical evidence. This integrative treatment approach has the promise to improve patients' disease activity and overall well-being.

Acknowledgments: We thank Jenna Arruda for assistance with literature search and writing, and Srisindu Vellanki for assistance with literature search.

Author Contributions: A.W., A.M.Y., and B.G wrote the manuscript and commented on the manuscript at all stages.

Conflicts of Interest: The authors declare no conflict of interest.

References

1. Cho, J.H. The genetics and immunopathogenesis of inflammatory bowel disease. *Nat. Rev. Immunol.* **2008**, *8*, 458–466. [CrossRef] [PubMed]
2. Mackner, L.M.; Greenley, R.N.; Szigethy, E.; Herzer, M.; Deer, K.; Hommel, K.A. Psychosocial issues in pediatric inflammatory bowel disease: Report of the North American Society for Pediatric Gastroenterology, Hepatology, and Nutrition. *J. Pediatr. Gastroenterol. Nutr.* **2013**, *56*, 449–458. [CrossRef] [PubMed]
3. Wilson, D.C.; Thomas, A.G.; Croft, N.M.; Newby, E.; Akobeng, A.K.; Sawczenko, A.; Fell, J.M.E.; Murphy, M.S.; Beattie, R.M.; Sandhu, B.K.; et al. Systematic review of the evidence base for the medical treatment of paediatric inflammatory bowel disease. *J. Pediatr. Gastroenterol. Nutr.* **2010**, *50* (Suppl. 1), S14–S34. [CrossRef] [PubMed]
4. Zachos, M.; Tondeur, M.; Griffiths, A.M. Enteral nutritional therapy for induction of remission in Crohn's disease. *Cochrane Database Syst. Rev.* **2007**. [CrossRef]
5. Day, A.S.; Whitten, K.E.; Lemberg, D.A.; Clarkson, C.; Vitug-Sales, M.; Jackson, R.; Bohane, T.D. Exclusive enteral feeding as primary therapy for Crohn's disease in Australian children and adolescents: A feasible and effective approach. *J. Gastroenterol. Hepatol.* **2006**, *21*, 1609–1614. [CrossRef] [PubMed]
6. Heuschkel, R.B.; Menache, C.C.; Megerian, J.T.; Baird, A.E. Enteral nutrition and corticosteroids in the treatment of acute Crohn's disease in children. *J. Pediatr. Gastroenterol. Nutr.* **2000**, *31*, 8–15. [CrossRef] [PubMed]
7. Cheifetz, A.S.; Gianotti, R.; Luber, R.; Gibson, P.R. Complementary and Alternative Medicines Used by Patients with Inflammatory Bowel Diseases. *Gastroenterology* **2017**, *152*, 415–429.e15. [CrossRef] [PubMed]
8. Complementary, Alternative, or Integrative Health: What's in a Name? Available online: https://nccih.nih.gov/health/integrative-health (accessed on 10 February 2017).
9. Mind and Body Practices. Available online: https://nccih.nih.gov/health/mindbody (accessed on 15 February 2017).

10. Serpico, M.; Boyle, B.; Kemper, K.J.; Kim, S. Complementary and Alternative Medicine Use in Children with Inflammatory Bowel Diseases: A Single Center Survey. *J. Pediatr. Gastroenterol. Nutr.* **2016**, *63*, 651–657. [CrossRef] [PubMed]
11. Mayer, E.A.; Tillisch, K. The brain–gut axis in abdominal pain syndromes. *Annu. Rev. Med.* **2011**, *62*, 381–396. [CrossRef] [PubMed]
12. Maunder, R.G.; Levenstein, S. The role of stress in the development and clinical course of inflammatory bowel disease: Epidemiological evidence. *Curr. Mol. Med.* **2008**, *8*, 247–252. [CrossRef] [PubMed]
13. Levenstein, S.; Prantera, C.; Varvo, V.; Scribano, M.L.; Berto, E.; Andreoli, A.; Luzi, C. Psychological stress and disease activity in ulcerative colitis: A multidimensional cross-sectional study. *Am. J. Gastroenterol.* **1994**, *89*, 1219–1225. [PubMed]
14. Bonaz, B.L.; Bernstein, C.N. Brain–gut interactions in inflammatory bowel disease. *Gastroenterology* **2013**, *144*, 36–49. [CrossRef] [PubMed]
15. Bitton, A.; Dobkin, P.L.; Edwardes, M.D.; Sewitch, M.J.; Meddings, J.B.; Rawal, S.; Cohen, A.; Vermeire, S.; Dufresne, L.; Franchimont, D.; et al. Predicting relapse in Crohn's disease: A biopsychosocial model. *Gut* **2008**, *57*, 1386–1392. [CrossRef] [PubMed]
16. Duffy, L.C.; Zielezny, M.A.; Marshall, J.R.; Weiser, M.M.; Phillips, J.F.; Byers, T.E.; Calkins, B.M.; Graham, S.; Ogra, P.L. Lag time between stress events and risk of recurrent episodes of inflammatory bowel disease. *Epidemiology* **1991**, *2*, 141–145. [CrossRef] [PubMed]
17. Collins, S.M. Stress and the Gastrointestinal Tract IV. Modulation of intestinal inflammation by stress: Basic mechanisms and clinical relevance. *Am. J. Physiol. Gastrointest. Liver Physiol.* **2001**, *280*, G315–G318. [PubMed]
18. Diederen, K.; Hoekman, D.R.; Hummel, T.Z.; de Meij, T.G.; Koot, B.G.P.; Tabbers, M.M.; Vlieger, A.M.; Kindermann, A.; Benninga, M.A. The prevalence of irritable bowel syndrome-type symptoms in paediatric inflammatory bowel disease, and the relationship with biochemical markers of disease activity. *Aliment. Pharmacol. Ther.* **2016**, *44*, 181–188. [CrossRef] [PubMed]
19. Halpin, S.J.; Ford, A.C. Prevalence of symptoms meeting criteria for irritable bowel syndrome in inflammatory bowel disease: Systematic review and meta-analysis. *Am. J. Gastroenterol.* **2012**, *107*, 1474–1482. [CrossRef] [PubMed]
20. Srinath, A.; Young, E.; Szigethy, E. Pain management in patients with inflammatory bowel disease: Translational approaches from bench to bedside. *Inflamm. Bowel Dis.* **2014**, *20*, 2433–2449. [CrossRef] [PubMed]
21. Bercik, P.; Verdu, E.F.; Collins, S.M. Is irritable bowel syndrome a low-grade inflammatory bowel disease? *Gastroenterol. Clin. N. Am.* **2005**, *34*, 235–245. [CrossRef] [PubMed]
22. Abdul Rani, R.; Raja Ali, R.A.; Lee, Y.Y. Irritable bowel syndrome and inflammatory bowel disease overlap syndrome: Pieces of the puzzle are falling into place. *Intest. Res.* **2016**, *14*, 297–304. [CrossRef] [PubMed]
23. Chung, C.-S.; Chang, P.-F.; Liao, C.-H.; Lee, T.-H.; Chen, Y.; Lee, Y.-C.; Wu, M.-S.; Wang, H.-P.; Ni, Y.-H. Differences of microbiota in small bowel and faeces between irritable bowel syndrome patients and healthy subjects. *Scand. J. Gastroenterol.* **2016**, *51*, 410–419. [CrossRef] [PubMed]
24. Shankar, V.; Reo, N.V.; Paliy, O. Simultaneous fecal microbial and metabolite profiling enables accurate classification of pediatric irritable bowel syndrome. *Microbiome* **2015**, *3*, 73. [CrossRef] [PubMed]
25. Putignani, L.; Del Chierico, F.; Vernocchi, P.; Cicala, M.; Cucchiara, S.; Dallapiccola, B.; Dysbiotrack Study Group. Gut Microbiota Dysbiosis as Risk and Premorbid Factors of IBD and IBS Along the Childhood–Adulthood Transition. *Inflamm. Bowel Dis.* **2016**, *22*, 487–504. [CrossRef] [PubMed]
26. Ricci, C.; Lanzarotto, F.; Lanzini, A. The multidisciplinary team for management of inflammatory bowel diseases. *Dig. Liver Dis.* **2008**, *40*, S285–S288. [CrossRef]
27. Goodhand, J.; Hedin, C.R.; Croft, N.M.; Lindsay, J.O. Adolescents with IBD: The importance of structured transition care. *J. Crohns Colitis* **2011**, *5*, 509–519. [CrossRef] [PubMed]
28. Regueiro, M.; Greer, J.B.; Szigethy, E. Etiology and Treatment of Pain and Psychosocial Issues in Patients with Inflammatory Bowel Diseases. *Gastroenterology* **2017**, *152*, 430–439.e4. [CrossRef] [PubMed]
29. Day, A.S.; Ledder, O.; Leach, S.T.; Lemberg, D.A. Crohn's and colitis in children and adolescents. *World J. Gastroenterol.* **2012**, *18*, 5862–5869. [CrossRef] [PubMed]

30. Cotton, S.; Humenay Roberts, Y.; Tsevat, J.; Britto, M.T.; Succop, P.; McGrady, M.E.; Yi, M.S. Mind–body complementary alternative medicine use and quality of life in adolescents with inflammatory bowel disease. *Inflamm. Bowel Dis.* **2010**, *16*, 501–506. [CrossRef] [PubMed]
31. Fuller-Thomson, E.; Sulman, J. Depression and inflammatory bowel disease: Findings from two nationally representative Canadian surveys. *Inflamm. Bowel Dis.* **2006**, *12*, 697–707. [CrossRef] [PubMed]
32. Kappelman, M.D.; Long, M.D.; Martin, C.; DeWalt, D.A.; Kinneer, P.M.; Chen, W.; Lewis, J.D.; Sandler, R.S. Evaluation of the patient-reported outcomes measurement information system in a large cohort of patients with inflammatory bowel diseases. *Clin. Gastroenterol. Hepatol.* **2014**, *12*, 1315–1323.e2. [CrossRef] [PubMed]
33. Mikocka-Walus, A.; Knowles, S.R.; Keefer, L.; Graff, L. Controversies Revisited: A Systematic Review of the Comorbidity of Depression and Anxiety with Inflammatory Bowel Diseases. *Inflamm. Bowel Dis.* **2016**, *22*, 752–762. [CrossRef] [PubMed]
34. Greenley, R.N.; Hommel, K.A.; Nebel, J.; Raboin, T.; Li, S.-H.; Simpson, P.; Mackner, L. A meta-analytic review of the psychosocial adjustment of youth with inflammatory bowel disease. *J. Pediatr. Psychol.* **2010**, *35*, 857–869. [CrossRef] [PubMed]
35. Keethy, D.; Mrakotsky, C.; Szigethy, E. Pediatric inflammatory bowel disease and depression: Treatment implications. *Curr. Opin. Pediatr.* **2014**, *26*, 561–567. [CrossRef] [PubMed]
36. Graff, L.A.; Walker, J.R.; Bernstein, C.N. Depression and anxiety in inflammatory bowel disease: A review of comorbidity and management. *Inflamm. Bowel Dis.* **2009**, *15*, 1105–1118. [CrossRef] [PubMed]
37. Gray, W.N.; Denson, L.A.; Baldassano, R.N.; Hommel, K.A. Treatment adherence in adolescents with inflammatory bowel disease: The collective impact of barriers to adherence and anxiety/depressive symptoms. *J. Pediatr. Psychol.* **2012**, *37*, 282–291. [CrossRef] [PubMed]
38. Goodhand, J.R.; Wahed, M.; Mawdsley, J.E.; Farmer, A.D.; Aziz, Q.; Rampton, D.S. Mood disorders in inflammatory bowel disease: Relation to diagnosis, disease activity, perceived stress, and other factors. *Inflamm. Bowel Dis.* **2012**, *18*, 2301–2309. [CrossRef] [PubMed]
39. Mittermaier, C.; Dejaco, C.; Waldhoer, T.; Oefferlbauer-Ernst, A.; Miehsler, W.; Beier, M.; Tillinger, W.; Gangl, A.; Moser, G. Impact of depressive mood on relapse in patients with inflammatory bowel disease: A prospective 18-month follow-up study. *Psychosom. Med.* **2004**, *66*, 79–84. [CrossRef] [PubMed]
40. Knowles, S.R.; Monshat, K.; Castle, D.J. The efficacy and methodological challenges of psychotherapy for adults with inflammatory bowel disease: A review. *Inflamm. Bowel Dis.* **2013**, *19*, 2704–2715. [CrossRef] [PubMed]
41. Timmer, A.; Preiss, J.C.; Motschall, E.; Rücker, G.; Jantschek, G.; Moser, G. Psychological interventions for treatment of inflammatory bowel disease. *Cochrane Database Syst. Rev.* **2011**. [CrossRef]
42. McCombie, A.; Gearry, R.; Andrews, J.; Mulder, R.; Mikocka-Walus, A. Does Computerized Cognitive Behavioral Therapy Help People with Inflammatory Bowel Disease? A Randomized Controlled Trial. *Inflamm. Bowel Dis.* **2016**, *22*, 171–181. [CrossRef] [PubMed]
43. Szigethy, E.; Bujoreanu, S.I.; Youk, A.O.; Weisz, J.; Benhayon, D.; Fairclough, D.; Ducharme, P.; Gonzalez-Heydrich, J.; Keljo, D.; Srinath, A.; et al. Randomized efficacy trial of two psychotherapies for depression in youth with inflammatory bowel disease. *J. Am. Acad. Child Adolesc. Psychiatry* **2014**, *53*, 726–735. [CrossRef] [PubMed]
44. Kendall, P.C.; Flannery-Schroeder, E.; Panichelli-Mindel, S.M.; Southam-Gerow, M.; Henin, A.; Warman, M. Therapy for youths with anxiety disorders: A second randomized clinical trial. *J. Consult. Clin. Psychol.* **1997**, *65*, 366–380. [CrossRef] [PubMed]
45. March, J.; Silva, S.; Petrycki, S.; Curry, J.; Wells, K.; Fairbank, J.; Burns, B.; Domino, M.; McNulty, S.; Vitiello, B.; et al. Fluoxetine, cognitive-behavioral therapy, and their combination for adolescents with depression: Treatment for Adolescents With Depression Study (TADS) randomized controlled trial. *JAMA* **2004**, *292*, 807–820. [PubMed]
46. Thompson, R.D.; Delaney, P.; Flores, I.; Szigethy, E. Cognitive-behavioral therapy for children with comorbid physical illness. *Child Adolesc. Psychiatr. Clin. N. Am.* **2011**, *20*, 329–348. [CrossRef] [PubMed]
47. Szigethy, E.; Whitton, S.W.; Levy-Warren, A.; DeMaso, D.R.; Weisz, J.; Beardslee, W.R. Cognitive-behavioral therapy for depression in adolescents with inflammatory bowel disease: A pilot study. *J. Am. Acad. Child Adolesc. Psychiatry* **2004**, *43*, 1469–1477. [CrossRef] [PubMed]

48. Szigethy, E.; Kenney, E.; Carpenter, J.; Hardy, D.M.; Fairclough, D.; Bousvaros, A.; Keljo, D.; Weisz, J.; Beardslee, W.R.; Noll, R.; et al. Cognitive-behavioral therapy for adolescents with inflammatory bowel disease and subsyndromal depression. *J. Am. Acad. Child Adolesc. Psychiatry* **2007**, *46*, 1290–1298. [CrossRef] [PubMed]

49. Keerthy, D.; Youk, A.; Srinath, A.I.; Malas, N.; Bujoreanu, S.; Bousvaros, A.; Keljo, D.; DeMaso, D.R.; Szigethy, E.M. Effect of Psychotherapy on Health Care Utilization in Children With Inflammatory Bowel Disease and Depression. *J. Pediatr. Gastroenterol. Nutr.* **2016**, *63*, 658–664. [CrossRef] [PubMed]

50. Levy, R.L.; van Tilburg, M.A.L.; Langer, S.L.; Romano, J.M.; Walker, L.S.; Mancl, L.A.; Murphy, T.B.; Claar, R.L.; Feld, S.I.; Christie, D.L.; et al. Effects of a Cognitive Behavioral Therapy Intervention Trial to Improve Disease Outcomes in Children with Inflammatory Bowel Disease. *Inflamm. Bowel Dis.* **2016**, *22*, 2134–2148. [CrossRef] [PubMed]

51. Van den Brink, G.; Stapersma, L.; El Marroun, H.; Henrichs, J.; Szigethy, E.M.; Utens, E.M.; Escher, J.C. Effectiveness of disease-specific cognitive-behavioural therapy on depression, anxiety, quality of life and the clinical course of disease in adolescents with inflammatory bowel disease: Study protocol of a multicentre randomised controlled trial (HAPPY-IBD). *BMJ Open Gastroenterol.* **2016**, *3*, e000071. [PubMed]

52. Shaw, L.; Ehrlich, A. Relaxation training as a treatment for chronic pain caused by ulcerative colitis. *Pain* **1987**, *29*, 287–293. [CrossRef]

53. Mizrahi, M.C.; Reicher-Atir, R.; Levy, S.; Haramati, S.; Wengrower, D.; Israeli, E.; Goldin, E. Effects of guided imagery with relaxation training on anxiety and quality of life among patients with inflammatory bowel disease. *Psychol. Health* **2012**, *27*, 1463–1479. [CrossRef] [PubMed]

54. Langhorst, J.; Mueller, T.; Luedtke, R.; Franken, U.; Paul, A.; Michalsen, A.; Schedlowski, M.; Dobos, G.J.; Elsenbruch, S. Effects of a comprehensive lifestyle modification program on quality-of-life in patients with ulcerative colitis: A twelve-month follow-up. *Scand. J. Gastroenterol.* **2007**, *42*, 734–745. [CrossRef] [PubMed]

55. Gerbarg, P.L.; Jacob, V.E.; Stevens, L.; Bosworth, B.P.; Chabouni, F.; DeFilippis, E.M.; Warren, R.; Trivellas, M.; Patel, P.V.; Webb, C.D.; et al. The Effect of Breathing, Movement, and Meditation on Psychological and Physical Symptoms and Inflammatory Biomarkers in Inflammatory Bowel Disease: A Randomized Controlled Trial. *Inflamm. Bowel Dis.* **2015**, *21*, 2886–2896. [CrossRef] [PubMed]

56. Smith, G.D.; Watson, R.; Roger, D.; McRorie, E.; Hurst, N.; Luman, W.; Palmer, K.R. Impact of a nurse-led counselling service on quality of life in patients with inflammatory bowel disease. *J. Adv. Nurs.* **2002**, *38*, 152–160. [CrossRef] [PubMed]

57. Milne, B.; Joachim, G.; Niedhardt, J. A stress management programme for inflammatory bowel disease patients. *J. Adv. Nurs.* **1986**, *11*, 561–567. [CrossRef] [PubMed]

58. García-Vega, E.; Fernandez-Rodriguez, C. A stress management programme for Crohn's disease. *Behav. Res. Ther.* **2004**, *42*, 367–383. [CrossRef]

59. Larsson, K.; Sundberg Hjelm, M.; Karlbom, U.; Nordin, K.; Anderberg, U.M.; Lööf, L. A group-based patient education programme for high-anxiety patients with Crohn disease or ulcerative colitis. *Scand. J. Gastroenterol.* **2003**, *38*, 763–769. [PubMed]

60. McCormick, M.; Reed-Knight, B.; Lewis, J.D.; Gold, B.D.; Blount, R.L. Coping skills for reducing pain and somatic symptoms in adolescents with IBD. *Inflamm. Bowel Dis.* **2010**, *16*, 2148–2157. [CrossRef] [PubMed]

61. Kabat-Zinn, J. *Wherever You Go, There You Are*; Hyperion: New York, NY, USA, 1994.

62. Baer, R.A. Mindfulness Training as a Clinical Intervention: A Conceptual and Empirical Review. *Clin. Psychol. Sci. Pract.* **2003**, *10*, 125–143. [CrossRef]

63. Jedel, S.; Hoffman, A.; Merriman, P.; Swanson, B.; Voigt, R.; Rajan, K.B.; Shaikh, M.; Li, H.; Keshavarzian, A. A randomized controlled trial of mindfulness-based stress reduction to prevent flare-up in patients with inactive ulcerative colitis. *Digestion* **2014**, *89*, 142–155. [PubMed]

64. Neilson, K.; Ftanou, M.; Monshat, K.; Salzberg, M.; Bell, S.; Kamm, M.A.; Connell, W.; Knowles, S.R.; Sevar, K.; Mancuso, S.G.; et al. A Controlled Study of a Group Mindfulness Intervention for Individuals Living With Inflammatory Bowel Disease. *Inflamm. Bowel Dis.* **2016**, *22*, 694–701. [CrossRef] [PubMed]

65. Schoultz, M.; Atherton, I.; Watson, A. Mindfulness-based cognitive therapy for inflammatory bowel disease patients: Findings from an exploratory pilot randomised controlled trial. *Trials* **2015**, *16*, 379. [CrossRef] [PubMed]

66. Segal, Z.; Williams, J.; Teasdale, J. *Mindfulness-Based Cognitive Therapy for Depression: A New Approach to Preventing Relapse*; The Guilford Press: New York, NY, USA, 2002.

67. Thomas, M.; Sadlier, M.; Smith, A. The effect of Multi Convergent Therapy on the psychopathology, mood and performance of Chronic Fatigue Syndrome patients: A preliminary study. *Couns. Psychother. Res.* **2006**, *6*, 91–99. [CrossRef]

68. Berrill, J.W.; Sadlier, M.; Hood, K.; Green, J.T. Mindfulness-based therapy for inflammatory bowel disease patients with functional abdominal symptoms or high perceived stress levels. *J. Crohns Colitis* **2014**, *8*, 945–955. [CrossRef] [PubMed]

69. Ali, A.; Weiss, T.R.; Dutton, A.; McKee, D.; Jones, K.D.; Kashikar-Zuck, S.; Silverman, W.K.; Shapiro, E.D. Mindfulness-Based Stress Reduction for Adolescents with Functional Somatic Syndromes: A Pilot Cohort Study. *J. Pediatr.* **2017**, *183*, 184–190. [CrossRef] [PubMed]

70. Lehrer, P.M.; Gevirtz, R. Heart rate variability biofeedback: How and why does it work? *Front. Psychol.* **2014**, *5*, 756. [CrossRef] [PubMed]

71. Stern, M.J.; Guiles, R.A.F.; Gevirtz, R. HRV biofeedback for pediatric irritable bowel syndrome and functional abdominal pain: A clinical replication series. *Appl. Psychophysiol. Biofeedback* **2014**, *39*, 287–291. [CrossRef] [PubMed]

72. Sowder, E.; Gevirtz, R.; Shapiro, W.; Ebert, C. Restoration of vagal tone: A possible mechanism for functional abdominal pain. *Appl. Psychophysiol. Biofeedback* **2010**, *35*, 199–206. [CrossRef] [PubMed]

73. Shaffer, F.; McCraty, R.; Zerr, C.L. A healthy heart is not a metronome: An integrative review of the heart's anatomy and heart rate variability. *Front. Psychol.* **2014**, *5*, 1040. [CrossRef] [PubMed]

74. Pagani, M.; Lombardi, F.; Guzzetti, S.; Rimoldi, O.; Furlan, R.; Pizzinelli, P.; Sandrone, G.; Malfatto, G.; Dell'Orto, S.; Piccaluga, E. Power spectral analysis of heart rate and arterial pressure variabilities as a marker of sympatho-vagal interaction in man and conscious dog. *Circ. Res.* **1986**, *59*, 178–193. [CrossRef] [PubMed]

75. Axelrod, S.; Lishner, M.; Oz, O.; Bernheim, J.; Ravid, M. Spectral Analysis of Fluctuations in Heart Rate: An Objective Evaluation of Autonomic Nervous Control in Chronic Renal Failure. *Nephron* **2004**, *45*, 202–206. [CrossRef]

76. Eckberg, D.L. Human sinus arrhythmia as an index of vagal cardiac outflow. *J. Appl. Physiol.* **1983**, *54*, 961–966. [PubMed]

77. Pal, G.K.; Adithan, C.; Ananthanarayanan, P.H.; Pal, P.; Nanda, N.; Durgadevi, T.; Lalitha, V.; Syamsunder, A.N.; Dutta, T.K. Sympathovagal Imbalance Contributes to Prehypertension Status and Cardiovascular Risks Attributed by Insulin Resistance, Inflammation, Dyslipidemia and Oxidative Stress in First Degree Relatives of Type 2 Diabetics. *PLoS ONE* **2013**, *8*, e78072. [CrossRef] [PubMed]

78. Jelenova, D.; Ociskova, M.; Prasko, J.; Hunkova, M.; Karaskova, E.; Kolarova, J.; Vydra, D.; Mihal, V. Heart rate variability in children with inflammatory bowel diseases. *Neuro Endocrinol. Lett.* **2015**, *36*, 72–79. [PubMed]

79. Twal, W.O.; Wahlquist, A.E.; Balasubramanian, S. Yogic breathing when compared to attention control reduces the levels of pro-inflammatory biomarkers in saliva: A pilot randomized controlled trial. *BMC Complement. Altern. Med.* **2016**, *16*, 294. [CrossRef] [PubMed]

80. Sharma, P.; Poojary, G.; Vélez, D.M.A.; Dwivedi, S.N.; Deepak, K.K. Effect of Yoga-Based Intervention in Patients with Inflammatory Bowel Disease. *Int. J. Yoga Ther.* **2015**, *25*, 101–112. [CrossRef] [PubMed]

81. Pascoe, M.C.; Bauer, I.E. A systematic review of randomised control trials on the effects of yoga on stress measures and mood. *J. Psychiatr. Res.* **2015**, *68*, 270–282. [CrossRef] [PubMed]

82. Hibbard, J.H.; Stockard, J.; Mahoney, E.R.; Tusler, M. Development of the Patient Activation Measure (PAM): Conceptualizing and Measuring Activation in Patients and Consumers. *Health Serv. Res.* **2004**, *39*, 1005–1026. [CrossRef] [PubMed]

83. Greene, J.; Hibbard, J.H. Why does patient activation matter? An examination of the relationships between patient activation and health-related outcomes. *J. Gen. Intern. Med.* **2012**, *27*, 520–526. [CrossRef] [PubMed]

84. Shah, S.L.; Siegel, C.A. Increasing Patient Activation Could Improve Outcomes for Patients with Inflammatory Bowel Disease. *Inflamm. Bowel Dis.* **2015**, *21*, 2975–2978. [CrossRef] [PubMed]

85. Evans, S.; Lung, K.C.; Seidman, L.C.; Sternlieb, B.; Zeltzer, L.K.; Tsao, J.C.I. Iyengar Yoga for Adolescents and Young Adults With Irritable Bowel Syndrome. *J. Pediatr. Gastroenterol. Nutr.* **2014**, *59*, 244–253. [CrossRef] [PubMed]

86. Kuttner, L.; Chambers, C.T.; Hardial, J.; Israel, D.M.; Jacobson, K.; Evans, K. A randomized trial of yoga for adolescents with irritable bowel syndrome. *Pain Res. Manag.* **2006**, *11*, 217–223. [CrossRef] [PubMed]

87. Schumann, D.; Anheyer, D.; Lauche, R.; Dobos, G.; Langhorst, J.; Cramer, H. Effect of Yoga in the Therapy of Irritable Bowel Syndrome: A Systematic Review. *Clin. Gastroenterol. Hepatol.* **2016**, *14*, 1720–1731. [CrossRef] [PubMed]
88. Sugarman, L.I. Hypnosis: Teaching children self-regulation. *Pediatr. Rev.* **1996**, *17*, 5–11. [CrossRef] [PubMed]
89. Ballou, S.; Keefer, L. Psychological Interventions for Irritable Bowel Syndrome and Inflammatory Bowel Diseases. *Clin. Transl. Gastroenterol.* **2017**, *8*, e214. [CrossRef] [PubMed]
90. Szigethy, E. Hypnotherapy for Inflammatory Bowel Disease Across the Lifespan. *Am. J. Clin. Hypn.* **2015**, *58*, 81–99. [CrossRef] [PubMed]
91. Section on Integrative Medicine. Mind–bodyTherapies in Children and Youth. *Pediatrics* **2016**, *138*, e20161896.
92. Keefer, L.; Taft, T.H.; Kiebles, J.L.; Martinovich, Z.; Barrett, T.A.; Palsson, O.S. Gut-directed hypnotherapy significantly augments clinical remission in quiescent ulcerative colitis. *Aliment. Pharmacol. Ther.* **2013**, *38*, 761–771. [CrossRef] [PubMed]
93. Keefer, L.; Keshavarzian, A. Feasibility and acceptability of gut-directed hypnosis on inflammatory bowel disease: A brief communication. *Int. J. Clin. Exp. Hypn.* **2007**, *55*, 457–466. [CrossRef] [PubMed]
94. Miller, V.; Whorwell, P.J. Treatment of inflammatory bowel disease: A role for hypnotherapy? *Int. J. Clin. Exp. Hypn.* **2008**, *56*, 306–317. [CrossRef] [PubMed]
95. Mawdsley, J.E.; Jenkins, D.G.; Macey, M.G.; Langmead, L.; Rampton, D.S. The effect of hypnosis on systemic and rectal mucosal measures of inflammation in ulcerative colitis. *Am. J. Gastroenterol.* **2008**, *103*, 1460–1469. [CrossRef]
96. Shaoul, R.; Sukhotnik, I.; Mogilner, J. Hypnosis as an adjuvant treatment for children with inflammatory bowel disease. *J. Dev. Behav. Pediatr.* **2009**, *30*, 268. [CrossRef] [PubMed]
97. Vlieger, A.M.; Menko-Frankenhuis, C.; Wolfkamp, S.C.S.; Tromp, E.; Benninga, M.A. Hypnotherapy for children with functional abdominal pain or irritable bowel syndrome: A randomized controlled trial. *Gastroenterology* **2007**, *133*, 1430–1436. [CrossRef] [PubMed]
98. Lowén, M.B.O.; Mayer, E.A.; Sjöberg, M.; Tillisch, K.; Naliboff, B.; Labus, J.; Lundberg, P.; Ström, M.; Engström, M.; Walter, S.A. Effect of hypnotherapy and educational intervention on brain response to visceral stimulus in the irritable bowel syndrome. *Aliment. Pharmacol. Ther.* **2013**, *37*, 1184–1197. [CrossRef] [PubMed]
99. Yapko, M. *Trancework: An Introduction to the Practice of Clinical Hypnosis*, 4th ed.; Routledge: New York, NY, USA, 2012.
100. *Bellybio Interactive Breathing*, version 1.1.3; RelaxLine, 2010.
101. *Breathe2Relax*, version 1.7; The National Center for Telehealth and Technology: Joint Base Lewis-McChord, WA, USA, 2016.

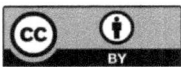

![children](children logo) **MDPI**

Commentary

Perspectives on Technology-Assisted Relaxation Approaches to Support Mind-Body Skills Practice in Children and Teens: Clinical Experience and Commentary

Timothy Culbert

PrairieCare Medical Group, Chaska, MN 55419, USA; tculbert@prairie-care.com; Tel.: +1-952-903-1380

Academic Editor: Hilary McClafferty
Received: 21 January 2017; Accepted: 19 March 2017; Published: 4 April 2017

Abstract: It has been well-established that a variety of mind-body (MB) techniques, including yoga, mental imagery, hypnosis, biofeedback, and meditation, are effective at addressing symptoms such as pain, anxiety, nausea, and insomnia, as well as helping with a wide variety of medical, emotional, and behavioral issues in pediatric populations. In addition, MB skills can also be health-promoting in the long-term, and with regular practice, could potentially contribute to longer attention spans, social skills, emotional regulation, and enhanced immune system functioning. Importantly, the benefits accrued from MB skills are largely dose-dependent, meaning that individuals who practice with some consistency tend to benefit the most, both in the short- and long-term. However, clinical experience suggests that for busy patients, the regular practice of MB skills can be challenging and treatment adherence commonly becomes an issue. This commentary reviews the concept of technology-assisted relaxation as an engaging and effective option to enhance treatment adherence (i.e., daily practice) for pediatric patients, for whom MB skills have been recommended to address physical and mental health challenges.

Keywords: technology; mind-body skills; biofeedback; mobile applications; meditation; multimedia; computer games; children; relaxation; stress; video games

1. Introduction

Interactive electronic devices can play a positive role in healthcare [1–17]. Technology-assisted relaxation is currently a very popular topic for healthcare consumers, including products which are available in the form of multimedia mobile applications for smartphones or tablets. Devices can be used in a variety of situations and are available in numerous formats, such as teaching relaxation techniques, providing interactive electronic physiological monitoring (biofeedback) which facilitates self-regulation, or stand-alone electrotherapeutic technologies, which can influence brainwave frequencies. Therapeutic technologies are rapidly emerging as a unique and effective way to provide health information and as a source for patient self-management tools. Recently, a number of new options for mind-body (MB) skills training have been developed, including technologies that support stress management approaches, emotional regulation strategies, and self-calming techniques. Although many healthcare providers are aware of the need for effective stress management strategies for patients of all ages, busy clinicians may not have the time to stay up-to-date with these new technological offerings. However, in many cases, companies are launching direct-to-consumer advertising of their product benefits, which allows patients and families direct access to, and use of, these approaches, as they seek attractive options for treating stress-mediated mental and physical challenges.

It is well-known that children are regularly utilizing interactive electronic media, such as smartphones or tablets, at home and school [18]. In a 2015 article in *Pediatrics* by Kabali et al. [19], the following was discovered about the use of mobile devices by children and families: "[a] cross-sectional study [was performed including] 350 children aged 6 months to 4 years, seen October to November 2014, at a pediatric clinic in an urban, low-income, minority community. The survey was adapted from Common Sense Media's 2013 nationwide survey...[and it was found that] most households had television (97%), tablets (83%), and smartphones (77%). At age 4, half the children had their own television and three-fourths [had] their own mobile device. Almost all children (96.6%) used mobile devices, and most started using before one years of age. Parents gave children devices when doing house chores (70%), to keep them calm (65%), and at bedtime (29%)." This study suggests that, even if not explicitly stated, many parents are currently utilizing technology with their children as a non-pharmacological option for purposes of calming and distraction.

After over twenty years working in the clinical practice of developmental/behavioral and integrative pediatrics, the author has witnessed the many benefits of teaching children a variety of MB skills, as an important therapeutic element in a comprehensive treatment plan. This commentary offers his opinions and perspectives on the way in which technology can enhance the process of learning and practicing MB skills for children and teens. Therefore, this paper is not intended to provide an exhaustive review of the literature on this subject, but instead is meant to reflect the author's clinical experience and what he has found to be useful in his own clinical practice.

One important goal of this commentary is to raise awareness of these technologies among clinicians, so that healthcare providers might better understand alternative therapeutic options and consequently discuss these options with their patients. An additional hope is that healthcare providers may creatively integrate these newer technology-assisted relaxation approaches, when indicated, into appealing treatment strategies for pediatric patients for whom MB skills are indicated.

1.1. Complementary Approaches and Pediatric Practice

Complementary and alternative medicine (CAM) is quite popular for children and teenagers seeking natural approaches [20–22] for a variety of medical and mental health issues, partly because families are now seeking out more natural and less invasive therapies. Many children and parents prefer non-pharmacological therapies, if available, for common complaints such as headaches, abdominal pain, insomnia, anxiety, stress, inattention, anger, or emotional dysregulation. Within the CAM domain, MB and self-regulation skills are particularly effective in managing a number of common symptoms of childhood with a very positive risk/benefit ratio in a safe, cost-effective, and time-efficient manner [23]. The attractiveness of these options can be seen in a recent review by Vohra and McClafferty et al., who note that MB therapies "are popular and ranked among the top ten complementary and integrative medicine practices reportedly used by adults and children" [1].

1.2. Chronic Over-Arousal

It is also reasonable to argue that, for most children and teenagers, the demands and exposures of modern life are increasingly leading to chronic autonomic nervous system (ANS) over-arousal, in a way that is often unrecognized by the majority of individuals, who commonly accept it as their normal baseline reference mode of experience. However, this constant over-arousal can cause physical and emotional regulation problems [24–26]. In fact, since this state of ANS imbalance (stress) is so often recognized as a normal baseline mood, individuals may feel uncomfortable with calmer, quieter states of mind and body, as these can feel unfamiliar or uncomfortable. Evidence suggests that this heightened baseline and continuous state of chronic stress may be depleting for the mind, body, and spirit, and when left unchecked, can lead to many physical and mental health problems [27]. For example, stress may serve as an epigenetic modifier [28,29], while accessing a relaxation response achieved from practicing MB techniques (i.e., dialing up parasympathetic nervous system activity and reducing sympathetic arousal), may counterbalance this stress-effect and help to turn on health-promoting genes and processes.

A chronic state of nervous system over-arousal can also contribute to the etiology and/or maintenance of a number of physical issues (inflammation, pain, immune dysregulation, insomnia) and mental health symptoms (anxiety, depression, inattention), for which medications are commonly prescribed [24–27]. For these reasons, it is important that all children and teenagers learn MB balancing skills early on, so that they might also have the option to utilize non-pharmacological alternatives that can facilitate the MB's natural healing capacity and perhaps address the causative issue at a more foundational level. It has also been well-established that the regular practice of a variety of MB techniques, including yoga, mental imagery, hypnosis, biofeedback, and meditation, are effective for re-balancing the ANS in pediatric populations and for addressing physical and emotional symptoms, such as pain, anxiety, insomnia, and gastrointestinal complaints [1,30–32]. Additionally, with regular practice, MB skills can be health-promoting in the long-term, contributing to better attention spans, social skills, emotional regulation, enhanced immune system function, and decreased inflammation [6,25,29,33].

1.3. Mind-Body Skills for Autonomic Nervous System Re-Balancing

Currently, there are no definitive studies detailing the exact amount of practice of MB skills required for optimal success, in terms of short-term symptom control (e.g., to reduce acute pain or anxiety), or long-term health and wellness improvements (e.g., baseline levels of stress, happiness, attention, inflammation). In clinical settings, some individuals do appear to achieve benefits—at least acutely—with only a single practice or a few experiences, but mastery and sustained change likely requires consistent practice of the skill, in order to use these skills effectively for the re-patterning of neurobiological processes and consequently create a new baseline. Therefore, it can be reasonably assumed that the benefits accrued from MB skills are likely dose-dependent. Despite the recognition that cost-efficient, safe, and effective MB techniques are readily available and can be used to address a variety of the aforementioned issues, children and teenagers often don't practice MB skills, and certainly not to an optimal level to be able to achieve the best possible therapeutic benefit.

Clinical experience suggests that: (1) although many kids are familiar with the concept of relaxation, few have learned any formal MB skills; (2) many kids, when asked how they relax, suggest alternative methods, such as to read a book, do an art project, play a video game, or watch TV, which may or may not be objectively relaxing in terms of ANS arousal; (3) kids that have learned MB skills don't practice them consistently in the appropriate situations; (4) kids that practice MB skills often get bored with that practice; (5) kids that understand and have practiced some form of MB skills are not necessarily applying them in a way that could be effective in-the-moment; and (6) kids often don't believe that a change in their thinking and feeling can really result in a physical change in the body.

1.4. Technology for Healing

The selective use of technology, although problematic in many ways, can be quite useful for children and teenagers to learn and practice MB skills, especially for those who have been reluctant to do so because it is perceived as another boring, non-preferred task, such as homework or household chores. Most individuals would prefer to interact with electronic media in the age of cellphones, computers, video game systems, or TV sets. This preference can be used to the advantage of healthcare providers, by becoming familiar with new "healing technologies", that can be harnessed to provide technology-assisted relaxation training and can make the process of learning and practicing effective MB skills much more engaging, playful, and user-friendly for kids.

Many studies have focused on the potential downside of technology, suggesting that too much exposure to electronic media and/or exposure to certain types of inappropriate electronic media content, may have negative impacts on the developing child, such as contributing to a short attention span, sedentary behavior, over-arousal, aggressive behavior, depression, insomnia, and unhealthy food choices related to advertisements. However, not enough attention has been paid to the concept of utilizing these interactive electronic multimedia devices in order to engage children and teenagers in constructive, health-promoting, self-care skill development and symptom management. In this commentary, concepts such as play, therapeutic play, self-regulation, and MB skills, and their relationship to new electronic media, are reviewed. This commentary also reviews some of the most helpful software and devices currently used in the field of technology-assisted relaxation.

2. Benefits of MB Skills

MB techniques typically focus on the interactions and connections between the brain, the body, and the subsequent behaviors. There are many ways in which emotional, spiritual, cognitive, and psychosocial phenomena can directly affect physical and mental health. A compilation of potential benefits of practicing MB skills is listed in Table 1.

Teaching self-regulation and/or MB skills of any kind often involves assisting individuals to achieve a state of improved MB health and healing by shifting the balance of: (1) the ANS (from sympathetic activity to parasympathetic activity); (2) emotions (from negative to positive); (3) thoughts (from unhelpful to helpful) and; (4) a sense of control over health status (from external to internal) [23,33].

Table 1. Potential benefits of mind-body (MB) skills training.

Eliciting the "Relaxation Response"
Autonomic Nervous System Balancing: decreasing sympathetic nervous system activity while dialing up parasympathetic nervous system activity
Enhanced Emotional Regulation
Training Attention and Cultivating Awareness
Stress Management
Modifying the central nervous system (CNS)
Performance Enhancement
Improved Social Interactions
Improved Decision Making
Increasing Peace and Happiness
Building Emotional and Physical Resilience
Pain and Symptom Management

3. The Interface of Video Games, Self-Regulation and Healing

Many healthcare providers know that, when teaching kids self-care skills, they are more effective and more likely to be practiced and operationalized, if the skills are customized to the child's interests and learning style, and delivered in a way that is playful, non-threatening, developmentally appropriate, and novel. Delivering treatments through "play" experiences or games, is an ideal, developmentally appropriate way to proceed in therapeutic interaction, and is often referred to as "therapeutic play." Over the past several years, playing video games, texting, and watching online videos have become popular activities for children and teens [34–36]. What exactly is it that seems to make video games so popular? One component of their appeal may involve the experience of "mastery" and being recognized as an expert. For a child with limited opportunities to experience success in activities such as sports, music, or theater, being talented at video games could have a positive impact on their self-esteem.

Additionally, video game designers also know what it takes to engage kids. In their 1983 book *Mind at Play: The Psychology of Video Games*, psychologists Loftus and Loftus describe the three elements that drive the design of successful, addictive video games and make them intrinsically motivating (i.e., curiosity, fantasy, and challenge) [37]. These concepts are still relevant and can therefore be used to inform the design of effective MB, self-care strategies for kids. In particular, children aged four to 13 years are developmentally driven towards mastery, have a rich fantasy life, move easily between real life and their imagination, and are engaged by experiences that are multimedia, interactive, and novel—thus evoking a strong sense of curiosity. The designers and marketers of computer games, mobile apps, and related software and gadgets have often exploited these elements in the design of popular multimedia entertainment that have become highly recognized brand names, such as *Final Fantasy*, *Angry Birds*, *Legend of Zelda*, and *Kingdom Hearts*, along with many games based on movies and cartoons, such as *Toy Story*, *Pokemon* and *Cars*. Interestingly, popular children's books are now among the top-sellers for mobile apps, but have also gone far beyond the book form—interactive elements have been added, such as gaming features and audio enhancements (i.e., entertaining sound effects).

Consequently, technology-assisted relaxation devices have been increasingly designed to harness the same power, absorption, and fun of these electronic games features and mobile applications, but for the service of health instead of strictly entertainment. Multimedia interactive game play can be utilized to connect with the imagistic, emotional, and sensory elements of the right brain for symptom management and healing. The following section will review the concept of MB skills, along with current electronics–based options for kids and teenagers that leverage the idea of "therapeutic play", in order to practice MB skills at home, at school, or in clinical settings. This listing is not complete, but has been gathered by the experience of the author, who has personally used the majority of these products in both inpatient and outpatient settings. Additionally, the paper will review common products that the author and his colleagues have found useful for supporting children in their regular, daily practice of MB skills. These products are organized by the type of technology involved: (1) mobile applications (for smart phones and tablet computers), which only involve software; (2) biofeedback devices (either stand-alone or computer-based), which involve hardware (a physiological sensor) and software; (3) other technology-assisted relaxation devices that are specialized portable technologies involving electrical stimulation.

4. Definitions of MB Skills

1. *Breathwork:* the conscious control of the rate, rhythm, and depth of breathing; a technique used in relaxation and meditative practices in order to reduce psychological stress and increase parasympathetic nervous system activity.
2. *Biofeedback*: a technique you can use to learn to control your body's functions, such as your heart rate, hand temperature, or muscle tension. With biofeedback, you're connected to electrical sensors or electromechanical devices that provide you with auditory and visual information about your body. This feedback helps you to then control a desired physiological function in a therapeutic direction, which provides the opportunity to more objectively observe the mind-body connection and understand how a change in thinking or feeling can directly correlate with a change in physiology.
3. *Guided and/or Mental Imagery/Self-hypnosis*: commonly invokes all of the five senses in journeys of imagination (and fantasy) and facilitates an intensification of focus, less attention to peripheral factors, more awareness of internal events/sensations, and enhanced suggestibility.
4. *Meditation and Mindfulness*: practices involving concentrated focus or intentional attention training, in order to increase awareness of the present moment or to reduce stress.
5. *Yoga*: a Hindu spiritual and ascetic discipline derived from the Sanskrit word *yuj*, meaning union. It includes body postures, breathwork, and meditative practices.

5. Electronic Mobile Applications for Smartphones and Tablet Computers

Mobile apps are often game-like in design and can include features of immersive, attention-maintaining properties of fantasy and imagery, offer interactivity and control, and can include useful behavioral change elements, such as symptom assessment, tailored messages, tracking progress, and goal setting.

5.1. Mobile Apps for Breathwork

5.1.1. Breathe2Relax

According to its website [38], "this (app) is a portable stress management tool which provides detailed information on the effects of stress on the body and instructions and practice exercises to help users learn the stress management skill called diaphragmatic breathing." This app also includes effective explanations and illustrations of the respiratory system.

5.1.2. Breathing Zone

This is a well-designed mobile app that basically serves as an interactive breath pacer. The user has the flexibility to pick the beginning breath pace, ending breath pace, and cueing audio for each breath (chime, water, voice, etc.), along with an optional timer.

5.1.3. Belly Bio Interactive Breathing

This is an interactive app for the iPhone that utilizes the phone's accelerometer to monitor proper diaphragmatic (belly) breathing techniques, by providing feedback about the movement of the user's stomach.

5.1.4. Breathing Bubbles

Breathing Bubbles is an app that helps kids to practice releasing worries and focus on pleasant feelings, while using a bubble as a visual representation for this release.

5.2. Mobile Apps for Meditation and Mindfulness

Meditation has been proven to be a helpful tool addressing medical and mental health issues, for both the pediatric and adult populations [2,31].

5.2.1. Take a Chill

According to the developers [39], "this mobile app offers mindfulness meditation exercises and texted practice reminders. As a teen, there are moments in your life when you're really stressed and just need to 'Take a Chill'." This app is full of tools to help manage that stress and incorporate mindful practices into a daily routine. Using quick mindful exercises and thoughtful activities, teenagers learn to begin to overcome those moments, whether it's studying for a test or preventing negative thoughts and patterns. Features in the app include:

1. Quick Exercises: two illustrated exercises for in-the-moment situations
2. Daily Dose: daily activities to help reinforce concepts and increase your mindful practice
3. Progress: see your progress and activity overtime
4. Reminders: keep yourself motivated with three types of Reminders
5. Motivational Quotes: receive a new motivational quote after each use

5.2.2. Stop, Breathe and Think

The creators [40] state that, "with this app, you can develop and apply awareness, kindness and compassion in your daily life through a meditative process called *Stop, Breathe and Think*: (1) Stop:

Stop what you are doing. Check in with what you are thinking, and how you are feeling; (2) Breathe: Practice mindful breathing to create space between your thoughts, emotions and reactions; (3) Think: Learn to broaden your perspective and strengthen your force field of peace and calm by practicing one of the meditations."

5.2.3. Smiling Mind

The creators of this app [41] state that, "*Smiling Mind* is a modern meditation approach, a unique web- and app-based program developed by psychologists and educators to help bring balance to people's lives by teaching meditation and related skills."

5.3. Mobile Apps for Yoga

Yoga can be used as another helpful tool to address a variety of psychological and physical conditions of childhood [30].

5.3.1. The Adventures of Superstretch

This is a mobile app [42] that teaches yoga with videos of real kids doing yoga postures, and animated narrators offering information, instructions, and insight. It is a helpful way to get sedentary kids moving in a fun, non-threatening process. The app's designers have declared that "kids don't have to be athletes, flexible or fit to do this. We've designed it to be non-competitive and even bring in partner activities to show we're all in this together. In yoga, there's no perfect. In each pose, the kids are just being kids—doing poses the best they can. No need to be perfect, to 'succeed' or do it 'right'. We are allowing ourselves to be present, in the moment. It's ok to fall out of poses. It's ok to laugh, to roar like a lion—in fact, that's the whole point. Be courageous, creative and just try."

5.3.2. Yoga by Teens

According to the developers [43], "within this app, kids can join yoga teens, Lauren, Emily and Jessica Parsons in a class that is designed and taught by teens. *Yoga by Teens* teaches basic hatha yoga poses that are fun, challenging and help to build strength and flexibility, as well as develop self-confidence and self-esteem. Its message is that yoga is for all ages and levels of ability, including people with special needs."

5.3.3. Kids Yogaverse: I Am Love

The website [44] claims, "this is a great app which allows kids to calm down and be ready for the day. It teaches individuals to always think about good things and always know that you are smart. It is beautifully hand-drawn and incorporates 13 yoga poses for children demonstrated by children. Get ready to open your heart, expand your mind and reveal that *you* are the real treasure to love. The yoga poses help you to stretch out and wake up your mind. The material on this app can be enjoyed by listening to the book, or reading the book." Additional interactive features include:

1. Animated Poses: follow the children as they do the real poses through the yoga journey
2. Breath Affirmations: press the Breath button on each page and you will hear a special message just for you
3. Guess What?: press the Guess What button and learn amazing new facts

5.4. Mobile Apps for Imagery, Movement and More

5.4.1. Healing Buddies Comfort Kit

The author has developed this free mobile app with the local children's hospital, called the *The Healing Buddies Comfort Kit*, for use in children's hospitals and clinical settings. It provides an interactive, game-like, colorful, multimedia way for kids and teens to learn a variety of integrative and holistic techniques in order to manage bothersome symptoms. It includes guided sessions of imagery, muscle relaxation, and breathing for a variety of symptoms that kids might experience at home, in hospitals, or anywhere, such as pain, nausea, fatigue, insomnia, and anxiety.

5.4.2. Me Moves

This app (now available as a digital download) is accessible on tablet computers, cellphones, and computers. The interaction involves using your arms and upper body to slowly follow and engage in graceful upper body movements, to the beat of a metronome and lovely background music. Kids with any kind of over-arousal or anxiety tendencies, including kids with autism and ADHD, can greatly benefit from this program. The developers [45] state that, "mirroring those on the screen, users are transformed by the music, images, movement, and the expressive features of emotion. This easy to use, interactive program has been widely praised by therapists, educators, and parents."

6. Biofeedback Devices (Stand-Alone, Computer-Based and Smartphone-Based)

Training MB self-regulation skills using biofeedback-based relaxation techniques and technologies can be quite engaging, interactive, and effective for treating a variety of conditions [1,3], which has been described by kids as "a videogame for your body". A therapist might use several different biofeedback methods. Determining the method that is right for your client depends on their specific health problems and goals. Biofeedback methods include:

1. *Brainwave*: also known as an electroencephalograph (EEG) and neurofeedback, this type of device uses head sensors to monitor brain wave frequencies.
2. *Heart rate*: this type of biofeedback uses an infrared finger or earlobe sensor, called a photoplethysmograph, to measure your heart rate and variability (HRV).
3. *Muscle*: electromyography (EMG) biofeedback, which involves placing sensors on skeletal muscles to measure the electrical activity that causes muscle contraction.
4. *Sweat glands*: sensors attached around your fingers or on your palm measure sweat gland activity (also called electrodermal activity; EDA).
5. *Temperature*: sensors read the temperature of your fingers/hands that is controlled by blood flow to the periphery (which is influenced by ANS balance).

6.1. HeartMath Products (Heart Rate Variability)

These products are available as a Mac- or PC-based program with game features (*emWave Pro* and *emWave Pro Plus*), as a mobile app for smartphones or tablet computers (called *Inner Balance*), or as a portable, handheld version (called *emWave2*, which features color changing LEDs that signal the user about ANS balance and an optimal state of psychophysiological harmony, termed "coherence".) The user receives information about the heart rate variability pattern as a proxy for ANS balance and emotional regulation. *HeartMath's emWave Pro* also contains video games, for example one game challenges the user to color in a picture that starts as black and white as they move into a more optimal ANS balance and shift to a positive emotional state. Another game format rewards the user with a hot air balloon ride over beautiful landscapes. With the newest game, dual drive, the user controls the speed and handling of a sports car by staying in optimal ANS balance. With the portable, handheld version (*emWave2*), the user can follow a breathing pacer and will then see a specific LED change from red (low coherence), to blue (medium coherence), to green (high coherence). Features of "Inner Balance" include the ability to customize screens with photographs and personally-selected music. This serves as a great tool for kids with any kind of chronic pain, anxiety, insomnia, tics, or anger management challenges.

6.2. Muse (Electrical Brain Activity)

The Muse is a brain-sensing headband that measures electrical brain signals using seven finely calibrated sensors—two on the forehead, two behind the ears, and three reference sensors. The headband uses information from these EEG sensors to measure whether your mind is calm and focused, or active and wandering, and translates that data into active sounds to guide you. There is a companion app for smartphones or tablets that provides audio and visual feedback to guide training.

6.3. The Pip (ElectroDermal Response)

The skin pores (sweat glands) on your fingertips are sensitive to changing levels of stress. *The Pip* accurately captures these changes, and through audio and visual feedback, allows you to be aware and change your response pattern. It achieves this by detecting variations in your EDA. This product comes with interactive software to provide audio and visual feedback and summary information about stress response patterns.

6.4. eSense (Peripheral Temperature Monitor)

According to its website [46], "*eSense* is a small sensor for measuring your skin temperature with the microphone input of your smartphone or tablet (Android or Apple iOS.). Hand warming training is an especially effective and common biofeedback method. The temperature of our hands is connected to our stress level: when we are stressed, we tend to have cold hands. Immediate feedback enables you to voluntarily increase the skin temperature in your fingers, thus increasing your peripheral blood circulation, leading to relaxation and stress reduction. *eSense* provides you, in various ways, with exact feedback about your momentary stress level (e.g., with measurement curves, video display and audio feedback features)."

6.5. Antense (Electromyography)

The developers [47] state that, "the *Antense* anti-tension device is a simple yet effective way to eliminate stress by helping you develop a greater sense of body awareness in the comfort and privacy of your home. A common cause of the discomfort associated with stress or tension is the contraction of your scalp, face and neck muscles. Learning how to relax these muscles is an essential step toward relief and prevention of this discomfort. Because these muscles are not normally under your conscious, direct control, a monitoring or guidance system is necessary to indicate or feedback to you their level of activity. EMG. The *Antense* biofeedback device provides this monitoring. The instrument continuously monitors and averages the EMG activity in the frontalis (forehead) muscle and converts it into a pleasant tone. Using patented technology, *Antense* measures these contractions and instantly converts the signal into a pleasant tone-pitch proportional to the level of muscle tension in your body. With the variations in the tone as a guide, you can quickly train your muscles to relax relieving the discomfort and preventing future problems related to tense facial muscles like headaches. By learning to feel how stress changes your body, you will quickly understand how to release that tension and stress and learn how to relax at will."

7. Other Technology-Assisted Relaxation Devices

As technology marches on, there are some additional, very promising gadgets that can assist individuals in achieving a deep relaxation response and decrease sympathetic nervous arousal, while enhancing parasympathetic nervous system activity. The available scientific literature regarding the use of these devices by children and teens is very limited, so they should be used with caution. However, these devices are generally safe and easy to use, and are available for anyone to purchase, without the prescription of a healthcare provider. Although there is still only limited research on the use of these technologies, they are worth considering and have shown promising preliminary results in adult populations [48–50].

7.1. Cranial Electrotherapeutic Stimulation (CES)

The concept of applying electrical stimulation for healing purposes has been in use for at least 2000 years. Machines that deliver a small, pulsed electric current across the head are now claiming efficacy for a variety of medical and mental health conditions. Cranial electrotherapeutic stimulation (CES) is a technology which applies small levels of electrical stimulation across the cranium, to benefit patients with issues such as anxiety, depression, insomnia, ADHD, and chronic pain [41,43,44].

One of the developers of a CES product called *alpha-stim* [51], states that, "our brain basically creates four different frequencies of brain waves each day: beta, alpha, theta and delta. Alpha waves are created when we are in a state of quiet, calm, focused contemplation, and are often associated with meditative states and practices. The CES device sends pulses of very low amperage (i.e., less than 1.0 milliampere) electricity through thin wires attached to electrodes clipped to the ear lobes or stuck to the skin over the bony prominences just to the front of, or behind each ear. The frequency of the electrical pulses can be adjusted—usually from 0.5 Hz to 100 Hz—depending on the treatment effect desired." You could think of these new gadgets that passively cultivate alpha waves as a passive form of meditation. Basically, you place small sensors on your earlobes, dial up the device (about the size of a thick cellphone), and passively enjoy the cultivation of alpha brain waves. Although the exact mechanisms of alpha wave stimulation are not known, some have claimed that these waves could promote the release of neurotransmitters, like serotonin, and the elicitation of alpha wave frequencies in the brain. In alpha wave states, people tend to feel calm, relaxed, and report an enhanced mental focus. Products include *alpha-stim*, *CES Ultra*, and *Fisher Wallace* (Table 2).

7.2. Audio-Visual Entertainment (AVE)

The brain is capable of being tuned in a remarkable variety of ways. For instance, certain music or light-pulsing colored sunglasses can significantly alter brain wave frequency, which affects different functions, depending upon the chosen frequency. Beta waves are associated with active problem solving, alpha waves with a calm, focused mind, theta with creative thinking, and delta waves with sleep. Brainwave entrainment refers to any practice intended to cause brain waves to fall into step—or certain frequencies—by using a periodic stimulus of some type. One potential desirable result of brainwave entrainment is to synchronize the two hemispheres of our brain with their brainwave frequency patterns. Potential benefits of hemisphere synchronization include promoting happiness, optimism, and contentment [52–54].

For simple audio entrainment, products include various music or nature sound CD's with embedded beats, vibration, and or therapeutic suggestions. Examples of this include CD's by Jeffrey Thompson, and holo-synch and hemi-synch recordings. When pulsing LED lights are added to audio entrainment, audio-visual entrainment is subsequently created: products include the *DAVID*, the *Dream Machine*, and *Proteus* (Table 2). Some of the benefits which have been seen from the use of brain entrainment include: healthier sleep patterns and more restful sleep each night; a greater ability to relax and meditate (some describe brain entrainment as the ultimate meditation tool); a lowering of situation-specific and overall stress levels; improvements in cognitive function and creativity; easing of negative emotions which affect health and happiness; and an overall sense of peace and well-being.

7.3. Transcutaneous (tc) Vagal Nerve Stimulation (tc-VNS)

The concept of influencing neurons with electricity has been used for over a century, when patients were treated with electro convulsive therapy as a treatment for severe depression. Additionally, and more recently, transcranial electromagnetic stimulation has also been gaining traction as a treatment for insomnia and other conditions [55,56]. The vagus nerve originates in the brain and vagal nerve stimulators electronically signal the vagus nerve (more specifically, they stimulate the afferent auricular branch of the vagus), which in turn stimulates the release of neurotransmitters in the brain, in order to generate a calming sensation. Stimulation of the vagal nerve also increases parasympathetic nervous system activity, which can potentially elicit a relaxation response. This can occur during the stimulation session, but also has longer lasting effects to decrease tension, if used daily. Surgically implantable vagal nerve stimulators are available and have been used to effectively treat seizures and depression. Wearable devices are now available that provide transcutaneous (tc) stimulation (and which do not require surgery). As of 2016, a device called *Nervana* offers an FDA-approved tc nerve stimulator, which combines music with vagal nerve stimulation in the ear canal, using ear buds.

8. Clinical Tips: Prescribing MB Skills Practice

One of the most important recommendations for prescribing the practice of MB skills to pediatric patients is to start small, such as a prescription for MB practice for only three to five minutes, once or twice a day. MB skills are best taught in an organized sequential manner, making certain that pediatric clients master each step along the way, as follows:

(1) Mind-Body Awareness

   a. Learn to discriminate (objectively) the mind-body differences between sympathetic nervous system arousal (stress) and parasympathetic nervous system dominant states (relaxation response).

(2) Mind-Body Self-Regulation

   a. Learn to modulate (first in a controlled environment) a given psychological or physiological function, in a therapeutic direction, consistently.

(3) Mind-Body Skill Transfer

   a. Apply this ability to self-regulate the mind and body in appropriate life situations, as needed, "in the moment".

(4) Mind-Body Reset

   a. Restructure (CNS) and rebalance (baseline ANS) with regular daily practice to a calmer, happier, emotionally resilient pattern long-term.

It is also necessary to prescribe daily practice in two different modes; consistent daily practices to reset the neurological baseline, along with recommending an "in-the-moment", brief application of techniques and technology, to manage acute situations in real life (e.g., feeling stressed, having a headache, trouble sleeping, getting angry). Have clients try and practice a variety of MB skills and gadgets so that they can figure out what works best for them. It is also ideal to have multiple options in one's "self-care toolkit" and to request that parents provide rewards for regular practice and effort shown. Clients should also focus on keeping a symptom diary, and describe practice frequency, length, and daily situations they find challenging, stating whether any MB skills that they had tried were helpful. A summary of potential MB resources to recommend to patients is listed in Table 2.

Table 2. List of MB resources.

Biofeedback	Other Technology-Assisted Relaxation Techniques	Mobile Apps
HRV Biofeedback www.heartmath.com	**AVE-Audio Entrainment** www.soundstrue.com www.centerpointe.com www.hemisynch.com	**Breathing** www.t2health.dcoe.mil www.breathing.zone www.bellybio.com
EDA Biofeedback www.thepip.com	**AVE-Audio Visual Entrainment** www.mindalive.com www.mindmachines.com www.deepakchopradreamweaver.com	**Me Moves** www.thinkingmoves.com
EMG Biofeedback www.lifematters.com	**CES** www.alpha-stim.com www.cesultra.com www.fisherwallace.com	**Healing Buddies Comfort Kit** www.healingbuddiescomfort.org

Table 2. *Cont.*

Biofeedback	Other Technology-Assisted Relaxation Techniques	Mobile Apps
TEMP Biofeedback www.mindfield.de	tc-VNS www.experiencenervana.com www.cerbomed.com	**Meditation** www.buddhify.com www.stopbreathethink.org www.stressedteens.com www.smilingmind.com.au
EEG Biofeedback www.choosemuse.com		**Yoga** www.adventuresofsuperstretch.com www.kidsyogaverse.com
MULTIMODAL BF www.wilddivine.com		

HRV: heart rate and variability; AVE: audio-visual entertainment; EDA: electrodermal activity; CES: cranial electrotherapeutic stimulation; EMG: electromyography; tc-VNS: transcutaneous vagal nerve stimulation; TEMP: temperature; EEG: electroencephalograph; BF: biofeedback.

9. Conclusions

The intention of this commentary was to provide an entertaining and informational perspective on the interface of technology, mind-body skills, and effective patient care for pediatric healthcare providers of all kinds. The reality is that computer games, interactive mobile apps, and other health-related gadgets are no longer just a trivial activity played by individuals for fun, but can now be utilized for various educational and therapeutic purposes. Consequently, the author intends to highlight the benefits of utilizing technology-assisted relaxation devices and strategies to enhance the practice of MB skills in children and youth in the service of healing and wellness promotion.

Well-designed computer games/apps have the potential to engage the player and are often designed to be intrinsically motivating, in order to encourage frequent use (the *Journey to Wild Divine* home biofeedback system serves as a good example of this) [57]. If technology-assisted relaxation devices and software provide positive reinforcement, mastery, and curiosity, kids and teens will be more willing to utilize them again, and therefore, therapeutic benefits can be gleaned from this approach. Although the use of technologies can be increasingly problematic in the life of children and teens, they can also be harnessed and adapted for therapeutic purposes. Technology-assisted relaxation can be quite useful (when carefully explained, prescribed, monitored, and utilized) as a culturally-syntonic vehicle to facilitate the regular practice of health-promoting MB therapies, such as breathwork, yoga, biofeedback-based relaxation, and mindfulness meditation. Therefore, healthcare providers should focus on understanding the latest technology available, and promoting self-regulation through MB skills training, which is known to provide benefits to humans of all ages.

In this age of rapid technological advancements, we could begin to imagine what the next frontier looks like: combining the best of the graphic design and multimedia arts, music, play, computerized hardware/software applications, and new miniaturized technologies for the creation of "therapeutic play" products, tools, and techniques for the next generation. Will the most effective therapists and pediatricians deliver their training on tablets and touch screen cellphones? Will clients check in regularly online via these devices? Will physiologic sensors be added into clothing or jewelry for additional information and options for more precise control of mind and body? As we continue to explore the interface of the arts, biomedical technologies, and healthcare endeavors in the service of healing, tremendous potential is available to develop new ways in which electronic media can enhance health and healing for kids and teenagers across a variety of settings, although vigilance is still needed to combat the potential downside to the overuse of technology [34].

Technology-assisted relaxation devices, in the form of computer games and electronic mobile apps, will certainly be part of the future of pediatric healthcare. Design features that optimize these healing technologies must take into account the specific client's play style, audio and visual preferences, developmental stage, and attention span. These products should support patients in a variety of ways, including promoting health literacy and improving self-regulatory abilities, both physically and psychologically. From a personalized healthcare perspective, computerized games utilized to promote health and wellness can provide a new source of information about patient preferences, health status, psychophysiological response patterns, and self-care abilities. Healthcare providers will hopefully find creative ways to utilize technology in care planning, as a way to enhance treatment adherence with recommendations to practice MB skills, and ultimately, to improve outcomes for the children, teenagers, and families we serve.

Author Contributions: Timothy Culbert is a developmental/behavioral pediatrician who is also board-certified in medical hypnosis, biofeedback, and holistic medicine. He has training in mindfulness meditation, functional medicine, nutrition, and clinical aromatherapy. Dr. Culbert is an author, lecturer, and product-developer in the area of natural therapies, self-regulation skills, and MB techniques for children, adults, and teens. Additionally, he has also written four books for children on holistic approaches for common problems, and co-edited the Oxford Series textbook "Integrative Pediatrics". He currently serves as Medical Director for Integrative Medicine at PrairieCare Medical Group in Minnesota.

Conflicts of Interest: Timothy Culbert, MD, is a lecturer for HeartMath LLC.

References

1. AAP Section On Integrative Medicine. Mind-body therapies in children and youth. *Pediatrics* **2016**, *138*, e20161896.
2. Sibinga, E.M.S.; Kemper, K.J. Complementary, Holistic, and Integrative. Meditation Practices for Pediatric Health. *Pediatr. Rev.* **2010**, *31*, e91. [CrossRef] [PubMed]
3. Culbert, T.; Banez, G. Pediatric Applications. In *Biofeedback: A Practitioner's Guide*; Schwartz, M.S., Andrasik, F., Eds.; Guilford Publications: New York, NY, USA, 2015.
4. Culbert, T.; Friedrichsdorf, S.; Kuttner, L. Mind-body skills for children in pain. *Clin. Pain Manag. Pract. Appl. Proced.* **2007**, *138*, e20161896.
5. Greenland, S.K. *The Mindful Child: How to Help Your Kid Manage Stress and Become Happier, Kinder, and More Compassionate*; Simon and Schuster: New York, NY, USA, 2010.
6. Rosenkranz, M.A.; Davidson, R.; MacCoon, D.; Sheridan, J.; Kalin, N.; Lutz, A. A comparison of mindfulness-based stress reduction and an active control in modulation of neurogenic inflammation. *Brain Behav. Immun.* **2013**, *27*, 174–184. [CrossRef] [PubMed]
7. Gruzelier, J.H. A review of the impact of hypnosis, relaxation, guided imagery and individual differences on aspects of immunity and health. *Stress* **2002**, *5*, 147–163. [CrossRef] [PubMed]
8. Nassau, J.H.; Tien, K.; Fritz, G.K. Review of the literature: Integrating psychoneuroimmunology into pediatric chronic illness interventions. *J. Pediatr. Psychol.* **2008**, *33*, 195–207. [CrossRef] [PubMed]
9. Saltzman, A. *A Still Quiet Place: A Mindfulness Program for Teaching Children and Adolescents to Ease Stress and Difficult Emotions*; New Harbinger Publications: Oakland, CA, USA, 2014.
10. McCallum, S. Gamification and serious games for personalized health. *Stud. Health Technol. Inform.* **2012**, *177*, 85–96. [PubMed]
11. McQueen, A.; Cress, C.; Tothy, A. Using a tablet computer during pediatric procedures: A case series and review of the "apps". *Pediatr. Emerg. Care* **2012**, *28*, 712–714. [CrossRef] [PubMed]
12. Luxton, D.D.; McCann, R.; Bush, N.; Mishkind, M.; Reger, G. mHealth for mental health: Integrating smartphone technology in behavioral healthcare. *Prof. Psychol. Res. Pract.* **2011**, *42*, 505. [CrossRef]
13. Donker, T.; Petrie, K.; Proudfoot, J.; Clarke, J.; Birch, M.R.; Christensen, H. Smartphones for smarter delivery of mental health programs: A systematic review. *J. Med. Internet Res.* **2013**, *15*, e247. [CrossRef] [PubMed]
14. Kato, P.M. Video games in health care: Closing the gap. *Rev. Gen. Psychol.* **2010**, *14*, 113. [CrossRef]
15. Baranowski, T. Playing for real: Video games and stories for health-related behavior change. *Am. J. Prev. Med.* **2008**, *34*, 74–82. [CrossRef] [PubMed]
16. Handel, M.J. mHealth (mobile health)—Using apps for health and wellness. *EXPLORE J. Sci. Heal.* **2011**, *7*, 256–261. [CrossRef] [PubMed]
17. O'Keeffe, G.S.; Clarke-Pearson, K. The impact of social media on children, adolescents, and families. *Pediatrics* **2011**, *127*, 800–804. [CrossRef] [PubMed]

18. Radesky, J.S.; Schumacher, J.; Zuckerman, B. Mobile and interactive media use by young children: The good, the bad, and the unknown. *Pediatrics* **2015**, *135*, 1–3. [CrossRef] [PubMed]

19. Kabali, H.K.; Irigoyen, M.M.; Nunez-Davis, R.; Budacki, J.G.; Mohanty, S.H.; Leister, K.P.; Bonner, R.L. Exposure and use of mobile media devices by young children. *Pediatrics* **2015**, *136*, 1044–1050. [CrossRef] [PubMed]

20. Kemper, K.J.; Vohra, S.; Walls, R. The use of complementary and alternative medicine in pediatrics. *Pediatrics* **2008**, *122*, 1374–1386. [CrossRef] [PubMed]

21. Barnes, P.M.; Bloom, B.; Nahin, R.L. Complementary and alternative medicine use among adults and children: United States, 2007. *Natl. Health Stat. Rep.* **2008**, *12*, 1–23.

22. Harris, P.E.; Cooper, K.; Relton, C.; Thomas, K. Prevalence of complementary and alternative medicine (CAM) use by the general population: A systematic review and update. *Int. J. Clin. Pract.* **2012**, *66*, 924–939. [CrossRef] [PubMed]

23. Sussman, G.D.; Culbert, T. Pediatric self-regulation (Chapter 91). In *Developmental-Behavioral Pediatrics*, 4th ed.; Carey, W.B., Crocker, A.C., Coleman, W.L., Elias, E.R., Feldman, H.M., Eds.; Saunders Elsevier: Philadelphia, PA, USA, 2009; pp. 911–922.

24. El-Sheikh, M.; Erath, S.; Buckhalt, J.; Granger, D.; Mize, J. Cortisol and children's adjustment: The moderating role of sympathetic nervous system activity. *J. Abnorm. Child Psychol.* **2008**, *36*, 601–611. [CrossRef] [PubMed]

25. Bauer, A.M.; Quas, J.A.; Boyce, W.T. Associations between physiological reactivity and children's behavior: Advantages of a multisystem approach. *J. Dev. Behav. Pediatr.* **2002**, *23*, 102–113. [CrossRef] [PubMed]

26. Wyller, V.B.; Eriksen, H.R.; Malterud, K. Can sustained arousal explain the Chronic Fatigue Syndrome? *Behav. Brain Funct.* **2009**, *5*, 10. [CrossRef] [PubMed]

27. Shonkoff, J.P.; Garner, A.; Siegel, B.; Dobbins, M.; Earls, M.; McGuinn, L.; Pascoe, J.; Wood, D. The lifelong effects of early childhood adversity and toxic stress. *Pediatrics* **2012**, *129*, e232–e246. [CrossRef] [PubMed]

28. Mathews, H.L.; Janusek, L.W. Epigenetics and psychoneuroimmunology: Mechanisms and models. *Brain Behav. Immun.* **2011**, *25*, 25–39. [CrossRef] [PubMed]

29. Zannas, A.S.; West, A.E. Epigenetics and the regulation of stress vulnerability and resilience. *Neuroscience* **2014**, *264*, 157–170. [CrossRef] [PubMed]

30. Birdee, G.S.; Yeh, G.Y.; Wayne, P.M.; Phillips, R.S.; Davis, R.B.; Gardiner, P. Clinical applications of yoga for the pediatric population: A systematic review. *Acad. Pediatr.* **2009**, *9*, 212–220. [CrossRef] [PubMed]

31. Black, D.S.; Milam, J.; Sussman, S. Sitting-meditation interventions among youth: A review of treatment efficacy. *Pediatrics* **2009**, *124*, e532–e541. [CrossRef] [PubMed]

32. Rosen, L.; French, A.; Sullivan, G. Complementary, Holistic, and Integrative Medicine: Yoga. *Pediatr. Rev./Am. Acad. Pediatr.* **2015**, *36*, 468. [CrossRef] [PubMed]

33. Barnes, A.J. Childhood Stress and Resilience. In *Health Promotion for Children and Adolescents*; Springer: New York, NY, USA, 2016; pp. 85–98.

34. AAP Council on Communications and Media. Media and young minds. *Pediatrics* **2016**, *138*, e20162591.

35. Buchman, D.D.; Funk, J.B. Video and computer games in the 90s: Children's time commitment and game preference. *Child. Today* **1996**, *24*, 12. [PubMed]

36. Gentile, D.A.; Walsh, D.A. A normative study of family media habits. *J. Appl. Dev. Psychol.* **2002**, *23*, 157–178. [CrossRef]

37. Loftus, G.R.; Loftus, E.F. *Mind at Play; The Psychology of Video Games*; Basic Books, Inc.: New York, NY, USA, 1983.

38. National Center for Telehealth and Technology. Available online: www.t2health.dcoe.mil/apps/breathe2relax.com (accessed on 21 January 2017).

39. Stressed Teens. Available online: www.stressedteens.com (accessed on 21 January 2017).

40. Stop, Breathe and Think App. Available online: www.stopbreathethink.org (accessed on 21 January 2017).

41. Smiling Mind. Available online: www.smilingmind.com.au (accessed on 21 January 2017).

42. The Adventures of Super Stretch. Available online: www.adventuresofsuperstretch.com (accessed on 21 January 2017).

43. Let It Go Yoga. Available online: www.letitgoyoga.com/yoga-by-teens/ (accessed on 21 January 2017).

44. Kids Yogaverse. Available online: www.kidsyogaverse.com (accessed on 21 January 2017).

45. Me Moves. Available online: www.thinkingmoves.com (accessed on 21 January 2017).

46. Mindfield Biosystems. Available online: www.mindfield.de (accessed on 21 January 2017).

47. Life Matters. Available online: www.lifematters.com/biofeedback-machines.asp (accessed on 21 January 2017).
48. Kirsch, D.L.; Nichols, F. Cranial electrotherapy stimulation for treatment of anxiety, depression, and insomnia. *Psychiatr. Clin. N. Am.* **2013**, *36*, 169–176. [CrossRef] [PubMed]
49. Kirsch, D.L.; Smith, R.B. The use of cranial electrotherapy stimulation in the management of chronic pain: A review. *NeuroRehabilitation* **2000**, *14*, 85–94. [PubMed]
50. Gilula, M.F.; Kirsch, D.L. Cranial electrotherapy stimulation review: A safer alternative to psychopharmaceuticals in the treatment of depression. *J. Neurother.* **2005**, *9*, 7–26. [CrossRef]
51. Alpha-Stim. Available online: www.alpha-stim.com (accessed on 21 January 2017).
52. Siever, D. Applying audio-visual entrainment technology for attention and learning. *Biofeedback Mag.* **2008**, *31*, 1–15.
53. Huang, T.L.; Charyton, C. A comprehensive review of the psychological effects of brainwave entrainment. *Altern. Ther. Health Med.* **2008**, *14*, 38. [PubMed]
54. Boersma, F.J.; Gagnon, C. The use of repetitive audiovisual entrainment in the management of chronic pain. *Med. Hypnoanal. J.* **1992**, *7*, 80–97.
55. Clancy, J.A.; Mary, D.; White, K.; Greenwood, J.; Deuchars, S.; Deuchars, J. Non-invasive vagus nerve stimulation in healthy humans reduces sympathetic nerve activity. *Brain Stimul.* **2014**, *7*, 871–877. [CrossRef] [PubMed]
56. George, M.S.; Sackeim, H.; Rush, J.; Marangell, L.; Nahas, Z.; Husain, M.; Lisanby, S.; Burt, T.; Goldman, J.; Ballenger, J. Vagus nerve stimulation: A new tool for brain research and therapy. *Biol. Psychiatry* **2000**, *47*, 287–295. [CrossRef]
57. Wild Divine. Available online: www.wilddivine.com (accessed on 21 January 2017).

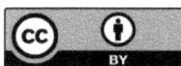

Review

A Mind–Body Approach to Pediatric Pain Management

Melanie L. Brown [1,2,*], Enrique Rojas [1] and Suzanne Gouda [1]

[1] Department of Pediatrics, The University of Chicago, Chicago, IL 60637, USA
erojas@peds.bsd.uchicago.edu (E.R.); Suzanne.Gouda@uchospitals.edu (S.G.)
[2] Department of Pain, Palliative Care and Integrative Medicine, Children's Hospitals and Clinics of Minnesota,
Minneapolis, MN 55404, USA
* Correspondence: melanie.brown@childrensmn.org

Academic Editor: Hilary McClafferty
Received: 1 March 2017; Accepted: 13 June 2017; Published: 20 June 2017

Abstract: Pain is a significant public health problem that affects all populations and has significant
financial, physical and psychological impact. Opioid medications, once the mainstay of pain therapy
across the spectrum, can be associated with significant morbidity and mortality. Centers for Disease
and Control (CDC) guidelines recommend that non-opioid pain medications are preferred for chronic
pain outside of certain indications (cancer, palliative and end of life care). Mindfulness, hypnosis,
acupuncture and yoga are four examples of mind–body techniques that are often used in the adult
population for pain and symptom management. In addition to providing significant pain relief,
several studies have reported reduced use of opioid medications when mind–body therapies are
implemented. Mind–body medicine is another approach that can be used in children with both acute
and chronic pain to improve pain management and quality of life.

Keywords: mind–body medicine; pain management; pediatrics; acupuncture; yoga; meditation; hypnosis

1. Introduction

Pain is a significant public health problem leading to lost days of school and increased use of
the healthcare system. Pain affects all populations and can significantly impact quality of life [1].
Over 11 million children have special health care needs and about 60% of them have difficulty
participating in any activity [2]. In one cross-sectional study of pain prevalence in a pediatric hospital,
the authors found that out of 241 patients, 27% had pain at the time of admission and 77% experienced
pain at some point during their admission; what is more, pain medication was found to be single-agent
and administered irregularly [3].

In recent years, opioid diversion, as well as the overuse and over prescription of opioid
medications, have come to the forefront as a significant public health concern. Integrative medicine uses
a patient centered approach to combine conventional medicine with evidence-based complementary
approaches. Integrative therapies such as mind–body medicine can provide a non-opioid and
nontoxic approach to pain management across the spectrum. Even in the case of end-of-life care [4,5],
integrative and mind–body therapies are recommended [4,5]. For example, the Hospice and Palliative
Nurses Association's most recent position statement supports and encourages the competent practice
of complementary therapies for the purpose of promoting holistic end-of-life-care.

2. The Problem

2.1. What Is Pain

Pain can be defined as an unpleasant sensation. In some cases, pain is a warning sign of actual or potential tissue damage. However, dysregulation of the nervous system can also lead to a pain sensation when there is no present danger [6,7]. In addition to the physical sensation, pain behaviors are also influenced by pain perception. In a recent randomized control trial, pain sensitivity was assessed in over 700 adult patients with major depression. It was found that those suffering from major depression had higher pain sensitivity even after adjusting for factors such as poor sleep and physical inactivity [8]. Severity of anxiety also predicted decreased pain threshold.

Chronic pain is known to be associated with changes in not only brain function, but also in brain structure. In 2013, researchers demonstrated that the brain areas that were activated in acute low back pain for example were limited to regions involving acute pain; in the chronic pain group, activity was found in the emotion-related circuitry of the brain [9].

Pain perception and experience in the pediatric population is complex and multi-faceted, including but not limited to the nidus of pain itself, the fear of pain, previously developed pain memories, and familial influence. Acute pain is usually classified as pain lasting less than three months with a sudden onset that is often related to tissue damage. When considering the development of chronic pain in pediatrics, typically defined as pain persisting beyond three months or beyond the expected duration of healing, a fear-avoidance response can emerge, leading to a self-fulfilling cycle made up of pain, emotional distress, and functional disability [10]. In pediatrics, there is also an added complexity when considering developmental stage and parental influence. Not only do parents often have to serve as the surrogate communicator for the patient, parents own magnification, rumination, and anxiety surrounding pain influences the child and vice versa, leading to increased pain sensitivity and fear-avoidance behaviors [11]. It is clear that pain is not as simple as a noxious stimulus to an extremity that sends a danger signal to the brain.

2.2. The Opioid Crisis

Increases in opioid prescriptions have been noted over the past decade [12–14]. The opioid overdose and death rates have also been noted to increase [15–20]. 2016 Centers for Disease and Control (CDC) guidelines state that that non-opioid therapy is preferred for chronic pain outside of active cancer, palliative and end-of-life care in patients over the age of 18 years. Inappropriate medication use and dosing can lead to death and disability [15–20]. At times, significant morbidity can result even when recommended dosage ranges are used [15–20]. For example, deaths have been described with the use of codeine despite dosages prescribed in the recommended range. In the case of codeine, the prodrug must be converted into morphine in the liver via the cytochrome P450 2D6 system and drug over or under conversion may be the result of genetic variation [21]. Furthermore, tolerance, withdrawal, and dependence present a problem even in the pediatric population and the neuropsychological effects of opioids may also be a cause for concern [22–25]. Opioid medications can play an important role in the treatment of pain; however, a pain management plan is not complete without including mind–body therapies.

2.3. Pain in Pediatrics

In pediatrics, pain, both acute and chronic, is often under-recognized and under-treated [26]. Studies have shown that up to 40% of children experience pain at least weekly, and conservative estimates say chronic pain affects 20% to 35% of children and adolescents around the globe [27]. Despite this significant prevalence, pain often goes under-addressed. A large-scale study involving eight pediatric hospitals observed inadequate pain assessment and management for patients undergoing painful procedures, reporting that less than one-third of patients had documentation of one or more pain management interventions [28]. When pain becomes chronic, significant physical and psychological tolls are experienced by both the patient and their families. Often the pain itself continues into adulthood, with 17% of adult chronic pain patients reporting a history of chronic pain in childhood/adolescence [29]. In addition, patients with chronic pain are at increased risk for several comorbidities, including many psychiatric disorders, hyperactivity disorders, social disability, and educational/occupational disability [10]. This patient population also has increased use of medical services, with healthcare costs for children with moderate to severe chronic pain averaging 19.5 billion annually [30]. Despite approximately 1.7 million children affected by chronic pain in the US alone with approximately 20% of cases having developed from acute post-operative pain, assessment and management of pain in pediatrics continues to be a challenge [26,31]. Mind–body medicine can provide a different approach. The mind–body approach is one in which the strengths of the patient and family are considered. In addition, this approach focuses on designing a treatment plan that is efficacious and minimizes the need for opioid medications. Mind–body remains a relatively novel approach in medicine. Although most of the current literature focuses on adult populations and on the more conventional psychological therapies (e.g.; cognitive behavioral therapy and dialectical behavioral therapy) that share similar inherent characteristics with mind–body approaches [32–34], there is a growing body of evidence that supports other mind–body therapies as effective and practical treatment approaches in pediatrics [35–39], particularly in the symptomatic treatment of cancer [4,40–45].

3. The Mind–Body Approach to Pain

3.1. The Use of Mind–Body Medicine in Pain Management

The American Academy of Pediatrics' clinical report on Mind–Body Therapies in Children and Youth describes mind–body therapies as those that focus on the interaction between the mind and the body, with the intent to use the mind to influence physical functions and directly affect health [46]. Mind–body therapies show promise as adjunct and at times primary treatment for pain in children and adults, and can be used across the spectrum. For example, diaphragmatic breathing stimulates the vagus nerve and promotes the relaxation response. The vagus nerve, an essential component of the autonomic nervous system, affects many of the body's internal organs including: the heart, lungs, liver, spleen, kidneys and gastrointestinal tract. As with many therapies, a development-based approach is essential. Teens can use complex imagery, while younger children can be taught diaphragmatic breathing techniques with simple imagery, such as blowing a balloon or blowing out candles. A toddler can be encouraged to engage in diaphragmatic breathing with the use of bubbles or pin wheels. For infants or children with severe cognitive disabilities, rocking and rhythmic womb or heartbeat sounds are techniques that can encourage diaphragmatic breathing.

These techniques are well tolerated in children [36,44,47,48] and can be used in a developmentally appropriate manner to serve as adjunct or primary pain management [47,48]. Furthermore, a reduction in opioid use may be seen. One study demonstrated a greater than 60% reduction of opioid-like medication usage following routine surgery when acupuncture was used [49–51]. Although more research is needed in the pediatric population, given the low risk and low cost of many of these techniques [52–54] for patients and potentially for insurance companies as well, their use is encouraged to enhance symptom management whenever feasible. In the next section, we give an overview of selected mind–body therapies and their function and applications in the management of pain in the pediatric population.

3.2. Selected Mind–Body Approaches

3.2.1. Meditation and Mindfulness

Over the past few decades, mindfulness has emerged as a fundamental component of numerous therapies and interventions for a wide spectrum of clinical aliments [55]. Mindfulness, described as "the awareness that emerges through paying attention on purpose, in the present moment, and non-judgmentally to the unfolding of experience moment by moment", is a meditation practice with ancient Buddhist origins that focuses on experiencing the present moment unobstructed by bias or judgmental thinking in an effort to improve cognitive and emotional well-being [56]. One such application of mindfulness is Kabat Zinn's Mindfulness-Based Stress Reduction (MBSR), a group intervention first introduced in 1990 that focuses on mindfulness meditation training as a complimentary therapy to the standard medical treatment of chronic pain and illness [57–64]. Research has suggested that mindfulness can improve symptoms associated with medical illnesses and increase quality of life [65]. From a neuroscientific perspective, magnetic resonance imaging (MRI) and functional magnetic resonance imaging (fMRI) studies have been conducted in hopes of identifying the neural mechanisms that are responsible for the efficacy of mindfulness meditation in pain relief [66–73]. In one study, thirteen skilled Zen mediators, each having had a minimum of 1000 hours of meditation experience, were recruited and experimentally exposed to pain via thermal stimuli while in an MRI [70]. During exposure to pain, the meditators exhibited increased brain activation in the insula, thalamus, and midcingulate cortex; areas associated with the sensory aspect of pain. Additionally, decreases in brain activity were observed within the hippocampus, amygdala, and caudate; areas responsible for the recollection, emotion, and appraisal components of pain, respectively. The authors concluded that the participants were completely aware of the sensation of pain but were able to inhibit the appraisal and emotional responses of pain. In other words, changes in the perception of pain were facilitated through the cognitive and affective components of the pain matrix rather than through the sensory properties of pain. Furthermore, the differences in brain activity were found to be inversely proportional to meditation skill level, establishing a correlation that supports the authors' hypothesis in regards to meditation's therapeutic effect on pain. As for neurophysiological findings, structural MRI results overlapped with the fMRI results: meditators were found to have thicker grey-matter in the same pain-related regions of the brain where changes in functional activity were observed [66,68,69].

In terms of overall clinical outcome research, controlled trials of adults suffering from various forms of chronic pain (chronic low back pain, chronic headache/migraine, chronic neck pain, arthritis, cancer, and fibromyalgia) have indeed demonstrated improved pain ratings in regards to multiple dimensions of pain including intensity, acceptance, functional limitations, quality of life, and psychological well-being [62]. Nonetheless, mindfulness as it relates to pain in children has not been extensively studied and although mindfulness meditation has shown to be beneficial in classroom and school settings for improving psychological distress [74–77], more research is required in order to determine whether the same effects can be translated in children and pediatric medicine.

3.2.2. Hypnosis

Hypnosis as a form of therapy has a long history and has been widely used across various disciplines of health care. While the current research establishes hypnosis as a beneficial treatment for the management of pain in regards to both acute medical conditions, such as trauma and post-operative care, and chronic medical conditions, such as cancer and sickle cell anemia [78–80]; it is only since the 1980s that it has been meaningfully applied to pediatric care [81,82].

In general, hypnosis includes three phases: induction, suggestion, and emergence [82]. During induction, the provider encourages patient relaxation by asking them to imagine a calm and serene setting on which they can focus all of their attention. Next, the patient is given therapeutic suggestions to achieve the desired effect. Lastly, the patient is asked to leave their imagined setting and to return to normal consciousness. Hypnosis for pain management follows this same protocol with a focus on suggestions that either turn down or decrease pain perception or increase pain thresholds [83].

Given the significance of the suggestion stage of hypnosis, an important factor in clinical outcomes is the degree to which an individual is responsive or susceptible to hypnotic suggestions—a trait that is often referred to as hypnotizability. Of note, studies that have attempted to measure hypnotizability among children via the Children's Hypnotic Susceptibility Scale and the Stanford Hypnotic Scale for Children have shown a positive correlation between hypnotizability [84,85] and age, thus suggesting that hypnosis may be an especially viable form of therapy for pain management in the pediatric population [82].

Taking a neuroscientific approach, neuro-imaging studies have attempted to measure the effects of hypnosis on the neuroanatomy and the neuro-cognitive functions of the brain in the context of pain [85–88]. In other words, many researchers have set out to investigate how hypnosis affects the brain's neural-networks and physiology that in turn, are responsible for the perception of pain within an individual. This "pain matrix", as it has been described, is comprised of specific areas of the brain that collectively produce the experience of pain. In the simplest summary of the current literature, the components of the pain matrix include: the prefrontal cortex, frontal lobes, anterior cingulate cortex, primary and secondary somatosensory cortices, thalamus and insula. The cerebellum, though not technically a component of the pain matrix, also plays a role. Using fMRIs to measure brain activity during hypnosis, researchers have concluded that by influencing activity in the various components of the pain matrix, hypnosis is indeed able to have a collective therapeutic effect on pain.

Research focusing on clinical and experimental outcomes has also yielded positive results. A meta-analysis performed in 2000 of 18 studies found hypnosis to have a moderate to large analgesic effect [78]. When compared to groups receiving standard treatment and groups receiving no treatment, 75% of participants receiving hypnotic suggestion experienced a greater analgesic effect. Furthermore, the effect was seen with both clinical and experimental pain with no significant difference between the two settings.

Hypnosis is a tool that carries minimal risk when used appropriately for pain management. It can be used by patients as well as practitioners. The goal is often to instruct the patient on the hypnotic technique so that hypnosis will become a tool of empowerment that the patient is able to use themselves at appropriate times for symptom management. It is important to note that hypnosis should only be performed by an appropriately trained practitioner and only to treat conditions that the practitioner is competent to treat.

3.2.3. Yoga

Yoga is another mind–body modality that should be considered in the management of pain. In brief, the ancient practice of yoga aims to unite the mind, body, and spirit through different isometric exercises, body poses, and mindful breathing. The goal is to optimize body functioning and reconditioning, skeletal realignment, and blood/lymph flow to the tissues [89]. Beyond the biophysical benefits, yoga is also inexpensive, can be practiced by people of any age and physical skill level, and can be performed almost anywhere. The side effects are minimal, with the most common being musculoskeletal injury, often resulting from inappropriate supervision and/or technique [90].

Growing research has shown yoga to be an effective therapy for chronic pain among adults, but studies remain limited for the pediatric population [91]. In a 2006 meta-analysis, when yoga was incorporated into school curricula, improvements in academic performance, behavior, concentration, emotional balance, and self-esteem were all seen [92]. Regular practice of yoga has been associated with improvement in mood and function in patients suffering from depression [93].

These same techniques can be of great benefit in the management of chronic pain in particular. One pilot study of a yoga program in pediatric patients with Irritable Bowel Syndrome (IBS) and functional abdominal pain, demonstrated significant decreases in pain frequency and intensity, as well as improved quality of life per parents report [94]. A study of 30 children, aged 11–18, with amplified pain syndromes enrolled in an intensive interdisciplinary pain rehabilitation program incorporating 5–6 h of yoga weekly demonstrated improved pain and functioning without the use of pharmacology therapy [95]. Positive effects have also been shown in pediatric patients with rheumatoid arthritis [96]. Current evidence is encouraging, but more large-scale research is still needed to determine the efficacy of yoga in the treatment of pediatric chronic pain [39].

3.2.4. Acupuncture

Acupuncture has been a focus of Traditional Chinese Medicine (TCM) for thousands of years and since its introduction into western medicine, it has become one of the most popular complementary and alternative medical (CAM) therapies in the US [97]. First acknowledged as a medical therapy by the National Institute of Health (NIH) in 1997, the number of licensed acupuncturists in the US has grown exponentially over the decades with over 27,000 licensed acupuncturists in 2013—a one hundred percent increase from 2000—and an estimated one million annual American consumers. In 2001, Battlefield Acupuncture, an auricular acupuncture procedure, was developed by Richard Niemtzow as a simple and effective method for rapid pain relief that can be performed with minimal training by non-licensed acupuncturists [98–100]. Since then, it has since been utilized in emergency rooms and has been taught to US military and North Atlantic Treaty Organization (NATO) personnel for use in both medical and battlefield environments [99,101].

Research into the efficacy of the therapy has also increased over the years with many studies demonstrating acupuncture to be more effective at treating chronic pain than placebo, standard care, and no care [102–112]. Acupuncture is a viable alternative for the treatment and management of acute and chronic pain across various illnesses [22,103,113–115]. One overview of Cochrane reviews concluded that acupuncture demonstrates effectiveness as a treatment for pain associated with migraines, tension headaches, neck disorders, arthritis, and low back pain [104].

Research studies aiming at understanding the physiological and neurological mechanisms that make acupuncture an effective therapy have produced interesting results that have served as the basis for several potential hypotheses [107,116–129]. Many researchers believe that acupuncture stimulates nerves and muscles located within the acupuncture points and trigger a release of neurochemicals endorphins such as serotonin, oxytocin, and endogenous opioid peptides and therefore result in an analgesic effect [117,123,127]. However, while substantial research has shown acupuncture to be an effective therapy for pain among the adult population, there is limited research on acupuncture in regards to the treatment of pain among pediatric patients. Nonetheless, what little research does exist concludes that acupuncture is an effective and feasible therapy option for pain in pediatric populations [48,103,130–134]. One study in the pediatric intensive care unit (PICU) that used acupuncture for acute post-operative pain in children showed that acupuncture was highly accepted and well tolerated without morbidity. In addition, the majority (70%) of patients and families surveyed believed that acupuncture helped their pain. This particular study used the Japanese form of acupuncture with fine needles for older children and Shonishin (a non-needling technique using special tools) for those who were younger than two years of age [135]. A number of other articles have also shown some perceived pain relief without significant adverse effects due to acupuncture. [136,137]

Though acupuncture is safe when administered by appropriately trained and credentialed practitioners, there are some children who have a fear of needles or for medical reasons such as low platelet count or immunodeficiency that may not be recommended to receive acupuncture. For those patients, other techniques such as Shonishin or acupressure can be employed.

4. Discussion: H.O.P.E, A New Paradigm

The use of mind–body techniques in pediatrics can be a powerful adjunct to empower patients and their families and to give them hope for a brighter future with improved quality of life. In partnership with their physicians, families can begin to uncover what is in their tool box for pain and symptom management. One such framework developed by us is the pneumonic: H.O.P.E. We have used H.O.P.E. with success in clinical practice with families as a strategy for approaching pain management. H.O.P.E. addresses four essential components in the evaluation of pain and of the treatment plan. It is described in more detail below.

- H: **How** has the pain affected you and impacted your quality of life? **How** have they addressed the pain in the past and what therapies have been used?

- O: **Observations** about previous management approaches. What have they **observed**? What worked and what did not? What makes the pain perception worse?
- P: **Plan** for the future, set goals and determine the treatment plan.
- E: **Evaluate** the **efficacy** of the plan and manage **expectations.**

In addition to understanding what pharmacologic, non-pharmacological and integrative options are available; it is also important for all parties involved to discuss goals of care. In fully unpacking the child and family's needs, appropriate recommendations for pain management can be made. Recommendations will be different based on the clinical condition and goals of care.

5. Conclusions

Mind–body medicine provides an important approach to the management of both acute and chronic pain in the pediatric population. There are many modalities that are underutilized in pediatrics including mindfulness, hypnosis, yoga and acupuncture. It is important to note that these can be of significant benefit with minimal risk. Mind–body approaches can be used alongside conventional treatment or in some cases as the primary treatment for pain. Though more research is needed; the mind–body approaches discussed are recommended for patients who have no underlying contraindications. As our understanding of pediatric pain and pain management continues to mature, mind–body medicine is an area that is ripe for future studies and investigations.

Acknowledgments: Special thank you to Brian Steiner for sharing the paper that he published in The Atlantic on treating chronic pain with meditation and for his input during the initial planning of this article.

Author Contributions: M.B. is primarily responsible for the conception and design of this article. M.B.; S.G. and E.R. drafted the text. All authors provided evaluation and revision of the manuscript and have given final approval of the manuscript.

Conflicts of Interest: M.B. is supported in part by the Coleman Foundation, the Oberweiler Foundation and the Patient-Centered Outcomes Research Institute (PCORI). E.R. is supported in part by PCORI. The funding sponsors had no role in the design of the article; in the collection, analysis, or interpretation of information; in the writing of the manuscript, or in the decision to publish.

References

1. Goldberg, D.S.; McGee, S.J. Pain as a global public health priority. *BMC Public Health* **2011**, *11*, 770. [CrossRef] [PubMed]
2. National Hospice and Palliative Care Organisation. *NHPCO's Facts and Figures: Hospice Care in America*; National Hospice and Palliative Care Organization: Alexandria, VA, USA, 2015.
3. Taylor, E.M.; Boyer, K.; Campbell, F.A. Pain in hospitalized children: A prospective cross-sectional survey of pain prevalence, intensity, assessment and management in a Canadian pediatric teaching hospital. *Pain Res. Manag.* **2008**, *13*, 25–32. [CrossRef] [PubMed]
4. Carlson, L.E.; Bultz, B.D. Mind-body interventions in oncology. *Curr. Treat. Options Oncol.* **2008**, *9*, 127–134. [CrossRef] [PubMed]
5. Lafferty, W.E.; Downey, L.; McCarty, R.L.; Standish, L.J.; Patrick, D.L. Evaluating CAM treatment at the end of life: A review of clinical trials for massage and meditation. *Complement. Ther. Med.* **2006**, *14*, 100–102. [CrossRef] [PubMed]
6. Elvey, R.L. Physical evaluation of the peripheral nervous system in disorders of pain and dysfunction. *J. Hand Ther.* **1997**, *10*, 122–129. [CrossRef]
7. Woolf, C.J. What is this thing called pain? *J. Clin. Invest.* **2010**, *120*, 3742–3744. [CrossRef] [PubMed]
8. Hermesdorf, M.; Berger, K.; Baune, B.T.; Wellmann, J.; Ruscheweyh, R.; Wersching, H. Pain Sensitivity in Patients With Major Depression: Differential Effect of Pain Sensitivity Measures, Somatic Cofactors, and Disease Characteristics. *J. Pain* **2016**, *17*, 606–616. [CrossRef] [PubMed]
9. Hashmi, J.A.; Baliki, M.N.; Huang, L.; Baria, A.T.; Torbey, S.; Hermann, K.M.; Schnitzer, T.J.; Apkarian, A.V. Shape shifting pain: Chronification of back pain shifts brain representation from nociceptive to emotional circuits. *Brain* **2013**, *136*, 2751–2768. [CrossRef] [PubMed]

10. Asmundson, G.J.; Noel, M.; Petter, M.; Parkerson, H.A. Pediatric fear-avoidance model of chronic pain: Foundation, application and future directions. *Pain Res. Manag.* **2012**, *17*, 397–405. [CrossRef] [PubMed]
11. Friedrichsdorf, S.; Giordano, J.; Dakoji, K.D.; Warmuth, A.; Daughtry, C.; Schulz, C. Chronic Pain in Children and Adolescents: Diagnosis and Treatment of Primary Pain Disorders in Head, Abdomen, Muscles and Joints. *Children* **2016**, *3*, 42. [CrossRef] [PubMed]
12. Dunn, K.M. Opioid prescriptions for chronic pain and overdose: A cohort study. *Ann. Intern. Med.* **2010**, *152*, 85–92. [CrossRef] [PubMed]
13. Kuehn, B.M. Opioid prescriptions soar: Increase in legitimate use as well as abuse. *JAMA* **2007**, *297*, 249–251. [CrossRef] [PubMed]
14. Volkow, N.D.; McLellan, T.A. Characteristics of opioid prescriptions in 2009. *JAMA* **2011**, *305*, 1299–1301. [CrossRef] [PubMed]
15. Bohnert, A.S.; Valenstein, M.; Bair, M.J.; Ganoczy, D.; McCarthy, J.F.; Ilgen, M.A.; Blow, F.C. Association between opioid prescribing patterns and opioid overdose-related deaths. *JAMA* **2011**, *305*, 1315–1321. [CrossRef] [PubMed]
16. McLellan, A.; Turner, B. Prescription opioids, overdose deaths, and physician responsibility. *JAMA* **2008**, *300*, 2672–2673. [CrossRef] [PubMed]
17. International Association for the Study of Pain: Unrelieved Pain Is a Major Global Healthcare Problem. Available online: http://www.iasp-pain.org/AM/Template.cfm?Section=Home&Template=/CM/ContentDisplay.cfm&ContentID=2908 (accessed on 20 June 2017).
18. Okie, S. A flood of opioids, a rising tide of deaths. *N. Engl. J. Med.* **2010**, *363*, 1981–1985. [CrossRef] [PubMed]
19. Dhalla, I.A.; Mamdani, M.M.; Sivilotti, M.L.A.; Kopp, A.; Qureshi, O.; Juurlink, D.N. Prescribing of opioid analgesics and related mortality before and after the introduction of long-acting oxycodone. *CMAJ* **2009**, *181*, 891–896. [CrossRef] [PubMed]
20. Manchikanti, L.; Damron, K.S.; Pampati, V.; Fellows, B. Increasing deaths from opioid analgesics in the United States: An evaluation in an interventional pain management practice. *J. Opioid Manag.* **2008**, *4*, 271–283. [PubMed]
21. Friedrichsdorf, S.J.; Nugent, A.P.; Strobl, A.Q. Codeine-associated pediatric deaths despite using recommended dosing guidelines: Three case reports. *J. Opioid Manag.* **2013**, *9*, 151–155. [CrossRef] [PubMed]
22. Anand, K.J.; Arnold, J.H. Opioid tolerance and dependence in infants and children. *Crit. Care Med.* **1994**, *22*, 334–342. [CrossRef] [PubMed]
23. Anand, K.J.S.; Willson, D.F.; Berger, J.; Harrison, R.; Meert, K.L.; Zimmerman, J.; Carcillo, J.; Newth, C.J.L.; Prodhan, N.P.; Dean, J.M.; et al. Tolerance and withdrawal from prolonged opioid use in critically ill children. *Pediatrics* **2010**, *125*, 1208–1225. [CrossRef] [PubMed]
24. Yaster, M.; Kost-Byerly, S.; Berde, C.; Billet, C. The management of opioid and benzodiazepine dependence in infants, children, and adolescents. *Pediatrics* **1996**, *98*, 135–140. [PubMed]
25. Jain, G.; Mahendra, V.; Singhal, S.; Dzara, K.; Pilla, T.; Manworren, R. Long-term neuropsychological effects of opioid use in children: A descriptive literature review. *Pain Physician* **2014**, *17*, 109–118. [CrossRef] [PubMed]
26. Mathews, L. Pain in children: Neglected, unaddressed and mismanaged. *Indian J. Palliat. Care* **2011**, *17*, S70–S73. [CrossRef] [PubMed]
27. King, S.; Chambers, C.T.; Huguet, A.; MacNevin, R.C.; McGrath, P.J.; Parker, L.; MacDonald, A.J. The epidemiology of chronic pain in children and adolescents revisited: A systematic review. *Pain* **2011**, *152*, 2729–2738. [CrossRef] [PubMed]
28. Stevens, B.J.; Abbott, L.K.; Yamada, J.; Harrison, D.; Stinson, J.; Taddio, A.; Barwick, M.; Latimer, M.; Scott, SD.; Rashotte, J.; et al. Epidemiology and management of painful procedures in children in Canadian hospitals. *CMAJ* **2011**, *183*, 403–410. [CrossRef] [PubMed]
29. Hassett, A.L.; Hilliard, P.E.; Goesling, J.; Clauw, D.J.; Harte, S.E.; Brummett, C.M. Reports of chronic pain in childhood and adolescence among patients at a tertiary care pain clinic. *J. Pain* **2013**, *14*, 1390–1397. [CrossRef] [PubMed]
30. Groenewald, C.B.; Essner, B.S.; Wright, D.; Fesinmeyer, M.D.; Palermo, T.M. The economic costs of chronic pain among a cohort of treatment-seeking adolescents in the United States. *J. Pain* **2014**, *15*, 925–933. [CrossRef] [PubMed]

31. Simons, L.E.; Smith, A.; Ibagon, C.; Coakley, R.; Logan, D.E.; Schechter, N.; Borsook, D.; Hill, J.C. Pediatric Pain Screening Tool: Rapid identification of risk in youth with pain complaints. *Pain* **2015**, *156*, 1511–1518. [CrossRef] [PubMed]

32. Robins, C.J. Zen principles and mindfulness practice in dialectical behavior therapy. *Cogn. Behav. Pract.* **2002**, *9*, 50–57. [CrossRef]

33. McCracken, L.M.; Gauntlett-Gilbert, J.; Vowles, K.E. The role of mindfulness in a contextual cognitive-behavioral analysis of chronic pain-related suffering and disability. *Pain* **2007**, *131*, 63–69. [CrossRef] [PubMed]

34. Morgan, D. Mindfulness-based cognitive therapy for depression: A new approach to preventing relapse. *Psychother. Res.* **2003**, *13*, 123–125. [CrossRef] [PubMed]

35. Ball, T.M.; Shapiro, D.E.; Monheim, C.J.; Weydert, J.A. A pilot study of the use of guided imagery for the treatment of recurrent abdominal pain in children. *Clin. Pediatr.* **2003**, *42*, 527–532. [CrossRef] [PubMed]

36. Burke, C.A. Mindfulness-Based Approaches with Children and Adolescents: A Preliminary Review of Current Research in an Emergent Field. *J. Child. Fam. Stud.* **2009**, *19*, 133–144. [CrossRef]

37. Barnes, P.M.; Bloom, B.; Nahin, R.L. Complementary and alternative medicine use among adults and children: United States, 2007. *Natl. Health Stat. Rep.* **2008**, *10*, 1–23.

38. Gerik, S.M. Pain management in children: Developmental considerations and mind-body therapies. *South. Med. J.* **2005**, *98*, 295–302. [CrossRef] [PubMed]

39. Galantino, M.L.; Galbavy, R.; Quinn, L. Therapeutic effects of yoga for children: A systematic review of the literature. *Pediatr. Phys. Ther.* **2008**, *20*, 66–80. [CrossRef] [PubMed]

40. Post-White, J.; Hawks, R.G. Complementary and Alternative Medicine in Pediatric Oncology. *Semin. Oncol. Nurs.* **2005**, *21*, 107–114. [CrossRef] [PubMed]

41. Zeltzer, L.; LeBaron, S. Hypnosis and nonhypnotic techniques for reduction of pain and anxiety during painful procedures in children and adolescents with cancer. *J. Pediatr.* **1982**, *101*, 1032–1035. [PubMed]

42. Kelly, K.M. Complementary and alternative medical therapies for children with cancer. *Eur. J. Cancer* **2004**, *40*, 2041–2046. [CrossRef] [PubMed]

43. Laengler, A.; Spix, C.; Seifert, G.; Gottschling, S.; Graf, N.; Kaatsch, P. Complementary and alternative treatment methods in children with cancer: A population-based retrospective survey on the prevalence of use in Germany. *Eur. J. Cancer* **2008**, *44*, 2233–2240. [CrossRef] [PubMed]

44. Molassiotis, A.; Cubbin, D. 'Thinking outside the box': Complementary and alternative therapies use in paediatric oncology patients. *Eur. J. Oncol. Nurs.* **2004**, *8*, 50–60. [CrossRef]

45. Favara-Scacco, C.; Smirne, G.; Schilirò, G.; Cataldo, A.D. Art therapy as support for children with leukemia during painful procedures. *Med. Pediatr. Oncol.* **2001**, *36*, 474–480. [CrossRef] [PubMed]

46. Section On Integrative Medicine. Mind-Body Therapies in Children and Youth. *Pediatrics* **2016**, *138*, e20161896.

47. Lee, A.A.; Renee, L. Treatment of children in an acupuncture setting: A survey of clinical observations. *J. Chin. Med.* **2006**, *82*, 21–27.

48. Jindal, V.; Ge, A.; Mansky, P.J. Safety and efficacy of acupuncture in children: A review of the evidence. *J. Pediatr. Hematol. Oncol.* **2008**, *30*, 431–442. [CrossRef] [PubMed]

49. Lin, J.; Lo, M.; Wen, Y.; Hsieh, C.; Tsai, S.; Sun, W. The effect of high and low frequency electroacupuncture in pain after lower abdominal surgery. *Pain* **2002**, *99*, 509–514. [CrossRef]

50. Wang, B.; Tang, J.; White, P.F.; Naruse, R.; Sloninsky, A.; Kariger, R.; Gold, J.; Wender, R.H. Effect of the intensity of transcutaneous acupoint electrical stimulation on the postoperative analgesic requirement. *Anesth. Analg.* **1997**, *85*, 406–413. [CrossRef] [PubMed]

51. Zheng, Z.; Guo, R.J.; Helme, R.D.; Muir, A.; Costa, C.; Xue, C.C. The effect of electroacupuncture on opioid-like medication consumption by chronic pain patients: A pilot randomized controlled clinical trial. *Eur. J. Pain* **2008**, *12*, 671–676. [CrossRef] [PubMed]

52. Friedman, R.; Sobel, D.; Myers, P.; Caudill, M.; Al, E. Behavioral medicine, clinical health psychology, and cost offset. *Health Psychol.* **1995**, *14*, 509–518. [CrossRef] [PubMed]

53. Sobel, D.S. The cost-effectiveness of mind-body medicine interventions. *Prog. Brain Res.* **2000**, *122*, 393–412. [PubMed]

54. Sobel, D.S. MSJAMA: Mind matters, money matters: The cost-effectiveness of mind/body medicine. *JAMA* **2000**, *284*, 1705. [CrossRef] [PubMed]

55. Ludwig, D.S.; Kabat-Zinn, J. Mindfulness in medicine. *JAMA* **2008**, *300*, 1350–1352. [CrossRef] [PubMed]
56. Thera, N. *The Heart of Buddhist Meditation*; Rider Co.: London, UK, 1962.
57. Grossman, P.; Niemann, L.; Schmidt, S.; Walach, H. Mindfulness-based stress reduction and health benefits. *J. Psychosom. Res.* **2004**, *57*, 35–43. [CrossRef]
58. Miller, J.J.; Fletcher, K.; Kabat-Zinn, J. Three-year follow-up and clinical implications of a mindfulness meditation-based stress reduction intervention in the treatment of anxiety disorders. *Gen. Hosp. Psychiatry* **1995**, *17*, 192–200. [CrossRef]
59. Kabat-Zinn, J.; Lipworth, L.; Burney, R. The clinical use of mindfulness meditation for the self-regulation of chronic pain. *J. Behav. Med.* **1985**, *8*, 163–190. [CrossRef] [PubMed]
60. Morone, N.E.; Greco, C.M.; Weiner, D.K. Mindfulness meditation for the treatment of chronic low back pain in older adults: A randomized controlled pilot study. *Pain* **2008**, *134*, 310–319. [CrossRef] [PubMed]
61. Kabat-Zinn, J. An outpatient program in behavioral medicine for chronic pain patients based on the practice of mindfulness meditation: Theoretical considerations and preliminary results. *Gen. Hosp. Psychiatry* **1982**, *4*, 33–47. [CrossRef]
62. Rosenzweig, S.; Greeson, J.M.; Reibel, D.K.; Green, J.S.; Jasser, S.A.; Beasley, D. Mindfulness-based stress reduction for chronic pain conditions: Variation in treatment outcomes and role of home meditation practice. *J. Psychosom. Res.* **2010**, *68*, 29–36. [CrossRef] [PubMed]
63. Kabat-Zinn, J.; Massion, A.O.; Kristeller, J.; Peterson, L.G.; Fletcher, K.E.; Pbert, L.; Lenderking, W.R.; Santorelli, S.F. Effectiveness of a meditation-based stress reduction program in the treatment of anxiety disorders. *Am. J. Psychiatry.* **1992**, *149*, 936–943. [PubMed]
64. Edenfield, T.M.; Saeed, S.A. An update on mindfulness meditation as a self-help treatment for anxiety and depression. *Psychol. Res. Behav. Manag.* **2012**, *5*, 131–141. [CrossRef] [PubMed]
65. Jastrowski Mano, K.E.; Salamon, K.S.; Hainsworth, K.R.; Anderson Khan, K.J.; Ladwig, R.J.; Davies, W.H.; Weisman, S.J. A randomized, controlled pilot study of mindfulness-based stress reduction for pediatric chronic pain. *Altern. Ther. Health Med.* **2013**, *19*, 8–14. [PubMed]
66. Grant, J.A.; Courtemanche, J.; Duerden, E.G.; Duncan, G.H.; Rainville, P. Cortical thickness and pain sensitivity in zen meditators. *Emotion* **2010**, *10*, 43–53. [CrossRef] [PubMed]
67. Hölzel, B.K.; Lazar, S.W.; Gard, T.; Schuman-Olivier, Z.; Vago, D.R.; Ott, U. How does mindfulness meditation work? Proposing mechanisms of action from a conceptual and neural perspective. *Perspect. Psychol. Sci.* **2011**, *6*, 537–559. [CrossRef] [PubMed]
68. Lazar, S.W.; Kerr, C.E.; Wasserman, R.H.; Gray, J.R.; Greve, D.N.; Treadway, M.T.; McGarvey, M.; Quinn, B.T.; Dusek, J.A.; Benson, H.; et al. Meditation experience is associated with increased cortical thickness. *Neuroreport* **2005**, *16*, 1893–1897. [CrossRef] [PubMed]
69. Hölzel, B.K.; Ott, U.; Gard, T.; Hempel, H.; Weygandt, M.; Morgen, K.; Vaitl, D. Investigation of mindfulness meditation practitioners with voxel-based morphometry. *Soc. Cogn. Affect. Neurosci.* **2008**, *3*, 55–61. [CrossRef] [PubMed]
70. Grant, J.A.; Courtemanche, J.; Rainville, P. A non-elaborative mental stance and decoupling of executive and pain-related cortices predicts low pain sensitivity in Zen meditators. *Pain* **2011**, *152*, 150–156. [CrossRef] [PubMed]
71. Grant, J.A.; Rainville, P. Pain sensitivity and analgesic effects of mindful states in Zen meditators: A cross-sectional study. *Psychosom. Med.* **2009**, *71*, 106–114. [CrossRef] [PubMed]
72. Zeidan, F.; Gordon, N.S.; Merchant, J.; Goolkasian, P. The effects of brief mindfulness meditation training on experimentally induced pain. *J. Pain* **2010**, *11*, 199–209. [CrossRef] [PubMed]
73. Zeidan, F.; Grant, J.; Brown, C.; Mchaffie, J.; Coghill, R. Mindfulness meditation-related pain relief: Evidence for unique brain mechanisms in the regulation of pain. *Neurosci. Lett.* **2012**, *520*, 165–173. [CrossRef] [PubMed]
74. Britton, W.B.; Lepp, N.E.; Niles, H.F.; Rocha, T.; Fisher, N.E.; Gold, J.S. A randomized controlled pilot trial of classroom-based mindfulness meditation compared to an active control condition in sixth-grade children. *J. Sch. Psychol.* **2014**, *52*, 263–278. [CrossRef] [PubMed]
75. Sibinga, E.M.; Perry-Parrish, C.; Chung, S.; Johnson, S.B.; Smith, M.; Ellen, J.M. School-based mindfulness instruction for urban male youth: A small randomized controlled trial. *Prev. Med.* **2013**, *57*, 799–801. [CrossRef] [PubMed]

76. Joyce, A.; Etty-Leal, J.; Zazryn, T.; Hamilton, A. Exploring a mindfulness meditation program on the mental health of upper primary children: A pilot study. *Adv. Sch. Ment. Health Prom.* **2010**, *3*, 17–25. [CrossRef]

77. Hooker, K.E.F.; Fodor, I.E. Teaching mindfulness to children. *Gestalt Rev.* **2008**, *12*, 75–91.

78. Montgomery, G.H.; DuHamel, K.N.; Redd, W.H. A meta-analysis of hypnotically induced analgesia: How effective is hypnosis? *Int. J. Clin. Exp. Hypn.* **2000**, *48*, 138–153. [CrossRef] [PubMed]

79. Potié, A.; Roelants, F.; Pospiech, A.; Momeni, M.; Watremez, C. Hypnosis in the Perioperative Management of Breast Cancer Surgery: Clinical Benefits and Potential Implications. *Anesthesiol. Res. Pract.* **2016**, *2016*, 2942416. [CrossRef] [PubMed]

80. Chaves, J.F. Recent advances in the application of hypnosis to pain management. *Am. J. Clin. Hypn.* **1994**, *37*, 117–129. [CrossRef] [PubMed]

81. Kohen, D.P.; Kaiser, P. Clinical hypnosis with children and adolescents—What? Why? How?: Origins, Applications, and Efficacy. *Children* **2014**, *1*, 74–98. [CrossRef] [PubMed]

82. Rogovik, A.L.; Goldman, R.D. Hypnosis for treatment of pain in children. *Can. Fam. Physician* **2007**, *53*, 823–825. [PubMed]

83. Chaves, J.F. Hypnosis in pain management. In *Handbook of Clinical Hypnosis*; Rhue, J.W., Lynn, S.J., Kirsch, I., Eds.; American Psychological Association: Washington, DC, USA, 1993; pp. 511–532.

84. Terhune, D.B.; Cardena, E. Heterogeneity in high hypnotic suggestibility and the neurophysiology of hypnosis. *Neurophysiol. Clin.* **2015**, *45*, 177–178. [CrossRef] [PubMed]

85. Mcgeown, W.J.; Mazzoni, G.; Vannucci, M.; Venneri, A. Structural and functional correlates of hypnotic depth and suggestibility. *Psychiatry Res.* **2015**, *231*, 151–159. [CrossRef] [PubMed]

86. Dillworth, T.; Mendoza, M.E.; Jensen, M.P. Neurophysiology of pain and hypnosis for chronic pain. *Transl. Behav. Med.* **2012**, *2*, 65–72. [CrossRef] [PubMed]

87. Rainville, P.; Hofbauer, R.K.; Paus, T.; Duncan, G.H.; Bushnell, M.C.; Price, D.D. Cerebral mechanisms of hypnotic induction and suggestion. *J. Cogn. Neurosci.* **1999**, *11*, 110–125. [CrossRef] [PubMed]

88. Rainville, P.; Hofbauer, R.K.; Bushnell, M.C.; Duncan, G.H.; Price, D.D. Hypnosis modulates activity in brain structures involved in the regulation of consciousness. *J. Cogn. Neurosci.* **2002**, *14*, 887–901. [CrossRef] [PubMed]

89. Vallath, N. Perspectives on yoga inputs in the management of chronic pain. *Indian J. Palliat. Care* **2010**, *16*, 1–7. [CrossRef] [PubMed]

90. National Center for Complimentary and Integrative Health: Yoga. 2014. Available online: http://nccam.nih.gov/health/yoga (accessed on: 20 June 2017).

91. Nahin, R.L.; Boineau, R.; Khalsa, P.S.; Stussman, B.J.; Weber, W.J. Evidence-based evaluation of complementary health approaches for pain management in the United States. *Mayo Clin. Proc.* **2016**, *91*, 1292–1306. [CrossRef] [PubMed]

92. Kraag, G.; Zeegers, M.P.; Kok, G.; Hosman, C.; Abu-Saad, H.H. School programs targeting stress management in children and adolescents: A meta-analysis. *J. Sch. Psychol.* **2006**, *44*, 449–472. [CrossRef]

93. Woolery, A.; Myers, H.; Sternlieb, B.; Zeltzer, L. A yoga intervention for young adults with elevated symptoms of depression. *Altern. Ther. Health Med.* **2004**, *10*, 60–63. [PubMed]

94. Brands, M.M.; Purperhart, H.; Deckers-Kocken, J.M. A pilot study of yoga treatment in children with functional abdominal pain and irritable bowel syndrome. *Complement. Ther. Med.* **2011**, *19*, 109–114. [CrossRef] [PubMed]

95. Hoffart, C.; Anderson, R.; Wallace, D. A155: Development of an intensive interdisciplinary pediatric pain rehabilitation program: Improving pain, functioning, and psychological outcomes. *Arthritis Rheum.* **2014**, *66*, S201. [CrossRef]

96. Evans, S.; Moieni, M.; Taub, R.; Subramanian, S.K.; Tsao, J.C.; Sternlieb, B.; Zeltzer, L.K. Iyengar yoga for young adults with rheumatoid arthritis: Results from a mixed-methods pilot study. *J. Pain Symptom. Manag.* **2010**, *39*, 904–913. [CrossRef] [PubMed]

97. Lu, D.P.; Lu, G.P. An historical review and perspective on the impact of acupuncture on U.S. medicine and society. *Med. Acupunct.* **2013**, *25*, 311–316. [CrossRef] [PubMed]

98. Niemtzow, R.C. Battlefield Acupuncture. *Med. Acupunct.* **2007**, *19*, 225–228. [CrossRef]

99. Niemtzow, R.C.; Belard, J.L.; Nogier, R. Battlefield Acupuncture in the U.S. Military: A Pain-Reduction Model for NATO. *Med. Acupunct.* **2015**, *27*, 344–348. [CrossRef]

100. Tsai, S.-L.; Misra, S. Auricular Battlefield Acupuncture at the 2016 Pediatric Academic Societies Meeting. *Med. Acupunct.* **2016**, *28*, 173–174. [CrossRef]
101. Tsai, S.; Fox, L.M.; Murakami, M.; Tsung, J.W. Auricular Acupuncture in Emergency Department Treatment of Acute Pain. *Ann. Emerg. Med.* **2016**, *68*, 583–585. [CrossRef] [PubMed]
102. Tsang, P.L. Treatment of chronic pain with acupuncture. *JAMA* **1975**, *232*, 1133–1135. [CrossRef]
103. Golianu, B.; Krane, E.; Seybold, J.; Almgren, C.; Anand, K. Non-pharmacological techniques for pain management in neonates. *Semin. Perinatol.* **2007**, *31*, 318–322. [CrossRef] [PubMed]
104. Lee, M.S.; Ernst, E. Acupuncture for pain: An overview of Cochrane reviews. *Chin. J. Integr. Med.* **2011**, *17*, 187–189. [CrossRef] [PubMed]
105. Manheimer, E.; White, A.; Berman, B.; Forys, K.; Ernst, E. Meta-analysis: Acupuncture for low back pain. *Ann. Intern. Med.* **2005**, *142*, 651–663. [CrossRef] [PubMed]
106. Ezzo, J.; Berman, B.; Hadhazy, V.A.; Jadad, A.R.; Lao, L.; Singh, B.B. Is acupuncture effective for the treatment of chronic pain? A systematic review. *Pain* **2000**, *93*, 198–199. [CrossRef]
107. Andersson, S.; Lundeberg, T. Acupuncture—from empiricism to science: Functional background to acupuncture effects in pain and disease. *Med. Hypotheses* **1995**, *45*, 271–281. [CrossRef]
108. Riet, G.T.; Kleunen, J.; Knipschild, P. Acupuncture and chronic pain: A criteria-based meta-analysis. *J. Clin. Epidemiol.* **1990**, *43*, 1191–1199. [CrossRef]
109. Thomas, M.; Eriksson, S.V.; Lundeberg, T. A comparative study of diazepam and acupuncture in patients with osteoarthritis pain: A placebo controlled study. *Am. J. Chin. Med.* **1991**, *19*, 95–100. [CrossRef] [PubMed]
110. Vickers, A.J.; Linde, K. Acupuncture for chronic pain. *JAMA* **2014**, *311*, 955–956. [CrossRef] [PubMed]
111. Jeanette, C.; Rico, R.C.; Trudnowski, R.J. Acupuncture and pain. *AANA J.* **1976**, *44*, 62–64.
112. Lund, I.; Lundeberg, T. Is acupuncture effective in the treatment of pain in endometriosis? *J. Pain Res.* **2016**, *9*, 157–165. [CrossRef] [PubMed]
113. Dumas, E.O.; Pollack, G.M. Opioid tolerance development: A pharmacokinetic/pharmacodynamic perspective. *AAPS J.* **2008**, *10*, 537. [CrossRef] [PubMed]
114. Han, B.; Compton, W.M.; Jones, C.M.; Cai, R. Nonmedical prescription opioid use and use disorders among adults aged 18 through 64 years in the United States, 2003–2013. *JAMA* **2015**, *314*, 1468–1478. [CrossRef] [PubMed]
115. Freitas, G.R.; Castro, C.G.; Castro, S.M.; Heineck, I. Degree of knowledge of health care professionals about pain management and use of opioids in pediatrics. *Pain Med.* **2014**, *15*, 807–819. [CrossRef] [PubMed]
116. Hui, K.K.; Marina, O.; Liu, J.; Rosen, B.R.; Kwong, K.K. Acupuncture, the limbic system, and the anticorrelated networks of the brain. *Auton. Neurosci.* **2010**, *157*, 81–90. [CrossRef] [PubMed]
117. Han, J.S. Acupuncture and endorphins. *Neurosci. Lett.* **2004**, *361*, 258–261. [CrossRef] [PubMed]
118. Wu, M. Neuronal Specificity of Acupuncture Response: A fMRI Study with Electroacupuncture. *NeuroImage* **2002**, *16*, 1028–1037. [CrossRef] [PubMed]
119. Biella, G.; Sotgiu, M.L.; Pellegata, G.; Paulesu, E.; Castiglioni, I.; Fazio, F. Acupuncture produces central activations in pain regions. *Neuroimage* **2001**, *14*, 60–66. [CrossRef] [PubMed]
120. Napadow, V.; Kettner, N.; Liu, J.; Li, M.; Kwong, K.K.; Vangel, M.; Makris, N.; Audette, J.; Hui, K.K. Hypothalamus and amygdala response to acupuncture stimuli in Carpal Tunnel Syndrome. *Pain* **2007**, *130*, 254–266. [CrossRef] [PubMed]
121. Dhond, R.P.; Yeh, C.; Park, K.; Kettner, N.; & Napadow, V. Acupuncture modulates resting state connectivity in default and sensorimotor brain networks. *Pain* **2008**, *136*, 407–418. [CrossRef] [PubMed]
122. Dhond, R.P.; Kettner, N.; Napadow, V. Do the neural correlates of acupuncture and placebo effects differ? *Pain* **2007**, *128*, 8–12. [CrossRef] [PubMed]
123. Wu, M.T.; Hsieh, J.C.; Xiong, J.; Yang, C.F.; Pan, H.B.; Chen, Y.C.; Tsai, G.; Rosen, B.R.; Kwong, K.K. Central nervous pathway for acupuncture stimulation: Localization of processing with functional MR imaging of the brain–preliminary experience. *Radiology* **1999**, *212*, 133–141. [CrossRef] [PubMed]
124. Carlsson, C. Acupuncture mechanisms for clinically relevant long-term effects—reconsideration and a hypothesis. *Acupunct. Med.* **2002**, *20*, 82–99. [CrossRef] [PubMed]
125. Melzack, R.; Stillwell, D.M.; Fox, E.J. Trigger points and acupuncture points for pain: Correlations and implications. *Pain* **1977**, *3*, 3–23. [CrossRef]

126. Hsieh, J.C.; Tu, C.H.; Chen, F.P.; Chen, M.C.; Yeh, T.C.; Cheng, H.C.; Wu, Y.T.; Liu, R.S.; Ho, L.T. Activation of the hypothalamus characterizes the acupuncture stimulation at the analgesic point in human: A positron emission tomography study. *Neurosci. Lett.* **2001**, *307*, 105–108. [CrossRef]

127. Lundeberg, T.; Stener-Victorin, E. Is there a physiological basis for the use of acupuncture in pain? *Int. Congress Ser.* **2002**, *12*, 3–10. [CrossRef]

128. Zhao, Z.Q. Neural mechanism underlying acupuncture analgesia. *Prog. Neurobiol.* **2008**, *85*, 355–375. [CrossRef] [PubMed]

129. Hui, K.K.; Liu, J.; Makris, N.; Gollub, R.L.; Chen, A.J.; Moore, C.I.; Kennedy, D.N.; Rosen, B.R.; Kwong, K.K. Acupuncture modulates the limbic system and subcortical gray structures of the human brain: Evidence from fMRI studies in normal subjects. *Hum. Brain Mapp.* **2000**, *9*, 13–25. [CrossRef]

130. Adams, D.; Cheng, F.; Jou, H.; Aung, S.; Yasui, Y.; Vohra, S. The safety of pediatric acupuncture: A systematic review. *Pediatrics* **2011**, *128*, e1575–e1587. [CrossRef] [PubMed]

131. Kemper, K.J.; Sarah, R.; Silver-Highfield, E.; Xiarhos, E.; Barnes, L.; Berde, C. On pins and needles? Pediatric pain patients' experience with acupuncture. *Pediatrics* **2000**, *105*, 941–947. [PubMed]

132. Waterhouse, M.W.; Stelling, C.; Powers, M.; Levy, S.; Zeltzer, L.K. Acupuncture and hypnotherapy in the treatment of chronic pain in children. *Clin. Acupunct. Oriental Med.* **2000**, *1*, 139–150. [CrossRef]

133. Zeltzer, L.K.; Tsao, J.C.; Stelling, C.; Powers, M.; Levy, S.; Waterhouse, M. A phase I study on the feasibility and acceptability of an acupuncture/hypnosis intervention for chronic pediatric pain. *J. Pain Symptom. Manag.* **2002**, *24*, 437–446. [CrossRef]

134. Slover, R.; Neuenkirchen, G.L.; Olamikan, S.; Kent, S. Chronic pediatric pain. *Adv. Pediatr.* **2010**, *57*, 141–162. [CrossRef] [PubMed]

135. Wu, S.; Sapru, A.; Stewart, M.A.; Milet, M.J.; Hudes, M.; Livermore, L.F.; Flori, H.R. Using acupuncture for acute pain in hospitalized children. Pediatric critical care medicine. *Pediatr. Crit. Care Med.* **2014**, *10*, 291–296. [CrossRef] [PubMed]

136. Ochi, J.W. Acupuncture instead of codeine for tonsillectomy pain in children. *Int. J. Pediatr. Otorhinolaryngol.* **2013**, *77*, 2058–2062. [CrossRef] [PubMed]

137. Cho, H.K.; Park, I.J.; Jeong, Y.M.; Lee, Y.J.; Hwang, S.H. Can perioperative acupuncture reduce the pain and vomiting experienced after tonsillectomy? A meta-analysis. *Laryngoscope* **2016**, *126*, 608–615. [CrossRef] [PubMed]

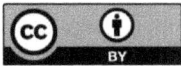

children

MDPI

Review

Review of Randomized Controlled Trials of Massage in Preterm Infants

Anna-Kaisa Niemi

Department of Pediatrics, Division of Neonatal & Developmental Medicine, Stanford University, Palo Alto, CA 94304, USA; annakaisa.niemi@gmail.com; Tel.: +1-650-723-5711

Academic Editor: Hilary McClafferty
Received: 1 February 2017; Accepted: 27 March 2017; Published: 3 April 2017

Abstract: Preterm birth affects about 10% of infants born in the United States. Massage therapy is being used in some neonatal intensive care units for its potential beneficial effects on preterm infants. This article reviews published randomized controlled trials on the effects of massage in preterm infants. Most studies evaluating the effect of massage in weight gain in premature infants suggest a positive effect on weight gain. Increase in vagal tone has been reported in infants who receive massage and has been suggested as a possible mechanism for improved weight gain. More studies are needed on the underlying mechanisms of the effects of massage therapy on weight gain in preterm infants. While some trials suggest improvements in developmental scores, decreased stress behavior, positive effects on immune system, improved pain tolerance and earlier discharge from the hospital, the number of such studies is small and further evidence is needed. Further studies, including randomized controlled trials, are needed on the effects of massage in preterm infants.

Keywords: infant massage; preterm; premature; newborn; neonate; weight gain; hyperbilirubinemia; mind–body; randomized controlled trial; tactile-kinesthetic stimulation

1. Introduction

Preterm birth (birth at <37 weeks of gestation) affects about 10% of infants born in the USA [1]. Premature infants often spend weeks or months in intensive care unit due to immaturity and need for intensive medical care, with hospital stay often prolonged by feeding immaturity and slow weight gain. Massage therapy is being used in some neonatal intensive care units for its possible beneficial effects with minimal side effects. This article reviews published randomized controlled trials on the effects of massage in preterm infants.

A PubMed search was performed for randomized controlled trials (RCTs) of massage in preterm infants. RCTs in English and indexed in PubMed by January 2017 were included. Studies assessing the effects of massage on caregivers only were excluded. A total of 34 randomized controlled trials on the effects of massage in preterm infants are reviewed [2–35].

2. Results

The outcome most commonly assessed on randomized controlled trials of massage in preterm infants (Table 1) was weight gain, either as primary or secondary outcome [2,5,8–10,12,15–19,21,26,28–31,33–35]. Other outcomes assessed in RCTs of massage in preterm infants include levels of transcutaneous bilirubin [3], sleep [4,26], calorie intake [5,17,19,30,33–35], vagal activity [5,19,24,26,29,30], gastric motility or number of stools [3,24,30], heart rate variability (HRV) [6,7,19,24,30], immunologic parameters [12], bone metabolism [11,32], changes in electroencephalogram (EEG) [13], behavior and/or neurodevelopment [14,15,23,26,28,29,31,34,35], pain [25], length of hospital stay [12,16,18] and levels of serum markers such as insulin-like growth factor I (IGF-1) [8,19], adiponectin [8], and serum triglycerides [9,27,31].

Most randomized controlled trials compared massage to standard care [2–4,6–9,11–14,16–35], while some compared oil massage to massage without oil [10], tactile massage to kinesthetic stimulation [5] and massage to light still touch [15]. While the type of massage used varied between studies, most studies assessed the effects of the tactile-kinesthetic stimulation (TKS) type of infant massage originally described by Field et al. in 1986 [36] or a modified version of TKS (Table 1). Modifications of TKS included shorter or longer duration of massage as well as elimination of kinesthetic range of movement exercise with only tactile stimulation provided. Other massage types evaluated include oil massage combined with either TKS or other standardized technique [2,9,10,27,28,31], Vimala massage [17] and acupressure and meridian massage [21].

In the following sections the outcomes of these studies as well as limitations are briefly reviewed. For number of study participants, gestational age, age at the time of study entry, and duration of massage intervention see Table 1.

2.1. Weight Gain

Weight gain, either as primary or secondary outcome is the most commonly assessed outcome in randomized controlled trials of massage in preterm infants [2,5,8–10,12,15–19,21,26,28–31,33–35]. Most studies have demonstrated a significantly greater daily or overall weight gain during the study period in massage group compared to control group [2,9,10,12,17,19,21,26,28,30,33–35] while some studies did not show a statistically significant difference in weight gain between groups [5,8,15,16,18,29,31]. Massaro et al. [16] evaluated the effects of massage or massage + kinesthetic stimulation on weight gain and length of hospital stay in a study of 59 infants who were randomized to massage only (n = 19), massage and kinesthetic stimulation (n = 20) or control group (n = 20). After controlling for covariates (birth weight, gestational age, caloric intake, etc.) the infants whose birth weight was >1000 g benefited from massage with a significantly higher average daily weight gain with more pronounced effects in infants who received massage + kinesthetic stimulation ($p = 0.012$) [16]. To study the possible contribution to weight gain of medium chain triglyceride (MCT) oil used in massage therapy (via absorption of oil through the skin) Saeidi et al. compared the effects of massage with MCT oil to massage without oil and controls (with no massage) and demonstrated a significantly higher weight gain during the 7-day study in the group that received massage with MCT oil compared to massage only ($p = 0.002$) and controls ($p = 0.000$) [2]. The mean weight gain during the study period in the MCT oil massage group was 105 ± 1.3 grams compared to a gain of 52 ± 0.1 grams in the massage only group and loss of 54 ± 1.3 grams in the control group [2].

2.2. Caloric Intake and Expenditure

Some studies have evaluated the effects of massage on caloric intake [5,8,17,19,30,33–35] and its possible connection to weight gain in preterm infants. Most studies did not show a difference in caloric intake between infants who received massage compared controls despite statistically significant higher weight gains in infants who received massage [8,17,19,30,33,34]. A study by Diego et al. showed increased calorie intake in infants who received kinesthetic stimulation compared to those who received tactile stimulation only, no difference in weight gain between the two groups [5]. Scafidi et al. evaluated factors that predict higher weight gain in infants who receive massage and a higher caloric intake was one of the factors that predicted weight gain [35]. One study evaluated energy expenditure in preterm infants, which was reported to be lower after a 5-day study period in infants who received massage compared to controls [22] suggesting that a decrease in energy expenditure may be in part responsible for the enhanced growth caused by massage therapy.

Table 1. Randomized controlled trials of massage in preterm infants.

Year	First Author	Number of Infants (Cases, Controls)	Gestational Age (Age at the Time of Study)	Massage Type	Intervention	Outcomes Measured	Results
2015	Basiri-Moghadam [3]	40 (20 massage, 20 controls)	34–36 weeks (<1 week)	N/A	20 min of massage twice daily for 4 days	Number of defecations Transcutaneous bilirubin level	Massage group had higher number of defecations ($p = 0.002$) and lower levels of transcutaneous bilirubin ($p = 0.003$)
2015	Saeadi [2]	121 (40 oil massage, 40 massage, 41 controls)	<37 weeks (<28 days)	N/A	5 min of massage 4 times a day for 7 days	Weight gain	The MCT oil-massage group gained more weight than massage ($p = 0.002$) and control groups ($p = 0.000$)
2014	Yates [4]	23 (cross-over study)	28–37 weeks (34–48 PMA)	TKS (modified, no kinesthetic component)	13 infants received a massage on day 1 and no massage on day 2 (10 infants received a massage on day 2)	Sleep efficiency Number of infants asleep at the end of massage	No significant difference in sleep efficiency ($p = 0.13$)
2014	Diego [5]	30 (15 tactile, 15 kinesthetic stimulation)	28–32 weeks; (15–60 days)	TKS (tactile or kinesthetic stimulation)	15 infants received tactile and 15 received kinesthetic stimulation 10 min a day for 5 days (no control group without massage)	Weight gain Calorie intake Vagal activity	No difference in weight gain. Increased calorie intake in kinesthetic group ($p < 0.05$). Increased vagal tone in tactile group ($p = 0.01$), decreased vagal tone in kinesthetic group.
2013	Fallah [10]	54 (17 oil massage, 17 massage alone) LBW infants	33–37 weeks (<10 days)	Moderate pressure	17 received moderate pressure massage alone, 17 received massage with sunflower oil 3 times a day for 14 days (no control group without massage)	Weight gain at 14 days, 1 month, 2 months	The oil massage group had a higher mean weight at ages 1 month ($p = 0.04$) and 2 months ($p = 0.005$) than the massage alone group.
2013	Smith [6]	21 (10 massage, 11 controls)	28–33 weeks (mean 31 weeks PMA)	Moderate pressure strokes with kinesthetic movement of extremities	20 min of massage twice daily for 4 weeks	Heart rate variability (HRV)	Significant group × time × sex interaction effect ($p < 0.05$) with male infants who received massage demonstrating higher HRV indicating increased vagal tone.
2013	Smith [7]	37 (17 massage, 20 control)	29–32 weeks	Soft-tissue compression strokes with following range of motion to arms and legs	20 min massage twice daily for 4 weeks	HRV	HRV improved in massage group but not in controls ($p < 0.05$). Male infants who received massage had a greater improvement in HRV than females ($p < 0.05$).

Table 1. *Cont.*

Year	First Author	Number of Infants (Cases, Controls)	Gestational Age (Age at the Time of Study)	Massage Type	Intervention	Outcomes Measured	Results
2013	Moyer-Mileur [8]	44 (22 massage, 22 controls)	29–32 weeks (32–33 weeks PMA)	Soft-tissue strokes with following range of motion to arms and legs	Twice-daily massage 6 days a week for 4 weeks	Energy and protein intake, body circumference, weight, length, ponderal index (PI), skinfold thickness (triceps, mid-thigh, subscapular), and IGF-1, leptin and adiponectin levels	Male infants in the massage group had smaller PI and skinfold thickness than control males ($p < 0.05$). Females in the massage group had larger subscapular skin fold increase than control females ($p < 0.05$). Adiponectin increased in control males ($p < 0.01$) and correlated to PI ($r = 0.39$, $p < 0.01$).
2013	Kumar [9]	48 (25 oil massage, 23 controls)	<35 weeks (<48 h)	20 strokes in: shoulders starting from neck with baby prone, upper back to the waist. Then limbs in supine position	10 min 4 times a day for 28 days	Weight, length, head circumference, serum triglyceride levels	At 7 days the massage group had less weight loss compared to controls ($p = 0.003$). At 28 days massage group had greater weight compared to controls ($p < 0.05$). No significant difference in serum triglycerides and other measured parameters.
2012	Haley [11]	40 (20 massage, 20 controls)	29–32 weeks, (mean 32 weeks PMA)	TKS	20 min twice daily, 6 days a week for 15 days	Tibial speed of sound (tSOS), urine markers of bone metabolism (pyridinium crosslinks and urinary osteocalcins (OC) U-MidOC and unOC)	Massage group had less decrease in tSOS than controls ($p < 0.05$). Urinary pyridinium crosslinks decreased in both massage and controls ($p < 0.005$). Massage group had greater increases in urinary osteocalcin (U-MidOC, $p < 0.001$ and unOC, $p < 0.05$) suggesting improved mineralization.
2012	Ang [12]	120 (58 massage, 62 controls)	Mean 30 weeks, range 25–33 (mean 32 weeks PMA, range 28–33)	TKS	5 days a week until hospital discharge for a maximum of 4 weeks	Immunologic parameters (absolute natural killer (NK) cells, T and B cells, T cell subsets, NK cytotoxicity), weight, number of infections, length of hospital stay	NK cytotoxicity was higher in the massage group, particularly in those who received ≥ 5 consecutive days of massage ($p = 0.04$). Infants in the massage group weighed more ($p = 0.05$) and had greater daily weight gain ($p = 0.01$) compared to controls. Other parameters, did not differ between the groups.
2011	Guzzetta [13]	20 (10 massage, 10 controls)	30–33 weeks (10 days)	TKS	10 min of massage 3 times a day for 12 days during a 2-week period	Changes in EEG spectral activity (before and after study period)	Significant difference in EEG spectral power.
2010	Procianoy [14]	73 (35 massage, 38 controls)	<32 weeks (48 h of life)	TKS (modified)	Massage and skin to skin care 15 min 4 times a day during hospital stay (skin to skin only)	Neurodevelopment (PDI, MDI) and growth at 2 years of corrected age	Massage group had higher MDI scores ($p = 0.035$). PDI scores and growth did not differ significantly.

Table 1. *Cont.*

Year	First Author	Number of Infants (Cases, Controls)	Gestational Age (Age at the Time of Study)	Massage Type	Intervention	Outcomes Measured	Results
2010	Ho [15]	24 (12 massage, 12 controls) VLBW infants	<34 weeks (34 weeks PMA)	TKS (modified)	15 min of massage daily, 5 days/week for 4 weeks (light still touch)	Test of Infant Motor Performance (TIMP) score gain, weight gain, post-conceptional age at discharge	No significant difference in TIMP score gain and weight gain when all subjects were analyzed. Those who had below-average pre-massage TIMP score and received massage had higher TIMP score gain ($p = 0.043$) and earlier discharge ($p = 0.045$) than controls.
2009	Massaro [16]	60 (20 massage with kinesthetic stimulation, 20 massage, 20 controls)	<32 weeks, mean 29 weeks for massage groups, 27 weeks for controls (30 weeks PMA)	TKS	15 min of massage ± kinesthetic stimulation (KS) twice daily from study enrollment until discharge	Weight gain Length of stay (LOS)	Average daily weight gain and LOS did not differ between the groups except for infants with BW > 1000 g, in whom average daily weight gain was higher in massage + KS group compared to control.
2009	Gonzalez [17]	60 (30 massage, 30 controls)	<35 weeks, mean 31 weeks (30–35 weeks PMA, mean 33)	Vimala massage	15–20 min twice daily massage for 10 days	Weight, head circumference, caloric intake, nutritional method, hospital stay	Massage group had higher weight gain ($p < 0.001$) and shorter hospital stay ($p = 0.03$) than controls.
2008	Field [19]	42 (N/A)	Mean 29–30 weeks (mean 34.8 weeks PMA)	TKS	15 min per day for 5 days	Weight gain, caloric consumption, vagal activity (high frequency component of HRV), serum insulin and IGF-1	Vagal activity increased during massage ($p < 0.001$). Massage group had greater increase in weight gain ($p = 0.02$), insulin ($p = 0.001$) and IGF-1 ($p = 0.05$). No difference in caloric consumption was noted between groups.
2008	Mendes [18]	104 (52 massage, 52 controls) VLBW infants	<32 weeks, mean 29 weeks (48 h)	TKS (modified)	15 min 4 times a day until discharge	Length of hospital stay (primary). Other outcomes: weight, length, head circumference, growth rate, ponderal index, age of partial and total enteral feeding, age of partial and total oral feeding, incidence of late onset sepsis, necrotizing enterocolitis (NEC), bronchopulmonary dysplasia (BPD)	Massage group had a higher probability of earlier hospital discharge ($p = 0.023$). Incidence of late-onset sepsis was lower in the massage group ($p = 0.005$).
2008	Chen [21]	40 (20 massage, 20 controls)	<34 weeks (>7 days)	Acupressure and meridian massage	15 min 3 times a day for 10 days	Weight gain	During 14-day study period the massage group gained more weight ($p = 0.008$) There was no significant difference in weight gain in the first week ($p = 0.384$). In the second week, the massage group had higher weight gain than controls ($p = 0.035$).

Table 1. Cont.

Year	First Author	Number of Infants (Cases, Controls)	Gestational Age (Age at the Time of Study)	Massage Type	Intervention	Outcomes Measured	Results
2008	Diego [20]	72 (abstract) or 48 (methods)(N/A)	Mean 29 weeks (N/A)	TKS	15 min of massage once	Temperature (15 min before, during massage and 15 min after)	Massage group had a greater increase in temperature
2007	Lahat [22]	10 (cross over)	Mean 32 weeks (29–34 weeks PMA, mean 3 weeks)	TKS (modified)	15 min 3 times a day for 5 days (5 infants received a massage for 5 days and no massage for 5 days, opposite sequence for 5 infants)	Energy expenditure by indirect calorimetry	Energy expenditure was lower in infants after the 5 days massage therapy than after the period with no massage ($p = 0.05$).
2007	Diego [24]	70 (36 massage, 34 controls)	Mean 29 weeks (mean 30 days)	TKS	15 min 3 times a day for 5 days	Vagal activity (HRV). Gastric motility (by ECG) measurements performed on days 1 and 5 of study 15 min before, during and 15 min after massage	Group-by-time analysis revealed significant increase in vagal activity that peaked during massage ($p < 0.001$); a significant increase in gastric motility that peaked 15 min after massage ($p < 0.01$) in the massage group. No changes in basal vagal activity or gastric motility were noted.
2007	Hernandez-Reif [23]	32 (16 massage, 16 controls)	28–32 weeks (15–60 days)	TKS	15 min 3 times a day for 5 days	Stress behavior (crying, grimacing, yawning, jerky arm or leg movement, sneezing, startles, finger flaring). Activity (movement of the limbs, torso or gross body movement of any kind)	Group-by-time analysis showed reduction in duration of stress behaviors in massage group ($p < 0.05$) and reduction in overall movement for the massage group ($p < 0.05$). No change in controls in these parameters were observed.
2006	Field [26]	68 (N/A)	28–32 weeks, mean 30 weeks (15–60 days), mean 23	TKS	15 min 3 times a day for 5 days of moderate vs. light pressure massage (no control group without massage)	Behavior state, stress behaviors, heart rate, weight gain	Moderate pressure massage group had a higher increase in weight gain ($p < 0.02$), less decrease in deep sleep ($p < 0.05$), less increase in active sleep ($p < 0.05$), less increase in fussing ($p < 0.01$, $p < 0.02$), less increase in crying ($p < 0.02$), less increase in gross movement ($p < 0.05$), less increase in stress behavior ($p < 0.01$), greater decrease in heart rate ($p < 0.01$), and greater increase in vagal tone ($p < 0.05$).
2006	Jain [25]	23 (crossover)	<37 weeks (1–7 days)	Slow massage of outer aspect of the leg	2-min massage of the ipsilateral leg prior to heel stick (n = 13) and no massage prior to next heel stick 2–7 days later (10 infants had reverse order)	Neonatal Infant Pain Scale NIPS (primary outcome). Heart rate, respiratory rate, oxygen saturation	NIPS ($p < 0.001$) and heart rate ($p = 0.03$) were higher after a heel stick with no massage.

Table 1. *Cont.*

Year	First Author	Number of Infants (Cases, Controls)	Gestational Age (Age at the Time of Study)	Massage Type	Intervention	Outcomes Measured	Results
2005	Arora [31]	69 (23 oil massage, 23 massage, 23 controls) VLBW infants	<37 weeks	Standardized technique for the study as described in article	10 min 4 times a day	Weight gain at 28 days after enrolment (primary), length, head circumference triceps skin fold thickness, neurobehavior (NBAS), serum triglycerides.	No significant differences in any of the measured parameters. Trend for increased weight gain/day in massage group ($p = 0.07$).
2005	Sankaranara-yanan [28]	112 (38 coconut oil, 37 mineral oil, 37 controls)	Mean 34.8 weeks (day 2 of life)	TKS	Four times a day for 31 days.	Weight gain velocity over the first 31 days of life (primary), length gain velocity, head growth, neuro-behavioral outcome, incidence of adverse events	Coconut oil massage group had a greater weight gain velocity compared to mineral oil ($p < 0.05$) and control groups ($p < 0.05$). Infants receiving coconut oil massage also showed a greater length gain velocity compared to controls ($p < 0.05$). No significant difference in other measures.
2005	Diego [30]	48 (16 massage, 16 light pressure sham massage, 16 controls)	22–37 weeks, mean ~30 (9–76 days, mean 29–34, no significant N difference between groups)	TKS	15 min 3 times a day for 5 days	Weight gain, vagal activity (HRV), gastric motility (EGG), days to discharge, caloric intake	Massage group had greater weight gain ($p < 0.01$), increased vagal tone ($p < 0.05$) and increased gastric motility ($p < 0.01$) during and after treatment. Weight gain was significantly related to gastric motility ($p < 0.01$) and vagal tone ($p < 0.01$). No differences in other parameters.
2005	Lee [29]	26 (13 massage, 13 controls)	<36 weeks (second day after starting enteral feeds)	TKS	15 min massage twice daily for 10 days	Weight, vagal tone, heart rate, oxygen saturation, and behavioral responses (behavioral states, motor activity, behavioral distress)	Massage group had significantly higher vagal tone after massage ($p = 0.05$) no change in controls. Massage group had higher scores for awake state ($p = 0.000$), fidgeting or crying ($p = 0.04$), and motor activity ($p = 0.04$) than controls.
2005	Solanki [27]	120 (40 coconut oil, 40 safflower oil, 40 no oil)	Three groups: GA < 34 weeks, GA 34–37 weeks, GA > 37 weeks	Not specified	5 mL of oil massaged for 10 min 4 times a day for 5 days	Serum triglycerides, serum fatty acid profile (linoleic, arachidonic, alpha linolenic acid, docosahexaemic acids and saturated fats)	Serum triglyceride values were significantly higher after massage in all groups compared to baseline (coconut oil $p < 0.001$, safflower oil $p < 0.001$, controls $p < 0.05$). There was a significant rise in linoleic and arachidonic acid in the safflower oil group ($p < 0.001$) and saturated fats in the coconut oil group ($p < 0.001$).

Table 1. *Cont.*

Year	First Author	Number of Infants (Cases, Controls)	Gestational Age (Age at the Time of Study)	Massage Type	Intervention	Outcomes Measured	Results
2004	Aly [32]	30 (15 massage, 15 controls)	28–35 weeks (<2 weeks)	TKS	Daily massage until infant reached 1.8 kg of weight	Serum type I collagen C-terminal propeptide (PICP) and urinary pyridinoline crosslinks of collagen (Pyd)	Serum PICP increased in massage group (p < 0.01) and decreased in control group (p < 0.01) compared to baseline, and this change differed significantly between massage group and controls (p = 0.0001). Urinary Pyd increased in both groups compared to baseline (p < 0.01 for both) but did not differ between the groups.
2002	Ferber [33]	57 (21 massage by mother, 17 massage by professional, 19 controls)	26–34 weeks, mean 31 weeks (mean 12–17 days)	TKS (modified)	15 min massage 3 times a day for 10 days	Weight gain Caloric intake	Infants massaged by either their mother or professional gained more weight than controls (p = 0.03). No significant difference in caloric intake.
1993	Wheeden [34]	30 (15 massage, 15 controls) All cocaine exposed infants	<37 weeks, mean 30 weeks (mean 16 days in controls, 20 days in massage group, NS)	TKS	15 min massage 3 times a day for 10 days	Weight gain, calorie intake, stress behavior, behavior (NBAS)	Massage group had greater weight gain per day (p = 0.009) than controls. There was no difference in feed type or caloric intake. Massage group had fewer postnatal complications (p = 0.005) and stress behaviors (p = 0.05) and more mature motor behaviors at the end of the 10-day study period (p = 0.02) than controls.
1993	Scafidi [35]	93 (50 massage, 43 controls)	26–36 weeks, mean 30 weeks (mean 15 days)	TKS	15 min massage 3 times a day for 10 days	Weight gain, calorie intake, stress behavior, behavior (NBAS)	Massage group had greater average daily weight gain (p < 0.01) than controls. Factors that predicted higher weight gain were history of obstetric complications, higher caloric intake and longer stay in intermediate nursery.

Controls received standard care unless otherwise noted. Statistically significant differences are noted in "Results" column, for other outcomes measured the difference was not statistically significant. BW = birth weight, EEG = electroencephalogram, EGG = electrogastrogram, GA = gestational age, HRV = heart rate variability, IGF-1 = insulin-like growth factor I, LBW = low birth weight, MCT = medium chain triglycerides, MDI = mental development index, NBAS = Brazelton's neonatal behavior assessment scale, NS = , PDI = Psychomotor Development Index, PMA = post-menstrual age, TKS = tactile/kinesthetic stimulation, a massage technique originally described by Field in 1986 [36], U-MidOC = urine osteocalcin midfragments, unOC = undercarboxylated form of osteocalcin, VLBW = very low birth weight.

2.3. Vagal Tone

Increased vagal activity induced by massage has been suggested as one potential mechanism for higher weight gain in infants who receive massage therapy. Vagal activity in most studies is assessed by measuring heart rate variability (HRV) with increased high frequency (HF) variability indicating higher vagal tone [37]. All studies that evaluated vagal activity demonstrated an increase in vagal tone in infants who receive massage [5–7,19,24,26,29,30]. However, in two studies, the increased vagal effect was more pronounced in male infants [6] or was demonstrated only in males [7]. In a study by Diego et al. comparing the effects of tactile to kinesthetic stimulation (the two components of TKS massage [36]), an increase in vagal tone measured by HRV was only noted in in the tactile group in group-by-time analysis ($p = 0.01$), whereas a decreased vagal tone was noted in infants receiving kinesthetic range of motion excercises only [5].

2.4. Gastric Motility

Massage-induced increases in vagal activity may lead to increased gastric motility, which has also been suggested as a possible mechanism for increased weight gain in infants who receive massage therapy. Gastric motility or number of stools have been assessed in three studies [3,24,30]. In infants who received massage therapy, significantly increased gastric motility during and immediately after massage and decreased tachygastria has been reported [24,30]. This increase in gastric motility was significantly correlated with increased weight gain and vagal tone [24,30]. During a 4-day study which evaluated the effects of massage on transcutaneous bilirubin levels and stool frequency, a significantly increased stool frequency was reported in the massage group compared to controls during the entire study period (day 1: $p = 0.001$, day 2: $p = 0.02$, day 3: $p = 0.01$ and day 4: $p = 0.04$) [3].

2.5. Immunological Effects

Two randomized controlled studies have reported on the effects of massage in immunological parameters and incidence of infections in preterm infants [12,18]. Absolute number of natural killer (NK) cells, white blood cells, B and T cells, and T-cell subsets were not statistically different between the groups. Number of infections did not differ between the groups. While the mean absolute NK cell number was not statistically different between the massage and control group, the adjusted mean NK cell cytotoxicity was higher in the massage group ($p = 0.05$) [12]. Mendes et al. reported on significantly lower incidence of late-onset sepsis in massage group ($p = 0.005$) [18]. The incidence of late-onset sepsis was 38.3% (18/47 infants) in controls compared to 10.9% (5/46 infants) in massage group. No serum immunological markers were reported in this latter study.

2.6. Bone Metabolism

Preterm infants have increased morbidity from osteopenia [38]. Physical activity stimulates bone formation. Two studies have evaluated the effects of massage therapy with physical activity on bone metabolism in preterm infants (Table 1) [11,32]. Physical activity was defined either as kinesthetic movement part of TKS massage [11] or a similar daily range of motion exercise, with gentle compression and extension/flexion to both upper and lower extremities [32]. Aly et al. reported an increase in serum type I collagen C-terminal propeptide (PICP, marker of bone formation) in the massage group ($p < 0.01$) compared to baseline, while PICP decreased in controls group ($p < 0.01$). This change differed significantly between the groups ($p = 0.0001$), suggesting increased bone formation in massage group. Furthermore, serum parathyroid hormone (PTH) level increased in the massage group while it decreased in the control group ($p < 0.001$).

2.7. Behavior, Sleep and Neurodevelopment

Yates et al. studied the effects of TKS massage on sleep efficiency in preterm infants in a crossover study [4] and found no significant difference between groups for sleep efficiency ($p = 0.13$). More infants were reported to sleep on the non-massage day (p = 0.026) [4]. Several studies have assessed the effects of massage on behavior and/or neurodevelopment of preterm infants [14,15,23,26,28,29,31,34,35]. Most studies have reported on immediate behavioral effects of massage [15,23,26,28,29,31,34,35] and only one randomized controlled trial has reported on long term neurodevelopmental outcome [14]. Massage groups were reported to have significantly less stress-related behaviors (crying, fidgeting) than controls in three studies [23,26,34], no difference between the groups in two [28,31], and one study reported increased crying and fidgeting in infants who received massage [29]. Ho et al. reported on a higher gain in motor performance score (Test of Infant Motor Performance, TIMP) in very low birth weight (VLBW) infants who received massage and who had a below-average pre-study score compared to a control group who received light touch (p = 0.043) suggesting that massage may have positive effects in motor outcomes in a subgroup of VLBW infants who have low motor performance [15]. Procianoy et al. compared neurodevelopmental outcomes (Psychomotor Development Index, PDI and Mental Development Index, MDI) at 2 years of age between preterm infants who had received massage intervention during hospital stay and controls [14]. Infants who had been randomly assigned to massage therapy group or control group during their hospital stay both received skin-to-skin care. Growth and neurodevelopmental outcome were evaluated in both groups at 2 years corrected age. Growth at 2 years corrected age did not differ between the groups. The massage group had slightly but not significantly higher PDI score (p = 0.072) and significantly higher MDI scores (p = 0.035) than controls [14].

2.8. Length of Hospital Stay

Length of hospital stay (LOS) was reported to be similar in the massage group and controls in one study [12], and in one there was a significant difference between groups [16] but this difference disappeared after controlling for gestational age, gender, sepsis and birth weight. Two studies have reported shorter duration of hospitalization in infants who received massage compared to controls [17,18]. A study by Gonzalez et al. evaluating the effects of Vimala massage in preterm infants reported a shorter hospital stay in infants of massage group (15.36 ± 5.41 days) compared to controls (19.33 ± 7.92 days (p = 0.03) [17]. A study by Mendez et al. on VLBW infants reported that those who received massage had a 1.85 times higher (95% confidence interval (CI): 1.09 to 3.13; p = 0.023) probability of earlier hospital discharge than control group [18].

2.9. Serum Markers

Levels of serum markers of growth and metabolism such as IGF-1 [8,19], adiponectin [8], serum triglycerides [9,27,31] have been studied in small randomized controlled trials. Moyer-Mileur et al. studied IGF-1, leptin, and adiponectin levels in infants who received massage and controls and correlated them with skin fold thickness, weight gain and ponderal index (PI) [8]. Serum leptin levels correlated significantly with weight gain, PI, triceps skin-fold thickness and mid-thigh skin-fold thickness [8]. Serum adiponectin level correlated with PI. There was no difference in weight gain however in this study between massage and control groups. In a study by Field et al. the massage group had a greater increase in weight gain (p = 0.02), and a greater increase in both insulin (p = 0.001) and IGF-1 (p = 0.05) levels [19] and weight gain correlated with increased insulin (p = 0.05) and IGF-1 (p = 0.02) levels [19]. Three randomized controlled trials have evaluated the effects of oil massage on serum triglycerides [9,27,31]. The primary objective of Solanki et al. was to assess transcutaneous absorption of massage oils by assessing serum lipid profiles in infants assigned to a massage without oil, or with safflower oil (rich in essential fatty acids, EFAs) or coconut oil (rich in saturated fats and medium chain triglycerides, MCTs) [27]. No weight gain was measured in this study. Serum triglyceride levels were significantly higher after massage compared to baseline in all groups (coconut oil p < 0.001, safflower oil p < 0.001, controls p < 0.05) though the rise was significantly higher in oil groups compared to controls (p < 0.05). In infants randomized to massage with safflower oil, a significant rise was seen in the essential fatty acids linoleic and arachidonic acid (p < 0.001) after massage. In those who received a massage with coconut oil an increase in serum saturated fats was reported ($p < 0.001$). In the control group who received a massage without oil a small but significant increase in serum linoleic ($p < 0.05$) and total saturated fats was seen ($p < 0.05$) [27]. The other two studies that assessed serum triglyceride levels used sunflower oil in the massage group evaluated serum triglyceride levels as a secondary outcome and reported no significant difference between massage group and controls [9,31].

2.10. Bilirubin levels, markers of brain maturation, pain

Basiri-Moghadam et al. reported significantly lower transcutaneous bilirubin levels ($p = 0.003$) in the massage group compared to controls after four days of massage [3]. Guzzetta et al. reported differences in EEG spectral power (an index of brain maturation) in massaged infants compared to controls suggesting a process of brain maturation in those who received massage [13]. Jain et al. reported in a cross-over study higher scores in Neonatal Infant Pain Scale (primary outcome) ($p < 0.001$) and heart rate ($p = 0.03$) in infants who had a blood sampling via a heel stick without a preceding 2-min massage of the ipsilateral leg compared to infants who had a massage prior to heel stick [25]. Respiratory rate, oxygen saturation and serum cortisol levels did not differ [25].

3. Discussion

Preterm birth (birth at <37 weeks of gestational age) is the leading cause of neonatal morbidity and mortality in the United States [39,40] and affects 10% of infants born in the USA [1]. Slow weight gain and poor oral-motor ability to feed are common factors delaying discharge from hospital in infants born prematurely. Interventions that improve either weight gain or oral-motor function may lead to shorter hospital stay and cost savings. Improved weight gain is the most commonly and consistently reported effect of massage in preterm infants with significantly greater daily or overall weight gain found in infants who received massage compared to controls [2,9,10,12,17,19,21,26,28,30,33–35]. While one study reported increased gain in an infant motor performance score in VLBW infants who received massage suggesting positive effects on motor development [15], oral–motor coordination and ability to feed was not evaluated. To date there are no randomized controlled trials evaluating the effects of massage on oral–motor coordination or feeding ability offering an area of future studies.

A recent meta-analysis by Wang et al. concluded that massage improved daily weight gain by 5.32 g (95% CI 4.15, 6.49 g, $p < 0.00001$) and reduced length of hospital stay by 4.41 days (95% CI 2.81, 6.02 days, $p < 0.00001$) [41]. A Cochrane systematic review by Vickers et al. also concluded that massage improved daily weight gain by 5.1 g (95% CI 3.5, 6.7 g) and appeared to reduce length of hospital stay by 4.5 days (95% CI 2.4, 6.5 days) [42], consistent with meta-analysis by Wang et al. [41]. Furthermore, a review by Field et al also suggested that infant massage leads to 3–6 days shorter length of hospital stay and, consequently, significant cost-savings up to $10,000 per infant [43].

The mechanism by which massage improves weight gain in preterm infants is not well understood. One suggested mechanism is that massage leads to higher consumption of calories. However, studies have not shown a difference in caloric intake between infants who received massage compared controls [8,17,19,30,33,34]. Another possible mechanism is increased vagal tone which may promote food absorption and anabolism. Increase in vagal activity has indeed been consistently reported in infants who receive massage in all randomized controlled trials that evaluated vagal tone [5–7,19,24,26,29,30]. Levels of serum anabolic hormones insulin and IGF-1 have been reported to be higher in infants who had received massage and correlated with weight gain [19] suggesting a possible anabolic effect. Field et al. postulate in more detail potential mechanisms for improved weight gain in preterm infants who received massage, including increased vagal tone and IGF-1 levels [44].

Furthermore, increased weight gain in preterm infants who receive massage with oil may be due to transcutaneous absorption of oils and contribution to caloric intake. While Solanki et al. reported a significant increase in serum essential fatty acids and saturated fats in infants massaged with safflower and coconut oil, respectively, their study did not assess weight gain [27]. Thus, the possible effects of transcutaneous absorption of oil in weight gain could not be evaluated. Study by Saeidi et al. did demonstrate a significantly higher weight gain in infants who received massage with MCT oil compared to massage only or controls [2] suggesting that MCT oil, possibly via transcutaneous absorption, may partly contribute to weight gain.

Improved weight gain and decreased length of hospital stay are important measures on the effects of massage in preterm infants and may lead to significantly lower health care costs [43]. Yet little is known about the long-term effects of early massage on infant development. Only one small study (n = 73) has assessed the long-term effects of massage given during neonatal hospital stay and compared neurodevelopmental scores between infants who received massage therapy to controls [14] and reported on a slightly higher PDI score and significantly higher MDI scores in the massage group, suggesting massage may induce long-term effects in neural modeling and neurodevelopment.

Overall, several studies as well as meta-analyses have suggested beneficial effects of massage in preterm infants with regards to improved weight gain and shortening the length of hospital, the latter of which has potential for significant cost-savings. Limitations and challenges of current randomized controlled trials on the effects of massage in preterm infants include small sample size in most studies, lack of studies in extremely premature infants, and lack of studies in infants with congenital anomalies or congenital heart disease who often have poor weight gain. The provider of the massage is also not consistent between studies. Massage has been variably provided by licensed massage therapists, trained nurses, or by a mother trained in massage technique. Although one study assessed the effects of massage in weight gain in infants massaged by either the mother or a professional gained and reported more weight gain in both groups compared to controls ($p = 0.03$) suggesting that different providers provide equally effective massage. There is limited information available on side effects of massage therapy with most of the studies not reporting side effects or quoting massage as "safe" or "relatively safe". However, given lack of reported side effects it is likely safe to conclude that massage is "relatively safe" in the infant groups in which it has been studied. There is not enough evidence to recommend massage for all preterm infants but it may be beneficial in selected clinically-stable preterm infants with slow weight gain.

4. Conclusions

In summary, randomized controlled trials on the effects of massage in preterm infants suggest improved weight gain and shortened length of hospital stay. Improved weight gain may be mediated through increase in vagal tone but more studies are needed on the underlying mechanisms of the effects of massage. Further randomized controlled studies are needed on the effects of massage on outcomes such as neurodevelopment, stress behavior, immune system, and pain tolerance.

Conflicts of Interest: The author declares no conflict of interest.

References

1. Hamilton, B.E.; Martin, J.A.; Osterman, M.J.; Curtin, S.C.; Matthews, T.J. Births: Final data for 2014. *Natl. Vital Stat. Rep.* **2015**, *64*, 1–64. [PubMed]
2. Saeadi, R.; Ghorbani, Z.; Shapouri Moghaddam, A. The effect of massage with medium-chain triglyceride oil on weight gain in premature neonates. *Acta Med. Iran.* **2015**, *53*, 134–138. [PubMed]
3. Basiri-Moghadam, M.; Basiri-Moghadam, K.; Kianmehr, M.; Jani, S. The effect of massage on neonatal jaundice in stable preterm newborn infants: A randomized controlled trial. *J. Pak. Med. Assoc.* **2015**, *65*, 602–606. [PubMed]
4. Yates, C.C.; Mitchell, A.J.; Booth, M.Y.; Williams, D.K.; Lowe, L.M.; Whit Hall, R. The effects of massage therapy to induce sleep in infants born preterm. *Pediatr. Phys. Ther.* **2014**, *26*, 405–410. [CrossRef] [PubMed]
5. Diego, M.A.; Field, T.; Hernandez-Reif, M. Preterm infant weight gain is increased by massage therapy and exercise via different underlying mechanisms. *Early Hum. Dev.* **2014**, *90*, 137–140. [CrossRef] [PubMed]
6. Smith, S.L.; Lux, R.; Haley, S.; Slater, H.; Beachy, J.; Moyer-Mileur, L.J. The effect of massage on heart rate variability in preterm infants. *J. Perinatol.* **2013**, *33*, 59–64. [CrossRef] [PubMed]

7.   Smith, S.L.; Haley, S.; Slater, H.; Moyer-Mileur, L.J. Heart rate variability during caregiving and sleep after massage therapy in preterm infants. *Early Hum. Dev.* **2013**, *89*, 525–529. [CrossRef] [PubMed]
8.   Moyer-Mileur, L.J.; Haley, S.; Slater, H.; Beachy, J.; Smith, S.L. Massage improves growth quality by decreasing body fat deposition in male preterm infants. *J. Pediatr.* **2013**, *162*, 490–495. [CrossRef] [PubMed]
9.   Kumar, J.; Upadhyay, A.; Dwivedi, A.K.; Gothwal, S.; Jaiswal, V.; Aggarwal, S. Effect of oil massage on growth in preterm neonates less than 1800 g: A randomized control trial. *Indian J. Pediatr.* **2013**, *80*, 465–469. [CrossRef] [PubMed]
10. Fallah, R.; Akhavan Karbasi, S.; Golestan, M.; Fromandi, M. Sunflower oil versus no oil moderate pressure massage leads to greater increases in weight in preterm neonates who are low birth weight. *Early Hum. Dev.* **2013**, *89*, 769–772. [CrossRef] [PubMed]
11. Haley, S.; Beachy, J.; Ivaska, K.K.; Slater, H.; Smith, S.; Moyer-Mileur, L.J. Tactile/kinesthetic stimulation (TKS) increases tibial speed of sound and urinary osteocalcin (U-MidOC and unOC) in premature infants (29–32 weeks PMA). *Bone* **2012**, *51*, 661–666. [CrossRef] [PubMed]
12. Ang, J.Y.; Lua, J.L.; Mathur, A.; Thomas, R.; Asmar, B.I.; Savasan, S.; Buck, S.; Long, M.; Shankaran, S. A randomized placebo-controlled trial of massage therapy on the immune system of preterm infants. *Pediatrics* **2012**, *130*, e1549–e1558. [CrossRef] [PubMed]
13. Guzzetta, A.; D'Acunto, M.G.; Carotenuto, M.; Berardi, N.; Bancale, A.; Biagioni, E.; Boldrini, A.; Ghirri, P.; Maffei, L.; Cioni, G. The effects of preterm infant massage on brain electrical activity. *Dev. Med. Child Neurol.* **2011**, *53* (Suppl. 4), 46–51. [CrossRef] [PubMed]
14. Procianoy, R.S.; Mendes, E.W.; Silveira, R.C. Massage therapy improves neurodevelopment outcome at two years corrected age for very low birth weight infants. *Early Hum. Dev.* **2010**, *86*, 7–11. [CrossRef] [PubMed]
15. Ho, Y.B.; Lee, R.S.; Chow, C.B.; Pang, M.Y. Impact of massage therapy on motor outcomes in very low-birthweight infants: Randomized controlled pilot study. *Pediatr. Int.* **2010**, *52*, 378–385. [CrossRef] [PubMed]
16. Massaro, A.N.; Hammad, T.A.; Jazzo, B.; Aly, H. Massage with kinesthetic stimulation improves weight gain in preterm infants. *J. Perinatol.* **2009**, *29*, 352–357. [CrossRef] [PubMed]
17. Gonzalez, A.P.; Vasquez-Mendoza, G.; Garcia-Vela, A.; Guzman-Ramirez, A.; Salazar-Torres, M.; Romero-Gutierrez, G. Weight gain in preterm infants following parent-administered vimala massage: A randomized controlled trial. *Am. J. Perinatol.* **2009**, *26*, 247–252. [CrossRef] [PubMed]
18. Mendes, E.W.; Procianoy, R.S. Massage therapy reduces hospital stay and occurrence of late-onset sepsis in very preterm neonates. *J. Perinatol.* **2008**, *28*, 815–820. [CrossRef] [PubMed]
19. Field, T.; Diego, M.; Hernandez-Reif, M.; Dieter, J.N.; Kumar, A.M.; Schanberg, S.; Kuhn, C. Insulin and insulin-like growth factor-1 increased in preterm neonates following massage therapy. *J. Dev. Behav. Pediatr.* **2008**, *29*, 463–466. [CrossRef] [PubMed]
20. Diego, M.A.; Field, T.; Hernandez-Reif, M. Temperature increases in preterm infants during massage therapy. *Infant Behav. Dev.* **2008**, *31*, 149–152. [CrossRef] [PubMed]
21. Chen, L.L.; Su, Y.C.; Su, C.H.; Lin, H.C.; Kuo, H.W. Acupressure and meridian massage: Combined effects on increasing body weight in premature infants. *J. Clin. Nurs.* **2008**, *17*, 1174–1181. [CrossRef] [PubMed]
22. Lahat, S.; Mimouni, F.B.; Ashbel, G.; Dollberg, S. Energy expenditure in growing preterm infants receiving massage therapy. *J. Am. Coll. Nutr.* **2007**, *26*, 356–359. [CrossRef] [PubMed]
23. Hernandez-Reif, M.; Diego, M.; Field, T. Preterm infants show reduced stress behaviors and activity after 5 days of massage therapy. *Infant Behav. Dev.* **2007**, *30*, 557–561. [CrossRef] [PubMed]
24. Diego, M.A.; Field, T.; Hernandez-Reif, M.; Deeds, O.; Ascencio, A.; Begert, G. Preterm infant massage elicits consistent increases in vagal activity and gastric motility that are associated with greater weight gain. *Acta Paediatr.* **2007**, *96*, 1588–1591. [CrossRef] [PubMed]
25. Jain, S.; Kumar, P.; McMillan, D.D. Prior leg massage decreases pain responses to heel stick in preterm babies. *J. Paediatr. Child Health* **2006**, *42*, 505–508. [CrossRef] [PubMed]
26. Field, T.; Diego, M.A.; Hernandez-Reif, M.; Deeds, O.; Figuereido, B. Moderate versus light pressure massage therapy leads to greater weight gain in preterm infants. *Infant Behav. Dev.* **2006**, *29*, 574–578. [CrossRef] [PubMed]
27. Solanki, K.; Matnani, M.; Kale, M.; Joshi, K.; Bavdekar, A.; Bhave, S.; Pandit, A. Transcutaneous absorption of topically massaged oil in neonates. *Indian Pediatr.* **2005**, *42*, 998–1005. [PubMed]

28. Sankaranarayanan, K.; Mondkar, J.A.; Chauhan, M.M.; Mascarenhas, B.M.; Mainkar, A.R.; Salvi, R.Y. Oil massage in neonates: An open randomized controlled study of coconut versus mineral oil. *Indian Pediatr.* **2005**, *42*, 877–884. [PubMed]

29. Lee, H.K. The effect of infant massage on weight gain, physiological and behavioral responses in premature infants. *Taehan Kanho Hakhoe Chi* **2005**, *35*, 1451–1460. [CrossRef] [PubMed]

30. Diego, M.A.; Field, T.; Hernandez-Reif, M. Vagal activity, gastric motility, and weight gain in massaged preterm neonates. *J. Pediatr.* **2005**, *147*, 50–55. [CrossRef] [PubMed]

31. Arora, J.; Kumar, A.; Ramji, S. Effect of oil massage on growth and neurobehavior in very low birth weight preterm neonates. *Indian Pediatr.* **2005**, *42*, 1092–1100. [PubMed]

32. Aly, H.; Moustafa, M.F.; Hassanein, S.M.; Massaro, A.N.; Amer, H.A.; Patel, K. Physical activity combined with massage improves bone mineralization in premature infants: A randomized trial. *J. Perinatol.* **2004**, *24*, 305–309. [CrossRef] [PubMed]

33. Ferber, S.G.; Kuint, J.; Weller, A.; Feldman, R.; Dollberg, S.; Arbel, E.; Kohelet, D. Massage therapy by mothers and trained professionals enhances weight gain in preterm infants. *Early Hum. Dev.* **2002**, *67*, 37–45. [CrossRef]

34. Wheeden, A.; Scafidi, F.A.; Field, T.; Ironson, G.; Valdeon, C.; Bandstra, E. Massage effects on cocaine-exposed preterm neonates. *J. Dev. Behav. Pediatr.* **1993**, *14*, 318–322. [CrossRef] [PubMed]

35. Scafidi, F.A.; Field, T.; Schanberg, S.M. Factors that predict which preterm infants benefit most from massage therapy. *J. Dev. Behav. Pediatr.* **1993**, *14*, 176–180. [CrossRef] [PubMed]

36. Field, T.M.; Schanberg, S.M.; Scafidi, F.; Bauer, C.R.; Vega-Lahr, N.; Garcia, R.; Nystrom, J.; Kuhn, C.M. Tactile/kinesthetic stimulation effects on preterm neonates. *Pediatrics* **1986**, *77*, 654–658. [PubMed]

37. Task Force of the European Society of Cardiology and the North American Society of Pacing and Electrophysiology. Heart rate variability: Standards of measurement, physiological interpretation and clinical use. *Circulation* **1996**, *93*, 1043–1065.

38. American Academy of Pediatrics, Committee on Nutrition. Nutritional needs of low-birth-weight infants. *Pediatrics* **1985**, *75*, 976–986.

39. Manuck, T.A.; Rice, M.M.; Bailit, J.L.; Grobman, W.A.; Reddy, U.M.; Wapner, R.J.; Thorp, J.M.; Caritis, S.N.; Prasad, M.; Tita, A.T.; et al. Preterm neonatal morbidity and mortality by gestational age: A contemporary cohort. *Am. J. Obstet. Gynecol.* **2016**, *215*, 103.e1–103.e14. [CrossRef] [PubMed]

40. Stoll, B.J.; Hansen, N.I.; Bell, E.F.; Walsh, M.C.; Carlo, W.A.; Shankaran, S.; Laptook, A.R.; Sanchez, P.J.; Van Meurs, K.P.; Wyckoff, M.; et al. Trends in care practices, morbidity, and mortality of extremely preterm neonates, 1993–2012. *JAMA* **2015**, *314*, 1039–1051. [CrossRef] [PubMed]

41. Wang, L.; He, J.L.; Zhang, X.H. The efficacy of massage on preterm infants: A meta-analysis. *Am. J. Perinatol.* **2013**, *30*, 731–738. [PubMed]

42. Vickers, A.; Ohlsson, A.; Lacy, J.B.; Horsley, A. Massage for promoting growth and development of preterm and/or low birth-weight infants. *Cochrane Database Syst. Rev.* **2004**, *2014*, CD000390.

43. Field, T.; Diego, M.; Hernandez-Reif, M. Preterm infant massage therapy research: A review. *Infant Behav. Dev.* **2010**, *33*, 115–124. [CrossRef] [PubMed]

44. Field, T.; Diego, M.; Hernandez-Reif, M. Potential underlying mechanisms for greater weight gain in massaged preterm infants. *Infant Behav. Dev.* **2011**, *34*, 383–389. [CrossRef] [PubMed]

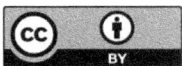

children MDPI

Review
Medical Yoga Therapy

Ina Stephens

Department of Pediatrics, University of Virginia Medical Center, Charlottesville, VA 22903, USA;
is8n@virginia.edu

Academic Editor: Hilary McClafferty
Received: 27 December 2016; Accepted: 3 February 2017; Published: 10 February 2017

Abstract: Medical yoga is defined as the use of yoga practices for the prevention and treatment of medical conditions. Beyond the physical elements of yoga, which are important and effective for strengthening the body, medical yoga also incorporates appropriate breathing techniques, mindfulness, and meditation in order to achieve the maximum benefits. Multiple studies have shown that yoga can positively impact the body in many ways, including helping to regulate blood glucose levels, improve musculoskeletal ailments and keeping the cardiovascular system in tune. It also has been shown to have important psychological benefits, as the practice of yoga can help to increase mental energy and positive feelings, and decrease negative feelings of aggressiveness, depression and anxiety.

Keywords: yoga; yogic practice; anxiety; depression; mindfulness; meditation; arthritis; ADHD; cardiovascular disease; inflammation

1. Introduction

Within the past decade, yoga has infiltrated not only Western culture, but also Western medicine. The more we learn about this ancient practice, the more we realize that its benefits go far beyond increased flexibility and muscle tone. A common misunderstanding is that yoga predominantly focuses on increasing flexibility; however, although Hatha Yoga, or the physical practice of yoga, does emphasize appropriate postural alignment, musculoskeletal strength and endurance as well as balance, the study and practice of yoga incorporates mindfulness-based practices such as mindful breathing techniques, focused concentration, meditation and self-reflection.

Modern medicine has made enormous progress in controlling communicable diseases over the past century, such that it is now the non-communicable diseases (NCDs) that have reached epidemic proportions and cause the majority of deaths worldwide. The World Health Organization (WHO) estimates that 80% of NCD deaths are due to four main disease types: cardiovascular disease, cancer, diabetes, and respiratory diseases [1]. Unfortunately, lifestyle is the major causative factor in NCDs, including tobacco use, sedentary lifestyle, lack of regular exercise, unhealthy diets and chronic psychosocial stress [1,2]. Chronic inflammation and stress is a common factor of many of the NCDs, and an area where yoga has been found to be extremely beneficial.

Recent research has shown that yogic and mindfulness-based practices can positively impact the body in many ways, including helping to regulate blood glucose levels and keeping the cardiovascular system healthy. It also has been shown to have important psychological benefits, as the practice of yoga can help to increase alertness and positive feelings, and decrease negative feelings of aggressiveness, depression and anxiety [3–8]. Some healthcare providers are responding to these positive findings—as well as the growing patient demand for an alternative approach to wellness that is natural, low-tech, relatively inexpensive and generally very safe—by incorporating medical yoga into their practices [1].

2. Prescription: Yoga

Medical yoga is defined as the use of yoga practices for the prevention and potential treatment of medical conditions. Beyond the physical elements of yoga, which are important and effective for strengthening the body, medical yoga also incorporates appropriate breathing techniques, mindfulness, meditation and self-reflection/study in order to achieve the maximum benefits. Medical Yoga Therapy or "Yoga Chikitsa" is the dynamic state of physical and mental ease, coupled with spiritual well-being. Yoga helps one to develop a positive state of health by not only treating illness, but also helping one to understand the underlying causes of disease. Medical yoga therapy, ideally, is an individualized, personalized and holistic approach that takes into account not only the patient's mind, body and spirit, but also their family, support network, work situation, and culture, as part of the patient's individualized treatment plan. As an example, if one is diagnosed with anxiety, a physician trained in medical yoga may prescribe specific breathing techniques (pranayamas), calming postures (asanas), mindfulness-based practices and/or meditation, as well as other lifestyle guidance. This type of therapy does not incur the potentially adverse effects of medications, and can produce benefits to the patient, long after their relationship with the health provider ends.

The mindfulness and meditation aspects of yoga are ways of training the mind so that one is not distracted and caught up in its endless churning thought stream. These practices build resilience, help the patient cope with stress and manage potential triggers for anxiety. They can also promote self-reflection that may uncover the source(s) of one's anxiety. If necessary, anti-anxiety medications and/or psychotherapy may be used in tandem; medical yoga in such cases is strongly adjunctive and complementary.

Yoga is most powerful when it changes the patient's general health outlook, changing the emphasis from reactive to proactive health management. The yogic definition of health or "svastha" is when the functions of the body and mind are in harmony so that they can turn inward to reach the goal of Self-realization. In yogic terms, when you are really your "Self", you are truly at "ease". It is the loss of the Self that creates "dis-ease". This is a bit different than the Western concept of health, which is often defined as "the absence of disease." In contrast, the yogic concept is that "disease is the absence of vibrant health". Accordingly, this way of thinking reaffirms the understanding that the nature of yoga is to find one's eternal Self of health, peace and well-being [1].

This review article will focus on: (1) The science behind medical yoga; (2) The relationship of stress to health and healing; (3) The yogic approach to health care; and (4) The research behind medical yoga therapy.

3. What Is Yoga

Yoga is not a particular denomination or religion, but an age-old practice based on a harmonizing system for the body, mind, and spirit to attain inner peace and liberation [9,10]. Yoga is a tool that can deepen and benefit anyone, of any religion. It does not conflict with personal beliefs; it is simply a vehicle to help one transform oneself by promoting conscious connection with oneself, the world, and the highest truth. There are many traditional paths of yoga, including tantra, mantra, kundalini, bhakti, jnana, karma, raja yoga, and others, all of which have their own techniques to awaken these connections. According to the classic text of the *Yoga Sutras of Patanjali*, "yoga" is the complete "inhibition of the modifications of the mind" [9] or quieting of the constant chatter in one's mind so that our True Selves can manifest, rest in our own true nature and be free of suffering. Disease, as described in the sutras, is said to be an impediment to spiritual practice, growth and freedom from suffering [9]. Traditional yogic practices include breath control and techniques (pranayama), meditation (including mindfulness), the adoption of specific bodily postures (asanas) and self-reflection (scriptural or self-study) [9,10].

As a mindfulness practice, yoga requires one to be fully aware in the present moment. This practice helps to diffuse anxiety (which largely concerns the future), and sadness (which largely concerns the past). All the yogic practices use present moment, non-judgmental awareness as the foundation.

Of course, such presence benefits the healthcare provider as much as the patient: if one can learn to pay attention to oneself, one can really pay attention to one's patients. One can then teach the patient to pay attention to him or herself as well.

4. Medical Yoga Prescription

Medical yoga as considered here comprises the use of traditional yogic practices to prevent, cure, and/or ameliorate disease. The ideal medical yoga prescription includes the yogic practices of breathing techniques, bodily postures, meditation techniques and self-reflection; a healthy, nourishing diet; reducing substances such as caffeine, tobacco, drugs and alcohol; healthy sleep hygiene and appropriate support, which may include family, spouse, children, friends and/or support groups, with or without psychotherapy. It is important that medical yoga therapy should start gently and with self-compassion.

For providers considering adding yoga to their therapeutic armamentarium, the best place to start is to consider yoga therapy as a complement to their patient's current medical treatment. Yoga alone should not be considered a substitute for appropriate medication or psychotherapy. However, in situations where a patient is at risk of an illness but does not currently need more intensive therapy, introduction of yogic practices may forestall or prevent progression to the point where medical therapy is needed. Patients whose daily activities produce back strain or who have inherently stressful lives may benefit from yoga as a prophylactic strategy, thereby potentially avoiding more intensive interventions. It is also important to remember that not all yoga is appropriate for all patients and that yoga therapy is different than simply taking a group yoga class where the yoga instructor may not be aware of an individual student's health concerns or problems. Most certified yoga teachers, or instructors, have received some training in anatomy and physiology; however, this training can be quite varied and is not equivalent to the training required by the yoga therapist or healthcare practitioner. As noted previously, yoga therapy, different from a yoga class, starts with a detailed history and physical examination and assessment from the health practitioner.

Yoga brings the autonomic nervous system into healthy balance by stimulating the parasympathetic nervous system [11,12]. The sympathetic nervous system, or our "emergency response system," is activated when our body or mind feels threatened or perceives being stressed, whether that be a "positive" or a "negative" stress. This "flight or fight" response results in vasoconstriction, causing decreased blood flow to the extremities and the digestive system in order to prepare one for survival [11]. One's heart rate and blood pressure increase, the liver converts glycogen to glucose and releases glucose into the bloodstream, the bronchioles dilate, and the blood flow pattern changes, leading to decreased digestive system activity and reduced urine output. In contrast, the parasympathetic system is stimulated when one relaxes; it is often called the "rest and digest" mechanism of our nervous system. The parasympathetic system stimulates blood flow to the digestive system, brain, extremities and sexual organs [11]. As many of us go through our day, what is happening on the "outside"—i.e., what we may think or what we may encounter—causes a constant interaction between the two facets of the nervous system. Yogic practices work by decreasing physiologic arousal and quieting down this continual play of the autonomic system. They can reduce one's heart rate and blood pressure, ease one's respirations and increase heart rate variability—all signs of improved parasympathetic tone [13].

5. Stress

Many in today's society live in "sympathetic overdrive." This occurs when the body perceives a continuous stressor, and the short-term sympathetic stress response persists all day long [11]. Unfortunately, our bodies were not really set up in a way to handle these continual stressors [12]. Due to the continued excitation, one of the major neuroendocrine systems of the body, the hypothalamic-pituitary-adrenal (HPA) axis is set in motion. The HPA axis regulates and helps to control many different bodily processes including one's reaction to stress, immune function, digestion and energy expenditure and storage. The axis is set in motion with release of corticotropin-releasing factor (CRF) from the hypothalamus. CRF then stimulates the anterior pituitary gland to release adrenocorticotropic hormone (ACTH), which subsequently stimulates the adrenal cortex to produce and release cortisol [14]. In response to the stress, cortisol functions by aiding in the metabolism of fat, protein, and carbohydrates by converting them to glucose through gluconeogenesis. This longer-term stress response subsequently raises blood glucose levels, suppresses the immune system, and causes retention of sodium and water by the kidneys, with subsequent increased blood volume and blood pressure. At a certain blood concentration, cortisol will exert a negative feedback to the hypothalamus and the pituitary gland with decreased discharging of both CRF and ACTH. At this point, homeostasis returns to the body and entire system. If, however, the body continues to be in a state of stress, real or perceived, this cycle perpetuates with subsequent sustained HPA axis activation [14,15].

Not all stress has unfavorable effects, of course. When the body is able to tolerate the stress, and can use it to boost one's performance, the positive effects are numerous and impressive. There are over >1400 biochemical reactions that the body has in response to stress, with subsequent effects on one's body, mind, emotions and behavior [12]. However, stress becomes negative when it exceeds one's ability to cope. At this point, the body systems can become fatigued, causing multiple problems, both physically and emotionally [15,16].

Chronic stress is experienced when there is a mismatch between a perceived demand and one's ability to cope with that demand; it includes one's emotional and mental response to the outside situation. When one is continually stressed, whether that stress is real or perceived, his or her nervous system can be shifted towards the state of sympathetic overdrive [11,12]. At this point, the actual activity of the sympathetic nervous system decreases with a decline in the release of epinephrine, but corticosteroid release continues to be activated at above-normal levels. In such a case, the individual may no longer even recognize that they are in a stressful state. Moreover, chronic stress can be precipitated by any number of factors and conditions, some regular and unavoidable: constant worry, daily life hassles, frustrations over one's job or family, traffic jams, finances, poor sleep or eating habits, demands on time, and challenging life situations all create stress [12]. Stress can even also be triggered by one's memory of difficult or scary past situations that have previously occurred. This state of high stress causing continuous sympathetic stimulation is epidemic in our society, from the corporate executive down to the young child on a busy school and activity schedule.

So stress is part of our lives—does it matter? In fact, the burden due to stress-related illness is quite concerning. The Centers for Disease Control and Prevention estimates that stress accounts for about 75% of all physician visits [12,16,17], and up to 80% of all visits to primary care providers are for stress-related complaints [12,17]. These involve a wide spectrum of complaints, including headache, back pain, hypertension, arrhythmias, irritable bowel syndrome, insomnia, depression, anxiety, skin problems, fatigue, obesity, migraines, hyperlipidemia and accidents.

Research has shown that continued and chronic stress can result in a generalized immunosuppressive effect that prevents the body to initiate a timely and appropriate immune reaction [16,18–20]. During acute stress, norepinephrine, epinephrine and ACTH are released, signaling certain kinds of cells to become mobilized into the bloodstream, potentially preparing the body for the "fight or flight" response [1]. Acute stress increases levels of pro-inflammatory cytokines in the bloodstream [21]. Whereas inflammation is a necessary short-term response for eliminating pathogens and initiating healing, chronic systemic inflammation causes dysregulation of the immune system and increases one's risk for chronic diseases [20–22]. Chronic stress, like acute stress, is associated with high levels of pro-inflammatory cytokines, but with potentially different health consequences [22]. Type 1 cytokine protective immune responses have been shown to be suppressed during times when the body is undergoing challenges of chronic stress, while pro-inflammatory and type-2 cytokine responses are activated [23,24]. Chronic or long-term stress can also suppress immunity by decreasing the number of immune cells as well as their function. These phenomenon may exacerbate pro-inflammatory diseases and thus potentially increase one's susceptibility to infections and possibly different types of cancer [24].

Chronically high levels of cortisol can also be neurotoxic [14]. These high levels have been associated with accelerated aging, cognitive inhibition, impaired memory and the ability to learn, increased anxiety and fear, as well as depression and anhedonia [25–27]. Areas of the brain, including the hippocampus and the prefrontal cortex (PFC), both with high cortisol receptors, can become impaired with high cortisol levels. Prolonged stress, both physiological and psychological, with continued high levels of blood cortisol can induce lowered metabolic rates and decreased synaptic densities in the hippocampus and the PFC [25,28–30]. Even perceived stress has been shown to negatively correlate with overall PFC volume, specifically in white matter volume of the PFC, specifically in the ventrolateral and dorsolateral PFC [31].

Cortisol activates the amygdala, the body's "threat center." The amygdala is an almond-shaped brain structure that is crucial in the stress response. An enlarged and hyperactive amygdala is often observed during stressful conditions placed on the body [14,32–35]. Of interest, studies performed on decreasing stress revealed that following stress-reduction interventions, where patients reported significantly reduced perceived stress, decreases basolateral amygdala gray matter density, as seen on Magnetic Resonance Imaging (MRI) scans [32,36].

Stress, of all kinds, is thought to play a significant role in the development of depression by depleting the body's "positive" neurotransmitters, such as gamma-aminobutyric acid (GABA), serotonin and dehydroepiandrosterone (DHEA) [37–42]. Dysregulation of the HPA axis is often seen and reported in those with depressive disorders. In addition, both the dopaminergic and serotonergic systems are thought to be involved in the development of depression if they become dysfunctional or dysregulated [43]. Studies done in rats have shown that chronic stress can induce a depressive state, along with notable dysregulation of both their HPA axes and their dopaminergic and serotonergic systems in the PFC. Release of GABA has also shown to be impaired in these rats as well [40,43]. Other mood disorders, including anxiety, are also thought to be aggravated by stress-induced modifications of the PFC. Of note, stress may impact the prefrontal GABA pathways. This can impair the function of the limbic structures, which are known to control one's emotions and behavior [44,45].

6. How Do Yogic Practices Work?

Yoga-based practices of postures (asanas) and movement sequences are usually taught in conjunction with some type of breathing and/or meditation technique [1]. This type of mindful movement with slow, rhythmic breathing is more likely to promote parasympathetic and vagal tone compared to other forms of exercise [1,11,46,47]. Improved vagal tone is reflected by increased heart rate variability (HRV), which is the variation in the time interval between heartbeats. This physiologic phenomenon can be predictive of how readily the heart rate returns to normal, or quiets down, after increasing in response to a stressor. Decreased HRV is associated with poorer myocardial function, often seen after a myocardial infarction, and is seen with increased sympathetic activity. Increased HRV with high frequency activity is associated with increased parasympathetic activity. Yogic breathing techniques—in particular, alternate nostril breathing, which involves breathing through the left and right nostril alternately—has been associated with increased parasympathetic activity, increased HRV and decreased systolic blood pressure [48]. Slow and rhythmic breathing has also been shown to promote the release of prolactin and the hormone oxytocin, which can foster feelings of friendship, calmness and bonding to others (released during childbirth which may help the mother relax and bond with her newborn during a very painful process) [1,49]. These yoga practices also reduce circulating levels of cortisol and have been demonstrated to reduce the manifestations of stress. With practice, there is decreased firing from the locus coeruleus, which is the principal site in the brain for synthesis of norepinephrine in response to stress and panic. This decreased norepinephrine output helps the body to relax and quiet down with reduced respiratory rates and heart rates. The decreased sympathetic output decreases the release of corticotropin releasing factor, with resultant decrease in cortisol output [50–52].

An open-label study from 2013 performed on a cohort of 54 outpatients with clinical depression at a tertiary care psychiatric hospital revealed that, as a group, this cohort had higher levels of serum cortisol compared to healthy controls [50]. These 54 subjects were offered yoga classes as adjunctive therapy for their depressive symptoms. The yoga module was taught to the group over a month's time and subjects were advised to practice daily at home. Antidepressant medication was prescribed in addition if advised by the subject's psychiatrist. The cohort was broken down into three groups: Group (G) 1 received conventional drug therapy (DT) alone (N-16), G2 received yoga therapy (YT) alone (N-19), and G3 received DT along with YT (N-19). A G4 group was used as healthy controls (N-18). The Hamilton Depression Rating Scale (HDRS) was used to rate subject's depressive symptoms, along with measurements of serum cortisol, obtained both at baseline and after three months of intervention. In the total sample, with good adherence, and irrespective of treatment method, the cortisol levels were found to be decreased significantly at the end of treatment in all subjects. Of interest, however, is that more subjects in the yoga groups (both YT and YT plus DT) had significantly greater drops in their cortisol levels as compared to the drug-only (DT) group ($p < 0.008$). In the YT-only group, there was also a high correlation between decreased cortisol levels and lower scores on the HDRS surveys, indicating a positive antidepressant effect as well ($p < 0.001$) [50].

7. Meditation

It appears that formal meditation practice can change both brain structure and function [53]. It has been found that people who do more meditation practice develop more robust brain structures in certain areas. Multiple studies have shown that yogic practices such as mindful meditation can increase both cortical thickness and gray matter, particularly in areas controlling emotional regulation and executive functioning. These regions notably include the insula, the ventromedial pre-frontal cortex and anterior cingulate cortex (ACC) [53,54]. The insula is involved with proprioception, self-awareness and emotional regulation. The ventromedial PFC is the brain's center for executive functioning, including planning, problem solving and emotional regulation. The ACC is the self-regulatory process center, giving one the ability to monitor attention conflicts and allow for more cognitive flexibility [55–58].

Meditation has been shown to increase the thickness of the left hippocampus, the region of the brain that functions in the formation of long-term memory, emotional regulation and cognition, as well as being a critical area of the brain that plays a vital role in the resiliency to chronic stress and depressive states, possibly due to expression of hippocampal neurotrophic protein (brain-derived neurotropic factor or BDNF) [59]. Resiliency to stress, stress-related depression and post-traumatic stress are housed in the hippocampus—multiple studies have shown that increased hippocampal activation correlated negatively with post-traumatic stress disorder (PTSD) and depression symptoms, and positively with resilience [25,55,60–62]. PTSD patients show considerable reduction in volume of the hippocampus, decreased ventromedial PFC activity and insufficient inhibition of the amygdala, all resulting in increased fear, persistent negative emotions, impulsivity, anxiety and depressive rumination.

Mindfulness meditation, particularly in long-term expert meditators, has been shown to diminish activity and size in anxiety-related areas of the brain such as the amygdala, as well as to increase the size of the PFC and insular cortex, both controlling emotional regulation. These meditators have also been shown to have diminished functional connections between the amygdala and the PFC, allowing for less reactivity to stressors [55,63,64]. Meditation also appears to be effective for PTSD and depression symptoms, although more high-quality studies are needed [65,66].

A recent study suggested that hatha yoga postures (asanas) alone can also improve stress and increase relaxation dispositions. This randomized controlled trial performed in 2015 among college students with high psychological stress assessed the effects of sun salutations or suryanamaskar (defined as a series of 12 physical postures) on relaxation dispositions (R-dispositions). Suryanamaskar is a traditional asana sequence that is a well-known yogic exercise; however, there are few studies on the physiologic effects of regular suryanamaskar practice [67,68]. In this study, the intervention group was to practice a daily suryanamaskar session for 14 days, which was composed of a short warm up, 13 rounds of suryanamaskar with mantras and breathing, followed by a cool down in a sitting position. The set of exercises took approximately 20 min to complete daily. No specific activity was given for the control arm to perform. After 14 days, the experimental group scored higher on multiple aspects on the surveys with increased points compared to the control group for: physical relaxation, mental calmness, feeling at ease and peace, being more well-rested and refreshed, improved strength, awareness and joy. In addition, the intervention group scored lower on fatigue, somatic stress, worry, and negative emotional feelings when compared with the control group [69].

8. Yoga and Neurotransmitters

Yoga practices can increase multiple neurotransmitters and hormones such as GABA, serotonin, and dopamine—all natural anti-depressants [11]. They have been shown to increase levels of melatonin, helping to initiate sleep, improving sleep quality and sleep regulation, as well as increasing levels of oxytocin, the "bonding hormone", thus helping with feelings of connectedness and "being seen and heard" [70–74].

GABA is one of the body's chief inhibitory neurotransmitters, working to reduce neuronal excitability and activity throughout the central nervous system (CNS). GABA acts as an important player in the body's response to stress, fear, depression, anxiety and sleep regulation. Lower-than-normal levels of GABA in the brain have been associated with schizophrenia, depression, anxiety, post-traumatic stress disorder, epilepsy and sleep disorders [73].

Multiple kinds of both anxiolytic and anti-depressant medications work by increasing GABA levels in the central nervous system. As mentioned earlier, yoga practices seem to be effective by bringing the parasympathetic and sympathetic systems into balance (often by increasing parasympathetic tone and decreasing sympathetic firing), and does this in large part by increasing GABA activity [75]. Meditation increases activity in the PFC as well as stimulates the thalamus (in particular, the reticular nucleus), which increases production and delivery of GABA throughout the CNS. Studies have shown that GABAergic inhibitory interneurons result in cortical inhibition which has been implicated in improved cognitive performance and enhanced emotional regulation capabilities [76]. Multiple studies have shown that the practice of yoga and meditation may work as well as other therapies in increasing GABA levels in the brain [77–79].

9. Yoga and Telomeres

As meditation, mindfulness practices and yoga have been moving more and more into the mainstream, it is becoming more apparent that these practices may work to keep our minds and bodies from withering with age by potentially stabilizing, and even lengthening telomeres. Telomeres are small, repetitive, chromosomal sequences found at the end of chromosomes which protect the chromosome from deterioration and cell death. They keep the chromosome stable. Telomere shortening, or unraveling, affects how quickly cells age. As they shorten, the chromosome's structural integrity weakens. Telomere length has been found to be a prognostic marker of aging, disease and premature morbidity in humans. Shorter telomeres are associated with cell aging, cell death, premature aging and a broad range of aging-related diseases, including cardiovascular disease, cancer, stroke, dementia, obesity, osteoporosis, Alzheimer's, macular degeneration, acquired immunodeficiency syndrome (AIDS), and osteoarthritis. They have also been associated with pediatric syndromes such as Progeria, Cri-du-chat, Down's syndrome, tuberous sclerosis, dyskeratosis congenita and Fanconi anemia. Telomere shortening is prevented by the enzyme telomerase. Of note, chronic stress may potentially speed up the aging process through decreased telomerase activity and telomere shortening [80].

In 2008, Dean Ornish found a significant association between comprehensive lifestyle changes (including yoga, meditation, breathing, stress management and a healthy whole-food, plant-based diet), and increased telomerase activity in human peripheral blood mononuclear cells. Of interest, the participants of this study also showed significant reductions in psychological distress and low-density lipoprotein cholesterol [81]. In 2013, a five-year follow-up study was completed on the same participants and controls. The participants were found to have persistently increased telomere length and telomerase activity over their age-matched controls. The study also compared blood samples from 2008 and 2013, evaluating both relative telomere length (RTL) and telomerase enzymatic activity per cell. Of interest, after five years, RTL was found to have increased in the lifestyle intervention group and to have decreased in the control group with the difference between the two groups as statistically significant [82]. This was the first controlled trial to show that any lifestyle intervention might lengthen telomeres over time.

Meditation has also been shown to be potentially protective regarding RTL. An intriguing study from 2013 evaluated a group of 15 subjects practicing Loving-Kindness Meditation (LKM) compared to a control group of non-meditators (n-22). LKM, or *Metta bhavana* from the Buddhist tradition, is a method of developing compassion by directing well-wishes towards others. It can be practiced by anyone, regardless of religious affiliation. It is a meditation of care, concern, friendship and compassion for oneself and others. Peripheral blood leukocytes were then measured for RTL in both groups. The LKM practitioners were found to have significantly longer RTLs than the control group, particularly for the women ($p = 0.007$). Although this study was limited by its small sample size, these results are exciting as they suggest that meditation—in particular, LKM practice—might increase RTL, a biomarker associated with aging and longevity [83].

10. Yoga and Inflammation

As noted above, inflammation is the body's natural immune response to infection, injury, and stress. However, inflammation can have serious health implications when it becomes prolonged and chronic. Chronic systemic inflammation may not be as apparent as acute inflammation, and can persist undetected at low levels for years. This can slowly damage the body, lead to the development of chronic diseases and increase one's risk for type II diabetes, atherosclerosis, cardiovascular disease, autoimmune disease and age-related diseases.

As previously discussed, yoga is beneficial for decreasing both acute and chronic stress levels. In multiple studies, yoga has been found to decrease inflammatory markers such as C-reactive protein and other inflammatory cytokines in the blood, while increasing levels of multiple immunoglobulins and natural killer cells [11,84–86]. Recent research has also shown that those who practice yoga regularly have higher levels of leptin and adiponectin in their bodies, both natural chemicals that work to alleviate inflammation in the body. Adiponectin has been found to be a key component of endothelial function and is cardioprotective [1,87,88].

A very interesting recent discovery is that even a small amount of practice may make a significant difference. A notable study by Yadav et al. in 2012 looked at how even a very brief (10-day) yoga-based lifestyle intervention can reduce the inflammatory markers of stress in patients with chronic diseases. In this trial, 86 patients (44 female/42 male) with chronic inflammatory diseases, including those who were overweight/obese received a ten-day yoga-based intervention program, including yoga asanas, pranayama and both individual and group stress management sessions. Statistically significant changes ($p < 0.05$) were seen after this short ten-day intervention with decreased cortisol, tumor necrosis factor-alpha (TNF-α) and interleukin-6 (IL-6) levels, and elevated levels of β-endorphins [89].

Another randomized, controlled clinical trial from 2014 also showed that practicing yoga for as little as three months can not only lower markers of inflammation, but can also make big differences in symptoms of fatigue in breast cancer survivors [90]. In this trial, 200 women were recruited and randomly assigned to either 12 weeks of 90-min hatha yoga classes twice per week, or a wait-list control. Breast cancer treatments were fully completed before the onset of the study.

Multiple inflammatory markers were evaluated as part of the outcome of this trial as well as multiple different surveys assessing both fatigue and depression. At three months post-treatment, comparing the yoga group to the control group, fatigue was found to be lower as well as a number of inflammatory markers such as IL-6, TNF-α and IL-1 β and scores for vitality were found to be higher (all statistically significant with $p < 0.05$) [90].

Of particular interest, this study also showed that the more yogic practices that the women did, the better their outcomes. Also significant was that the results were sustained: after six months post-intervention, both fatigue and inflammation were still lower in the intervention group as compared to controls (decreased by 57% and 20%, respectively) [90]. This suggests that yogic practices can continue to make significant sustained differences in signs and symptoms of inflammation even months later.

11. Yoga and Back Pain/Arthritis

The American College of Rheumatology states that exercise and physical activity is a necessary part of an effective treatment program for patients with both osteoarthritis and rheumatoid arthritis [91,92]. In these patients, exercise has been shown to have a vital role in promoting joint health without worsening disease. Patients suffering from arthritis who exercise regularly have less joint pain, more vitality, better sleep, reduced morning joint stiffness and improved daily living function. In particular, yoga incorporates important elements of body awareness such as proprioception, coordination, balance and postural alignment, all of which are particularly important in individuals with joint disease [93].

A comprehensive review of randomized controlled trials that evaluated yoga as an intervention for chronic low back pain (CLBP) supported the practices and found them to be efficacious on short-term improvements in functional disability [94]. In fact, yoga therapy has been shown to improve pain, back function, spinal mobility, depression and anxiety in patients with CLBP to a greater degree than physical therapy [95,96].

The largest, most rigorously conducted randomized controlled trial (RCT) of yoga and arthritis to date was published in 2015 by Moonaz et al. at Johns Hopkins University. Most importantly, this trial examined the safety, efficacy and feasibility of yoga for sedentary patients with both rheumatoid and osteoarthritis, with significant outcomes revealing important physical and mental health benefits in these individuals with regular yoga practice. After eight weeks of intervention, improvements were seen in physical pain, general health, vitality, ability to carry out Activities of Daily Living (ADLs), balance, upper body strength and mental health scales ($p < 0.05$). Of great interest, almost all benefits that were seen were still observable nine months after study completion [97].

12. Yoga and Cardiac Disease

Cardiovascular disease (CVD) encompasses a broad spectrum of syndromes, including atherosclerosis, stroke, arrhythmia, hypertension, hyperlipidemia, heart disease and peripheral vascular disease, and is the leading cause of mortality, morbidity and disability worldwide [1]. Although there have been tremendous advancements in medications, treatment plans and programs for both the prevention and treatment of CVD, there are still a number of challenges in implementation of these programs, and limitations of the treatments. Multiple risk factors are known to cause oxidative stress, leading to endothelial disruption and dysfunction. These include dyslipidemia, diabetes, hypertension, obesity, smoking and psychological stress, which can in turn start a cascade of events involving inflammatory and vasoactive mediators, in particular, interleukin-6, fibrinogen, C-reactive protein and tumor necrosis factor-alpha, that lead to the development of CVD [1]. Yoga therapy may be a significant and cost-effective therapy for CVD by interrupting a number of these different events along this cascade [1,11,88,98–100].

Of interest is a study done by Sarvottam et al. suggesting that even a short-term yoga-based program may reduce the risk for CVD. In this trial, a ten-day yoga intervention program was found to significantly reduce the body mass indices and systolic blood pressures in 51 overweight and obese men. These men were also found to have significant changes in certain inflammatory markers with decreases in IL-6 and elevation of adiponectin [88].

According to the American Heart Association, yoga practices can help to lower blood pressure, increase lung capacity, improve respiratory function and heart rate, improve circulation and boost muscle tone [101]. As previously discussed, yoga can reduce stress both by balancing the autonomic nervous system with increased parasympathetic and reduced sympathetic activities, respectively, thus optimizing and restoring the body's homeostasis (decreasing allostatic load), as well as decreasing the reactivity of the HPA axis. By decreasing both of these pathways, yoga can interrupt multiple different inflammatory events on the cascade toward CVD and enhance cardiovagal function [102].

An intriguing study by Krishna et al. in 2014 evaluated the effects of yoga therapy in patients with heart failure. Parameters including heart rate, blood pressure, heart rate variability (HRV) and rate pressure product (RPP) were measured before and after yoga intervention. As mentioned above, increased HRV is predictive of how readily the heart rate returns to normal, or quiets down, after increasing in response to a stressor—a sign of parasympathetic tone—and RRP is an index of myocardial O_2 consumption and load on the heart. Both of these are measures of cardiac autonomic function. In this trial of 130 heart failure patients, randomly assigned to receive either a yoga intervention program or standard medical therapy alone, heart rate (HR), blood pressure (BP), and measures of cardiac autonomic function were assessed before and after the 12-week intervention. The results were quite significant with p values all <0.05 regarding decreases in HR, BP and RPP in the yoga group compared to the controls. Sympathetic nervous system modulation (measured by Lfnu—low-frequency normalized unit) decreased significantly and parasympathetic nervous system modulation (measured by Hfnu—high frequency normalized unit) increased significantly as well in the intervention compared to the controls—both signs indicating improved HRV [103].

This study suggests that there could be a great benefit of yoga therapy as an adjunct to medical treatment in patients with heart failure. In addition, because it is important to consider that in patients with severe and/or decompensated heart failure physical exercise may not be well tolerated, yoga, particularly gentle asanas, breathing exercises and meditation, may be easily tolerated by these individuals [1].

As a complementary and integrative therapy, yoga for the management of hypertension has been studied in numerous randomized controlled trials. On average, the overall effect of yoga therapy results in a reduction of systolic BP of approximately 10 mmHg and approximately an 8 mmHg reduction in diastolic BP [75,104]. Of note, yoga seems to be efficacious only for hypertension, not for pre-hypertension. It is also important to recognize that at this time yoga therapy can only be recommended as an adjunct to antihypertensive pharmacological treatment, not as an alternative therapy alone. Breathing and meditation seem to be the important components of the yoga interventions as well rather than physical yoga asanas for hypertensive patients. These are the components of the yogic practice that can increase parasympathetic activity and decrease sympathetic tone, which counteracts the surplus of sympathetic activity associated with hypertension. In addition, the specific components of yoga practice may help one to self-regulate, so that the mind and body can work to bring one's physical, emotional, autonomic and psychological systems into balance, which is most critical when the body is under stress [105]. An interesting study conducted in 2013 on the effects of Iyengar yoga supports this theory. After an eight-week yoga program intervention, outcomes from surveys strongly suggested that the yoga practice helped to benefit self-regulation in terms of physical function, enriched sleep quality, dietary improvements with improved lifestyle choices, reduction of stress and anxiety and enhanced calm mental/emotional states in the study participants [106]. Despite the increasing evidence that yogic practices may reduce blood pressure, it is important to recognize that many of the studies done have also included diet modifications, exercise and/or supportive guidance and counseling—all part of the "yogic lifestyle". The exact mechanisms as to the potential benefits of yoga in controlling blood pressure remain unknown at this time. Additional rigorously controlled trials are needed to further investigate the potential benefits of yoga for improving blood pressure in those individuals with both pre-hypertension and hypertension to help determine optimal yogic practices, yoga program design and treatment plan [1,75,105,107].

Yoga therapy may also be quite useful as a complementary therapy for atrial fibrillation (AF). It is well known that the autonomic nervous system plays a pivotal role in the pathophysiology of AF, and it has been proposed that an imbalance in both the sympathetic and parasympathetic nervous systems contribute to the disease entity [108,109]. In a trial performed in 2013 by Lakkireddy et al. the impact of a three-month yoga intervention program was evaluated in 49 patients with paroxysmal AF. Both symptomatic and asymptomatic AF episodes were assessed for a three-month control period prior to the intervention, and during the intervention. Statistically significant decreases in both symptomatic and asymptomatic AF episodes were observed with p values < 0.001. Of interest, feelings of both depression and anxiety were also found to be reduced significantly in study subjects as well as improvements on several measures of quality of life including general health, physical functioning, vitality, social functioning and mental health [108]. The benefits of yoga therapy in these patients with AF are thought to be due to restoration of sympathetic and parasympathetic balance at the level of HPA axis as well as decreasing both inflammation and oxidative stress, resulting in the suppression of atrial remodeling, micro-reentry circuits and triggers for AF; however, the exact mechanism remains unknown [1,108].

13. Yoga for Pediatrics

A growing amount of evidence is showing that yoga and other mindfulness-based practices are paramount for today's children. Due to various new demands and standards in today's society, children and adolescents experience stress and mental health challenges that have not been seen in generations past. In a society exploding with technology, children now are confronted with many daily distractions and temptations, with resultant overstimulation and pressures from their peers. There are more stresses on families with reduced downtime and quiet time caused by the overscheduling of activities, overvaluing productive time and greater pressure to succeed academically. Recent research shows that the current generation of young adults is the most "stressed-out" generation, compared with their predecessors [110]. There is constant stimulation through technology, internet and social media, as well as extensive media usage by children and adolescents in today's world. Not only are children and young adults under more stress, but they also have fewer coping skills to manage these stressors. As with adults, when children internalize stress, it is often manifested physically, resulting in health issues such as insomnia, chronic abdominal pain, headaches, depression, anxiety and mood swings [103,111]. For the past number of years, schools have been cutting programs such as life skills courses and physical education classes. When these stress management skills are not learned at an early age, it only becomes harder to learn them as the children get older. Yoga may help children, adolescents and young adults cope with stress by teaching them self-regulation skills to control emotions and stress at a young age. These practices would, in turn, help their well-being and mental health, improve overall resiliency and help to positively keep their lives in balance. Yogic practices help the body to connect to the mind by helping one to focus on the present moment and clearing the mind of overwhelming thoughts. Even very young children can learn to benefit from yogic breathing techniques, which can help to calm and distract toddlers from a temper tantrum or help them to sleep. According to the National Institutes of Health, children who practice yoga have an increased sense of self-awareness and self-confidence. Concentration skills are enhanced [104,112]. These learned mind-body skills can also help a child reexamine a difficult, or even painful, experience into one that bolsters their sense of resiliency [105,113]. This, in turn, may contribute to improved attention, self-esteem, empowerment and good mental health [114–116].

According to the 2007 National Health Interview Survey (NHIS), mind-body therapies, including yoga, were the most favored complementary and alternative medicine (CAM) practices among children with behavioral, emotional or mental health problems. Per the 2012 NHIS, the use of yoga and yoga therapy in children had increased since 2007 from 2.5% to 3.2% (more than 400,000 children) [113]. Of note, older children between the ages of 13 and 17 were noted to use these mind-body therapies more often, and were more commonly used by female patients versus male patients (5.7% vs. 1.7%) [117].

Of interest, a survey taken in 2007 showed that in children and adolescents with chronic pain, over 60% of the subjects tried at least one CAM approach for pain. Of these practices, yogic practices and therapies were used by 32% as their first choice of CAM therapy [118].

Compared to research performed in adults, there is unfortunately a lack of good RCTs on the safety and efficacy of yoga among the pediatric population. In 2008, Galantino et al. performed a systematic review and found 24 studies of yoga for children which included case-control studies, pilot studies, cohort studies and RCTs. Although this review concluded that there was certainly positive evidence regarding the use of yoga in the pediatric population, more research is imperative [119,120]. Since then, there have been no recent systematic reviews of pediatric therapeutic yoga [114]; however, a growing number of RCTs are being performed. In a recent bibliometric analysis of yoga studies published between 1975 and 2014, there were 366 studies found with 31 of the studies (9.9%) including children [121]. In 2010, Kaley-Isley et al. performed a comprehensive review, and subsequently summarized applicable studies with children and adolescents treated with yoga therapy practices as an intervention. The majority of these studies showed benefit as well as very few adverse effects. Among these studies, the areas for which yoga was used for therapy in children include physical fitness, cardiac and respiratory symptoms, mental and behavioral health, developmental syndromes, irritable bowel syndrome, eating disorders including obesity, anorexia and bulimia, cancer and prenatal effects on birth outcomes [1]. In 2016, 14 individual controlled studies were evaluated, showing that yoga, as a CAM treatment and approach, appears to be an encouraging therapy and stress management intervention for children and adolescents, again with a very low rate of reported adverse effects. Yoga therapy can have significantly favorable effects on psychological and cognitive functioning, particularly in patients with emotional, mental and behavioral disorders [117]. Of note, many of the studies reviewed had methodological limitations, small sample sizes, lack of randomization and much variability between yoga practice intervention methods so that clear conclusions were not possible, and it was suggested that to obtain the most benefits from therapeutic yoga in children, more regulated research efforts are warranted [117,122].

There has been increasing interest in the use of mind-body techniques and therapies for children and adolescents with focusing, concentration and attention disorders. If yoga and mindfulness helps one to focus inward and pay attention, it would be only natural to assume that these types of therapies would be of great benefit to those who have difficulty with inattentiveness. Ideally, this increased focus would potentially increase attention naturally, even in children with challenging attention disorders.

In 2012, a systematic review of 124 trials examining the evidence for efficacy of yoga in the treatment of a number of different pediatric psychiatric disorders, of which 16 met appropriate criteria for the final review, showed emerging evidence (Grade B) to support a role for yoga in treating children with Attention Deficit and Hyperactivity Disorder (ADHD) in two RCTs [123]. Among these two RCTs was an intriguing randomized trial from 2004, published in the *Journal of Attention Disorders*, which showed that boys diagnosed with ADHD, on appropriate medication, reduced their symptoms in inattentiveness and behavior when practicing yoga regularly. In this trial, 16 boys with ADHD were randomized to receive either yoga therapy (YG) or cooperative activities (CG) in addition to their previously prescribed medications for a total of 20 weeks. The YG received one hour of hatha yoga per week along with breathing and relaxation techniques. Assessments were performed both pre- and post-intervention using the Conners' Parent and Teacher Rating Scales (CPRS and CTRS). Although there was improvement in both groups, the YG group showed significant improvement on five subscales of the CPRS. Positive changes on the CTRS were also seen in those who attended more yoga sessions and who engaged in more home practice. Although this was a small study, the trial did suggest that yoga may be a useful CAM therapy for adjunctive management, along with medical management, in children with ADHD. Larger and more collaborative studies on yoga's potential benefits for these children are needed [124].

Another trial from 2006 by Haffner et al. evaluated 19 children with ADHD and randomized them to receive either YG or conventional motor training (CG), along with their current medication regimens. The YG received 2 h of hatha yoga weekly for a period of 34 weeks. Outcome measures here included test scores on a task requiring focused attention, as well as both parent and teacher ratings of ADHD symptoms. Results from this trial revealed that the yoga training was superior to the conventional motor training. This pilot study also demonstrated that yoga can be an impressive adjunctive treatment for ADHD, though again limited by its small sample size. These researchers advocate for further research into the impact of yoga on children with ADHD [125].

What about the possibilities of yoga entering the school curriculum? It has become increasingly commonplace for large companies and offices to incorporate yoga and meditation facilities for their employees as a means to help improve concentration, refresh focus, improve motivation and counteract prolonged sitting at a desk orworkbench all work-day long. Schoolchildren, who also spend hours working and sitting all day, may benefit to the same degree.

There have been a few RCTs have evaluated the effects yoga within a school curriculum particularly in the prevention of mental health problems and enhancement of psychosocial well-being. One RCT from 2012 by Khalsa et al. studied 109 students randomly assigned to receive either an 11-week yoga education program versus regular physical education. In this trial, students were asked to self-report measures of mental health parameters including mood, anxiety, stress, and resilience both at baseline and post-intervention. Results were remarkable for statistically significant differences in measures of the students' feelings of anger control, fatigue and inertia [126]. Of note, this is one of a few trials that compares the effects of yoga to that of another form of exercise (in this case, physical education as an exercise control group). More studies comparing the yoga with standard exercise are warranted as benefits can certainly be seen for both.

Another interesting study from 2010 examined a school-based mindfulness and yoga intervention program in four inner city public schools in Baltimore, MD. Each of the schools was randomly assigned to undergo either a 12-week yoga/mindfulness intervention program or a wait-list control. Mental health parameters were also assessed in the trial including stress responses, feelings of depression, emotional arousal, control of thoughts and student social interactions. Positive outcomes were again seen in the intervention group compared to the controls in a number of these different psychological variables. Both of these studies are significant in that they suggest that mindfulness-based programs may be of great benefit for youths, especially in helping them to cope with daily stressors. In addition, both studies illustrate that a school-based mindfulness/yoga program is easily accessible, acceptable to students/staff and feasible to incorporate into schools that serve underprivileged and stressed youth [127].

A landmark study was recently performed in 2016, again in two inner-city public schools in Baltimore, MD. This large RCT examined in 300 students, randomized to receive either the Mindfulness Based Stress Reduction (MBSR) program, developed by Jon Kabat-Zinn, or a healthy education program (Healthy Topics (HT)) for an intervention period of 12 weeks. The two groups were comparable at baseline: average age was 12 years, 50.7% female, 99.7% African American, and 99% eligible for free lunch. After the 12-week intervention program, the results were quite significant with the MBSR students reporting lower levels of depression, self-hostility and other negative affective complaints than the group who received HT education ($p < 0.05$) [128]. These outcomes suggested that underprivileged, vulnerable and disadvantaged youths could significantly benefit from mindfulness-based programs in school, particularly with negative psychological symptoms and developing improved coping mechanisms for stress.

Of great significance is the impact that these positive outcomes may have as children mature—it is a well-appreciated fact that many adult diseases have their genesis in childhood, especially those due to high exposure to stress and trauma [128]. In a research review from 2014, Hagen et al. proposed that educational facilities including pre-schools, schools, and community centers offer yoga and mindfulness-based programs for children and adolescents. The authors suggested that these school-based programs may help students improve self-regulation of emotions, stress-coping skills, resiliency and overall mood. They concluded that for young people to start practicing mind-body techniques from an early age may prevent future generations from experiencing more stress in their adult lives. [114].

14. Conclusions

Ongoing research into yoga and mindfulness-based practices continues to reveal and uncover health benefits, supporting its use in health management.

Although there have been many published studies and research trials demonstrating and advocating yoga as a treatment and/or adjunct therapy for multiple disease entities, there are limitations that should be noted for a number of these studies. Many of these studies are single-center trials, have small and/or low-powered sample sizes and use non-standardized methodologies with short follow-up periods. It also should be noted that the field of yoga research encompasses the inherent dilemma of the wide variety of yogic practices used as interventional therapies. Larger, multi-centered studies using standardized yoga programs and uniform methodologies with long-term follow-up and outcomes are needed.

The practice of yoga is not as easy or as quick as taking medication, but mounting evidence suggests it is worth the effort and investment. Yoga helps one to reconnect with oneself. It can help to uncover why and how one's illness may have started, and can work with the body to start the recovery period from the ground up. The practice can help one to see how they may be reacting to the world around them, and may help them learn to respond from a different perspective. Slowing down, quieting our minds and connecting with our inner selves all help to bring one into the present moment. This can ultimately help to relieve one from the pressures and stressors from the hustle and bustle of this very busy world.

Conflicts of Interest: The author declares no conflict of interest.

References

1. Khalsa, S.B.; Cohen, L.; McCall, T.; Telles, S. *Principles and Practices of Yoga in Health Care*, 1st ed.; Handspring Publishing: Scotland, UK, 2016.
2. Hunter, D.J.; Reddy, K.S. Noncommunicable diseases. *NEJM* **2013**, *369*, 1336–1343. [CrossRef] [PubMed]
3. Miller, J.J.; Fletcher, K.; Kabat-Zinn, J. Three-year follow-up and clinical implications of a mindfulness meditation-based stress reduction intervention in the treatment of anxiety disorders. *Gen. Hosp. Psychiatry* **1995**, *17*, 192–200. [CrossRef]
4. Yadav, R.K.; Sarvottam, K.; Magan, D.; Yadav, R. A two-year follow-up case of chronic fatigue syndrome: substantial improvement in personality following a yoga-based lifestyle intervention. *Altern. Complement. Med.* **2015**, *21*, 246–249. [CrossRef] [PubMed]
5. Klainin-Yobas, P.; Oo, W.N.; Suzanne Yew, P.Y.; Lau, Y. Effects of relaxation interventions on depression and anxiety among older adults: A systematic review. *Aging Ment. Health* **2015**, *19*, 1043–1055. [CrossRef] [PubMed]
6. Amaranath, B.; Nagendra, H.R.; Deshpande, S. Effect of integrated Yoga module on positive and negative emotions in Home Guards in Bengaluru: A wait list randomized control trial. *Int. J. Yoga* **2016**, *9*, 35–43. [CrossRef] [PubMed]
7. DeBruin, E.; Formsma, A.R.; Frijstein, G.; Bogels, S.M. Mindful2Work: Effects of combined physical exercise, yoga and mindfulness meditations for stress relieve in employees. A proof of concept study. *Mindfulness* **2017**, *8*, 204–217. [CrossRef] [PubMed]
8. Danhauer, S.C.; Addington, E.L.; Sohl, S.J.; Chaoul, A.; Cohen, L. Review of yoga therapy during cancer treatment. *Support Care Cancer.* **2017**. [CrossRef] [PubMed]
9. Taimini, I.K. *The Science of Yoga: The Yoga-Sutras of Patanjali in Sanskrit*; Quest Books: New York, NY, USA, 1999.
10. Feuerstein, G. *The Yoga Tradition—Its History, Literature, Philosophy and Practice*; Hohm Press: Chino Valley, AZ, USA, 2008.
11. Penetrating Postures: The Science of Yoga. Available online: https://www.forbes.com/sites/alicegwalton/2011/06/16/penetrating-postures-the-science-of-yoga/?client=safari (accessed on 28 January 2017).

12. How Stress Cripples Your Digestive Health and Three Things to Do about It. Available online: http://www.coreconsciousliving.com/single-post/2015/06/29/How-Stress-Cripples-Your-Digestive-Health-3-Things-To-Do-About-It (accessed on 28 January 2017).
13. Stearns, M.N.; Stearns, R.N. *Yoga for Anxiety—Meditations and Practices for Calming the Body and Mind*; New Harbinger Publications, Inc.: Oakland, CA, USA, 2010.
14. Xiaoyun, L.; Li, H. The Role of Stress Regulation on Neural Plasticity in Pain Chronification. *Neural Plast.* **2016**. [CrossRef]
15. Gerra, G.; Somaini, L.; Manfredini, M.; Raggi, M.; Saracino, M.; Amore, M.; Leonardi, C.; Cortese, E.; Donnini, C. Dysregulated responses to emotions among abstinent heroin users: Correlation with childhood neglect and addiction severity. *Prog. Neuro-Psychopharmacol. Biol. Psychiatry* **2014**, *48*, 220–228. [CrossRef] [PubMed]
16. Mohd, R.S. Life event, stress and illness. *Malays. J. Med. Sci.* **2008**, *15*, 9–18.
17. Nerurkar, A.; Bitton, A.; Davis, R.; Phillips, R.; Yeh, G. When Physicians counsel about stress: Results of a National Study. *JAMA Intern. Med.* **2013**, *173*, 76–77. [CrossRef] [PubMed]
18. Nezi, M.; Mastorakos, G.; Mouslech, Z. Corticotropin Releasing Hormone and the Immune/Inflammatory Response; Endotext [Internet]; MDText.com, Inc.: South Dartmouth, MA, USA, 2000.
19. Zhao, J.; Liu, J.; Denney, J.; Li, C.; Li, F.; Chang, F.; Chen, M.; Yin, D. TLR2 Involved in Naive CD4+ T Cells Rescues Stress-Induced Immune Suppression by Regulating Th1/Th2 and Th17. *Neuroimmunomodulation* **2015**, *22*, 328–336. [CrossRef] [PubMed]
20. Morey, J.N.; Boggero, I.A.; Scott, A.B.; Segerstrom, S.C. Current Directions in Stress and Human Immune Function. *Curr. Opin. Psychol.* **2015**, *5*, 13–17. [CrossRef] [PubMed]
21. Steptoe, A.; Hamer, M.; Chida, Y. The effects of acute psychological stress on circulating inflammatory factors in humans: A review and meta-analysis. *Brain Behav. Immun.* **2007**, *21*, 901–912. [CrossRef] [PubMed]
22. Gouin, J.P.; Glaser, R.; Malarkey, W.B.; Beversdorf, D.; Kiecolt-Glaser, J. Chronic stress, daily stressors, and circulating inflammatory markers. *Health Psychol.* **2012**, *31*, 264–268. [CrossRef] [PubMed]
23. Glaser, R.; Kiecolt-Glaser, J.K. Stress-induced immune dysfunction: Implications for health. *Nat. Rev. Immunol.* **2005**, *5*, 243–251. [CrossRef] [PubMed]
24. Dhabhar, F.S. Enhancing versus Suppressive Effects of Stress on Immune Function: Implications for Immunoprotection and Immunopathology. *Neuroimmunomodulation* **2009**, *16*, 300–317. [CrossRef] [PubMed]
25. Carrion, V.G.; Wong, S.S. Can Traumatic Stress Alter the Brain? Understanding the Implications of Early Trauma on Brain Development and Learning. *J. Adolesc. Health* **2012**, *51*, S23–S28. [CrossRef] [PubMed]
26. Tomiyama, A.J.; O'Donovan, A.; Lin, J.; Puterman, E.; Lazaro, A.; Chan, J.; Dhabhar, F.S.; Wolkowitz, O.; Kirschbaum, C.; Blackburn, E.; et al. Does cellular aging relate to patterns of allostasis? An examination of basal and stress reactive HPA axis activity and telomere length. *Physiol. Behav.* **2012**, *106*, 40–45. [CrossRef] [PubMed]
27. Gotlib, I.H.; LeMoult, J.; Colich, N.L.; Foland-Ross, L.C.; Hallmayer, J.; Joormann, J.; Lin, J.; Wolkowitz, O.M. Telomere length and cortisol reactivity in children of depressed mothers. *Mol. Psychiatry* **2015**, *20*, 615–620. [CrossRef] [PubMed]
28. Carrion, V.G.; Weems, C.F.; Richert, K.; Hoffman, B.C.; Reiss, A.L. Decreased prefrontal cortical volume associated with increased bedtime cortisol in traumatized youth. *Biol. Psychiatry* **2010**, *68*, 491–493. [CrossRef] [PubMed]
29. Travis, S.G.; Coupland, N.J.; Hegadoren, K.; Silverstone, P.H.; Huang, Y.; Carter, R.; Fujiwara, E.; Seres, P.; Malykhin, N.V. Effects of cortisol on hippocampal subfields volumes and memory performance in healthy control subjects and patients with major depressive disorder. *J. Affect. Disord.* **2016**, *201*, 34–41. [CrossRef] [PubMed]
30. Reser, J.E. Chronic stress, cortical plasticity and neuroecology. *Behav. Process.* **2016**, *129*, 105–115. [CrossRef] [PubMed]
31. Moreno, G.L.; Bruss, J.; Denburg, N.L. Increased perceived stress is related to decreased prefrontal cortex volumes among older adults. *J. Clin. Exp. Neuropsychol.* **2016**, 1–13. [CrossRef] [PubMed]
32. Holzel, B.K.; Carmody, J.; Evans, K.C.; Hoge, E.A.; Dusek, J.A.; Morgan, L.; Pitman, R.K.; Lazar, S.W. Stress Reduction correlates with structural changes in the amygdala. *SCAN* **2010**, *5*, 11–17. [CrossRef] [PubMed]

33. Choi, J.; Kim, J.E.; Kim, T.K.; Park, J.Y.; Lee, J.E.; Kim, H.; Lee, E.H.; Han, P.L. TRH and TRH receptor system in the basolateral amygdala mediate stress-induced depression-like behaviors. *Neuropharmacology* **2015**, *97*, 346–356. [CrossRef] [PubMed]

34. Kim, T.K.; Han, P.L. Physical Exercise Counteracts Stress-induced Upregulation of Melanin-concentrating Hormone in the Brain and Stress-induced Persisting Anxiety-like Behaviors. *Exp. Neurobiol.* **2016**, *25*, 163–173. [CrossRef] [PubMed]

35. Tafet, G.E.; Nemeroff, C.B. The Links between Stress and Depression: Psychoneuroendocrinological, Genetic, and Environmental Interactions. *J. Neuropsychiatry Clin. Neurosci.* **2016**, *28*, 77–88. [CrossRef] [PubMed]

36. Doll, A.; Hölzel, B.K.; Mulej Bratec, S.; Boucard, C.C.; Xie, X.; Wohlschläger, A.M.; Sorg, C. Mindful attention to breath regulates emotions via increased amygdala-prefrontal cortex connectivity. *Neuroimage* **2016**, *134*, 305–313. [CrossRef] [PubMed]

37. Moriam, S.; Sobhani, M.E. Epigenetic effect of chronic stress on dopamine signaling and depression. *Genet. Epigenet.* **2013**, *5*, 11–16. [CrossRef] [PubMed]

38. Seo, J.S.; Wei, J.; Qin, L.; Kim, Y.; Yan, Z.; Greengard, P. Cellular and molecular basis for stress-induced depression. *Mol. Psychiatry* **2016**. [CrossRef] [PubMed]

39. Souza-Teodoro, L.H.; de Oliveira, C.; Walters, K.; Carvalho, L.A. Higher serum dehydroepiandrosterone sulfate protects against the onset of depression in the elderly: Findings from the English Longitudinal Study of Aging (ELSA). *Psychoneuroendocrinology* **2016**, *64*, 40–46. [CrossRef]

40. Ma, K.; Xu, A.; Cui, S.; Sun, M.R.; Xue, Y.C.; Wang, J.H. Impaired GABA synthesis, uptake and release are associated with depression-like behaviors induced by chronic mild stress. *Transl. Psychiatry* **2016**, *6*, e910. [CrossRef] [PubMed]

41. Dale, E.; Bang-Andersen, B.; Sánchez, C. Emerging mechanisms and treatments for depression beyond SSRIs and SNRIs. *Biochem. Pharmacol.* **2015**, *95*, 81–97. [CrossRef] [PubMed]

42. Usta, M.B.; Tuncel, O.K.; Akbas, S.; Aydin, B.; Say, G.N. Decreased dehydroepiandrosterone sulphate levels in adolescents with post-traumatic stress disorder after single sexual trauma. *Nord. J. Psychiatry* **2016**, *70*, 116–120. [CrossRef] [PubMed]

43. Mizoguchi, K.; Shoji, H.; Ikeda, R.; Tanaka, Y.; Tabira, T. Persistent depressive state after chronic stress in rats is accompanied by HPA axis dysregulation and reduced prefrontal dopaminergic neurotransmission. *Pharmacol. Biochem. Behav.* **2008**, *91*, 170–175. [CrossRef]

44. Shepard, R.; Page, C.E.; Coutellier, L. Sensitivity of the prefrontal GABAergic system to chronic stress in male and female mice: Relevance for sex differences in stress-related disorders. *Neuroscience* **2016**, *332*, 1–12. [CrossRef] [PubMed]

45. McKlveen, J.M.; Morano, R.L.; Fitzgerald, M.; Zoubovsky, S.; Cassella, S.N.; Scheimann, J.R.; Ghosal, S.; Mahbod, P.; Packard, B.A.; Myers, B.; et al. Chronic Stress Increases Prefrontal Inhibition: A Mechanism for Stress-Induced Prefrontal Dysfunction. *Biol. Psychiatry* **2016**, *80*, 754–764. [CrossRef] [PubMed]

46. Payne, P.; Crane-Godreau, M.A. Meditative movement for depression and anxiety. *Front. Psychiatry* **2013**, *4*, 71. [CrossRef] [PubMed]

47. Brown, R.P.; Gerbar, P.L. Sudarshan Kriya yogic breathing in the treatment of stress, anxiety and depression: Part 1—Neurophysiologic model. *J. Altern. Complement. Med.* **2005**, *11*, 189–201. [CrossRef] [PubMed]

48. Telles, S.; Sharma, S.K.; Balkrishna, A. Blood pressure and heart rate variability during yoga-based alternate nostril breathing practice and breath awareness. *Med. Sci. Mont. Basic Res.* **2014**, *20*, 184–193.

49. Torner, L.; Toschi, N.; Nava, G.; Clapp, C.; Neumann, L.D. Incresaed hypothalamic expression of prolactin in lactation: Involvement in behavioural and neuroendocrine stress responses. *Eur. J. Neurosci.* **2002**, *15*, 1381–1389. [CrossRef] [PubMed]

50. Thirthalli, J.; Naveen, G.H.; Rao, M.G.; Varambally, S.; Christopher, R.; Gangadhar, B.N. Cortisol and antidepressant effects of yoga. *Indian J. Psychiatry* **2013**, *55*, S405–S408. [CrossRef] [PubMed]

51. Naveen, G.H.; Varambally, S.; Thirthalli, J.; Rao, M.; Christopher, R.; Gangadhar, B. Serum cortisol and BDNF in patients with major depression-effect of yoga. *Int. Rev. Psychiatry* **2016**, *28*, 273–278. [CrossRef] [PubMed]

52. Riley, K.E.; Park, C.L. How does yoga reduce stress? A systematic review of mechanisms of change and guide to future inquiry. *Health Psychol. Rev.* **2015**, *9*, 379–396. [CrossRef] [PubMed]

53. Davidson, R.; Lutz, A. Buddha's Brain: Neuroplasticity and Meditation. *IEEE Signal Process. Mag.* **2008**, *25*, 176–174. [CrossRef] [PubMed]

54. Davidson, R.; Kabat-Zinn, J.; Schumacher, J.; Rosenkranz, M.; Muller, D.; Santorelli, S.; Urbanowski, F.; Harrington, A.; Bonus, K.; Sheridan, J. Alterations in Brain and Immune Function Produced by Mindfulness Meditation. *Psychosom. Med.* **2003**, *65*, 564–570. [CrossRef] [PubMed]
55. Ricard, M.; Lutz, A.; Davidson, R. Mind of the Meditator. *Sci. Am.* **2014**, *311*, 38–45. [CrossRef] [PubMed]
56. Hernández, S.E.; Suero, J.; Barros, A.; González-Mora, J.L.; Rubia, K. Increased Grey Matter Associated with Long-Term Sahaja Yoga Meditation: A Voxel-Based Morphometry Study. *PLoS ONE* **2016**, *11*, e0150757. [CrossRef] [PubMed]
57. Deepeshwar, S.; Vinchurkar, S.A.; Visweswaraiah, N.K.; Nagendra, H.R. Hemodynamic responses on prefrontal cortex related to meditation and attentional task. *Front. Syst. Neurosci.* **2015**, *8*, 252. [CrossRef] [PubMed]
58. Villemure, C.; Čeko, M.; Cotton, V.A.; Bushnell, M.C. Neuroprotective effects of yoga practice: Age-, experience-, and frequency-dependent plasticity. *Front. Hum. Neurosci.* **2015**, *9*, 281. [CrossRef] [PubMed]
59. Taliaz, D.; Loya, A.; Gersner, R.; Haramati, S.; Chen, A.; Zangen, A. Resilience to chronic stress is mediated by hippocampal brain-derived neurotrophic factor. *J. Neurosci.* **2011**, *31*, 4475–4483. [CrossRef] [PubMed]
60. Hariprasad, V.R.; Varambally, S.; Shivakumar, V.; Kalmady, S.V.; Venkatasubramanian, G.; Gangadhar, B.N. Yoga increases the volume of the hippocampus in elderly subjects. *Indian J. Psychiatry* **2013**, *55*, S394–S396. [PubMed]
61. Engström, M.; Pihlsgård, J.; Lundberg, P.; Söderfeldt, B. Functional magnetic resonance imaging of hippocampal activation during silent mantra meditation. *J. Altern. Complement. Med.* **2010**, *16*, 1253–1258. [CrossRef] [PubMed]
62. Van Rooij, S.J.; Stevens, J.S.; Ely, T.D.; Fani, N.; Smith, A.K.; Kerley, K.A.; Lori, A.; Ressler, K.J.; Jovanovic, T. Childhood Trauma and COMT Genotype Interact to Increase Hippocampal Activation in Resilient Individuals. *Front. Psychiatry* **2016**, *7*, 156. [CrossRef] [PubMed]
63. Desbordes, G.; Negi, L.T.; Pace, T.W.; Wallace, B.A.; Raison, C.L.; Schwartz, E.L. Effects of mindful-attention and compassion meditation training on amygdala response to emotional stimuli in an ordinary, non-meditative state. *Front. Hum. Neurosci.* **2012**, *6*, 292. [CrossRef] [PubMed]
64. Tang, Y.Y.; Hölzel, B.K.; Posner, M.I. The neuroscience of mindfulness meditation. *Nat. Rev. Neurosci.* **2015**, *16*, 213–225. [CrossRef] [PubMed]
65. Hilton, L.; Maher, A.R.; Colaiaco, B.; Apaydin, E.; Sorbero, M.E.; Booth, M.; Shanman, R.M.; Hempel, S. Meditation for Posttraumatic Stress: Systematic Review and Meta-analysis. *Psychol. Trauma* **2016**. [CrossRef] [PubMed]
66. *CADTH Rapid Response Reports. Mindfulness Interventions for the Treatment of Post-Traumatic Stress Disorder, Generalized Anxiety Disorder, Depression, and Substance Use Disorders: A Review of the Clinical Effectiveness and Guidelines*; Canadian Agency for Drugs and Technologies in Health: Ottawa, ON, USA, 2015.
67. Bhavanani, A.B.; Udupa, K.; Madanmohan Ravindra, P. A comparative study of slow and fast suryanamaskar on physiological function. *Int. J. Yoga* **2011**, *4*, 71–76. [CrossRef]
68. Sinha, B.; Ray, U.S.; Pathak, A.; Selvamurthy, W. Energy cost and cardiorespiratory changes during the practice of Surya Namaskar. *Indian J. Physiol. Pharmacol.* **2004**, *48*, 184–190. [PubMed]
69. Godse, A.S.; Shejwal, B.R.; Godse, A.A. Effects of suryanamaskar on relaxation among college students with high stress in Pune, India. *Int. J. Yoga* **2015**, *8*, 15–21. [CrossRef] [PubMed]
70. Harinath, K.; Malhotra, A.S.; Pal, K.; Prasad, R.; Kumar, R.; Kain, T.C.; Rai, L.; Sawhney, R.C. Effects of Hatha yoga and Omkar meditation on cardiorespiratory performance, psychologic profile, and melatonin secretion. *J. Altern. Complement. Med.* **2004**, *10*, 261–268. [CrossRef] [PubMed]
71. Tooley, G.A.; Armstrong, S.M.; Norman, T.R.; Sali, A. Acute increases in night-time plasma melatonin levels following a period of meditation. *Biol. Psychol.* **2000**, *53*, 69–78. [CrossRef]
72. Jayaram, N.; Varambally, S.; Behere, R.V.; Venkatasubramanian, G.; Arasappa, R.; Christopher, R.; Gangadhar, B.N. Effect of yoga therapy on plasma oxytocin and facial emotion recognition deficits in patients of schizophrenia. *Indian J. Psychiatry* **2013**, *55*, S409–S413. [PubMed]
73. Streeter, C.C.; Gerbarg, P.L.; Saper, R.B.; Ciraulo, D.A.; Brown, R.P. Effects of yoga on the autonomic nervous system, gamma-aminobutyric-acid, and allostasis in epilepsy, depression, and post-traumatic stress disorder. *Med. Hypotheses* **2012**, *78*, 571–579. [CrossRef] [PubMed]

74. Lipschitz, D.L.; Kuhn, R.; Kinney, A.Y.; Grewen, K.; Donaldson, G.W.; Nakamura, Y. An Exploratory Study of the Effects of Mind-Body Interventions Targeting Sleep on Salivary Oxytocin Levels in Cancer Survivors. *Integr. Cancer Ther.* **2015**, *14*, 366–380. [CrossRef] [PubMed]

75. Cramer, H. The Efficacy and Safety of Yoga in Managing Hypertension. *Exp. Clin. Endocrinol. Diabetes* **2016**, *124*, 65–70. [CrossRef] [PubMed]

76. Guglietti, C.L.; Daskalakis, Z.J.; Radhu, N.; Fitzgerald, P.B.; Ritvo, P. Meditation-related increases in GABAB modulated cortical inhibition. *Brain Stimul.* **2013**, *6*, 397–402. [CrossRef] [PubMed]

77. Streeter, C.C.; Jensen, J.E.; Perlmutter, R.M.; Cabral, H.J.; Tian, H.; Terhune, D.B.; Ciraulo, D.A.; Renshaw, P.F. Yoga Asana Sessions Increase Brain GABA Levels. *J. Altern. Complement. Med.* **2007**, *13*, 419–426. [CrossRef] [PubMed]

78. Streeter, C.C.; Whitfield, T.H.; Owen, L.; Rein, T.; Karri, S.K.; Yakhkind, A.; Perlmutter, R.; Prescot, A.; Renshaw, P.F.; Ciraulo, D.A.; et al. Effects of yoga versus walking on mood, anxiety, and brain GABA levels: A randomized controlled MRS study. *J. Altern. Complement. Med.* **2010**, *16*, 1145–1152. [CrossRef] [PubMed]

79. Naveen, G.H.; Thirthalli, J.; Rao, M.G.; Varambally, S.; Christopher, R.; Gangadhar, B.N. Positive therapeutic and neurotropic effects of yoga in depression: A comparative study. *Indian J. Psychiatry* **2013**, *55*, S400–S404. [PubMed]

80. Epel, E.S.; Blackburn, E.H.; Lin, J.; Dhabhar, F.S.; Adler, N.E.; Morrow, J.D.; Cawthon, R.M. Accelerated telomere shortening in response to life stress. *Proc. Natl. Acad. Sci. USA* **2004**, *101*, 17312–17315. [CrossRef]

81. Ornish, D.; Lin, J.; Daubenmier, J.; Weidner, G.; Epel, E.; Kemp, C.; Magbanua, M.; Marlin, R.; Yglecias, L.; Carroll, P.; et al. Increased telomerase activity and comprehensive lifestyle changes: A pilot study. *Lancet Oncol.* **2008**, *9*, 1048–1057. [CrossRef]

82. Ornish, D.; Lin, J.; Chan, J.M.; Epel, E.; Kemp, C.; Weidner, G.; Marlin, R.; Frenda, S.J.; Magbanua, M.J.; Daubenmier, J.; et al. Effect of comprehensive lifestyle changes on telomerase activity and telomere length in men with biopsy-proven low-risk prostate cancer: 5-year follow-up of a descriptive pilot study. *Lancet Oncol.* **2013**, *14*, 1112–1120. [CrossRef]

83. Hoge, E.A.; Chen, M.M.; Orr, E.; Metcalf, C.A.; Fischer, L.E.; Pollack, M.H.; de Vivo, I.; Simon, N.M. Loving-Kindness Meditation practice associated with longer telomeres in women. *Brain Behav. Immun.* **2013**, *32*, 159–163. [CrossRef] [PubMed]

84. Ross, A.; Thomas, S. The health benefits of yoga and exercise: A review of comparison studies. *J. Altern. Complement. Med.* **2010**, *16*, 3–12. [CrossRef] [PubMed]

85. Infante, J.R.; Peran, F.; Rayo, J.I.; Serrano, J.; Domínguez, M.L.; Garcia, L.; Duran, C.; Roldan, A. Levels of immune cells in transcendental meditation practitioners. *Int. J. Yoga* **2014**, *7*, 147–151. [CrossRef] [PubMed]

86. Bhargav, H.; Metri, K.; Raghuram, N.; Ramarao, N.H.; Koka, P.S. Enhancement of cancer stem cell susceptibility to conventional treatments through complementary yoga therapy: Possible cellular and molecular mechanisms. *J. Stem Cells* **2012**, *7*, 261–267. [PubMed]

87. Kiecolt-Glaser, J.K.; Christian, L.M.; Andridge, R.; Hwang, B.S.; Malarkey, W.B.; Belury, M.A.; Emery, C.F.; Glaser, R. Adiponectin, leptin, and yoga practice. *Physiol. Behav.* **2012**, *107*, 809–813. [CrossRef] [PubMed]

88. Sarvottam, K.; Magan, D.; Yadav, R.K.; Mehta, N.; Mahapatra, S.C. Adiponectin, interleukin-6, and cardiovascular disease risk factors are modified by a short-term yoga-based lifestyle intervention in overweight and obese men. *J. Altern. Complement. Med.* **2013**, *19*, 397–402. [CrossRef] [PubMed]

89. Yadav, R.K.; Magan, D.; Mehta, N.; Sharma, R.; Mahapatra, S.C. Efficacy of a short-term yoga-based lifestyle intervention in reducing stress and inflammation: Preliminary results. *J. Altern. Complement. Med.* **2012**, *18*, 662–667. [CrossRef] [PubMed]

90. Kiecolt-Glaser, J.K.; Bennett, J.M.; Andridge, R.; Peng, J.; Shapiro, C.L.; Malarkey, W.B.; Emery, C.F.; Layman, R.; Mrozek, E.E.; Glaser, R. Yoga's impact on inflammation, mood, and fatigue in breast cancer survivors: A randomized controlled trial. *J. Clin. Oncol.* **2014**, *32*, 1040–1049. [CrossRef] [PubMed]

91. Hochberg, M.C.; Altman, R.D.; April, K.T.; Benkhalt, M.; Guyatt, G.; McGowan, J.; Towheed, T.; Welch, V.; Wells, G.; Tugwell, P. American College of Rheumatology 2012 Recommendations for the Use of Nonpharmacologic and Pharmacologic Therapies in Osteoarthritis of the Hand, Hip, and Knee. *Arthritis Care Res.* **2012**, *64*, 465–474. [CrossRef]

92. Stenström, C.H.; Minor, M.A. Evidence for the benefit of aerobic and strengthening exercise in rheumatoid arthritis. *Arthritis Care Res.* **2003**, *49*, 428–434. [CrossRef] [PubMed]

93. Exercise and Arthritis. Available online: http://www.rheumatology.org/I-Am-A/Patient-Caregiver/ Diseases-Conditions/Living-Well-with-Rheumatic-Disease/Exercise-and-Arthritis#sthash.2dxYmjdw. dpufRA (accessed on 30 January 2017).

94. Holtzman, S.; Beggs, R.T. Yoga for chronic low back pain: A meta-analysis of randomized controlled trials. *Pain Res. Manag.* **2013**, *18*, 267–272. [CrossRef] [PubMed]

95. Tilbrook, H.E.; Cox, H.; Hewitt, C.E.; Kang'ombe, A.R.; Chuang, L.H.; Jayakody, S.; Aplin, J.D.; Semlyen, A.; Trewhela, A.; Watt, I.; et al. Yoga for chronic low back pain: A randomized trial. *Ann. Intern. Med.* **2011**, *155*, 569–578. [CrossRef] [PubMed]

96. Tekur, P.; Nagarathna, R.; Chametcha, S.; Hankey, A.; Nagendra, H.R. A comprehensive yoga programs improves pain, anxiety and depression in chronic low back pain patients more than exercise: An RCT. *Complement. Ther. Med.* **2012**, *20*, 107–118. [CrossRef] [PubMed]

97. Moonaz, S.H.; Bingham, C.O., 3rd; Wissow, L.; Bartlett, S.J. Yoga in Sedentary Adults with Arthritis: Effects of a Randomized Controlled Pragmatic Trial. *J. Rheumatol.* **2015**, *42*, 1194–1202. [CrossRef] [PubMed]

98. Chu, P.; Pandya, A.; Salomon, J.A.; Goldie, S.J.; Hunink, M.G. Comparative Effectiveness of Personalized Lifestyle Management Strategies for Cardiovascular Disease Risk Reduction. *J. Am. Heart Assoc.* **2016**, *5*, e002737. [CrossRef] [PubMed]

99. Manchanda, S.C. Yoga—A promising technique to control cardiovascular disease. *Indian Heat Assoc.* **2014**, *66*, 487–489. [CrossRef] [PubMed]

100. Dzau, V.J.; Antman, E.M.; Black, H.R.; Manson, J.E.; Plutzky, J.; Popma, J.J.; Stevenson, W. The cardiovascular disease continuum validated: Clinical evidence of improved patient outcomes: Part 1: Pathophysiology and clinical trial evidence (risk factors through stable coronary artery disease). *Circulation* **2006**, *114*, 2850–2870. [CrossRef] [PubMed]

101. Yoga and Heart Health. Available online: http://www.heart.org/HEARTORG/HealthyLiving/PhysicalActivity/ Yoga-and-Heart-Health_UCM_434966_Article.jsp# (accessed on 31 January 2017).

102. Innes, K.E.; Bourguignon, C.; Taylor, A.G. Risk indices associated with the insulin resistance syndrome, cardiovascular disease, and possible protection with yoga: A systematic review. *J. Am. Board Fam. Med.* **2005**, *18*, 491–519. [CrossRef]

103. Krishna, B.H.; Pal, P.; Pal, G.; Balachander, J.; Jayasettiaseelon, E.; Sreekanth, Y.; Sridhar, M.; Gaur, G. Effect of yoga therapy on heart rate, blood pressure and cardiac autonomic function in heart failure. *J. Clin. Diagn. Res.* **2014**, *8*, 14–16. [PubMed]

104. Thiyagarajan, R.; Pal, P.; Pal, G.K.; Subramanian, S.K.; Trakroo, M.; Bobby, Z.; Das, A.K. Additional benefit of yoga to standard lifestyle modification on blood pressure in prehypertensive subjects: A randomized controlled study. *Hypertens. Res.* **2015**, *38*, 48–55. [CrossRef] [PubMed]

105. Gard, T.; Noggle, J.J.; Park, C.L.; Vago, D.R.; Wilson, A. Potential self-regulatory mechanisms of yoga for psychological health. *Front. Hum. Neurosci.* **2014**, *8*, 770. [CrossRef] [PubMed]

106. Alexander, G.K.; Innes, K.E.; Selfe, T.K.; Brown, C.J. "More than I expected"; perceived benefits of yoga practice among older adults at risk for cardiovascular disease. *Complement. Ther. Med.* **2013**, *21*, 14–28. [CrossRef] [PubMed]

107. Hagins, M.; States, R.; Selfe, T.; Innes, K. Effectiveness of Yoga for Hypertension: Systematic Review and Meta-Analysis. *Evid. Based Complement. Altern. Med.* **2013**. [CrossRef] [PubMed]

108. Lakkireddy, D.; Atkins, D.; Pillarisetti, J.; Ryschon, K.; Bommana, S.; Drisko, J.; Vanga, S.; Dawn, B. Effect of yoga on arrhythmia burden, anxiety, depression, and quality of life in paroxysmal atrial fibrillation: The YOGA My Heart Study. *Am. Coll. Cardiol.* **2013**, *61*, 1177–1182. [CrossRef] [PubMed]

109. Mearns, B.M. Arrhythmias: Benefits of yoga in patients with atrial fibrillation. *Nat. Rev. Cardiol.* **2013**, *10*, 182. [CrossRef] [PubMed]

110. Sifferlin, A. The Most Stressed-Out Generation? Young Adults (2013). Available online: http://healthland. time.com/2013/02/07/the-most-stressed-out-generation-young-adults/ (accessed on 25 January 2017).

111. Yoga for Kids: How to Calm Little Minds. Available online: http://www.todaysparent.com/family/family- health/yoga-for-kids-how-to-calm-little-minds/ (accessed on 21 December 2016).

112. The Benefits of Yoga for Kids, One Downward Dog at a Time. Available online: http://www.good2grow.com/ healthy-living-library/the-benefits-of-yoga-for-kids-one-downward-dog-at-a-time#sthash.2nc91QVF.dpuf (accessed on 21 December 2016).

113. Rosen, L.; French, A.; Sullivan, G. Complementary, Holistic, and Integrative. *Pediatr. Rev.* **2015**, *36*, 468. [CrossRef] [PubMed]
114. Hagen, I.; Nayar, U.S. Yoga for Children and Young People's Mental Health and Well-Being: Research Review and Reflections on the Mental Health Potentials of Yoga. *Front. Psychiatry* **2014**, *5*, 35. [CrossRef] [PubMed]
115. Khalsa, S.B.S. Yoga in Schools Research: Improving Mental and Emotional Health. In Proceedings of the Second International Conference on Yoga for Health and Social Transformation, Haridwar, India, 7–10 January 2013.
116. Khalsa, S.B.; Butzer, B. Yoga in school settings: A research review. *Ann. N. Y. Acad. Sci.* **2016**, *1373*, 45–55. [CrossRef] [PubMed]
117. Vohra, S.; McClafferty, H. Mind-Body Therapies in Children and Youth, Section on integrative medicine. *Pediatrics* **2016**, *138*, e20161896.
118. Tsao, J.C.; Meldrum, M.; Kim, S.C.; Jacob, M.C.; Zeltzer, L.K. Treatment preferences for CAM in children with chronic pain. *Evid. Based Complement. Altern. Med.* **2007**, *4*, 367–374. [CrossRef] [PubMed]
119. Birdee, G.S.; Yeh, G.Y.; Wayne, P.M.; Phillips, R.S.; Davis, R.B.; Gardiner, P. Clinical Applications of Yoga for the Pediatric Population: A Systematic Review. *Acad. Pediatr.* **2009**, *9*, 212–220. [CrossRef] [PubMed]
120. Galantino, M.L.; Galbavy, R.; Quinn, L. Therapeutic effects of yoga for children: A systematic review of the literature. *Pediatr. Phys. Ther.* **2008**, *20*, 66–80. [CrossRef]
121. Cramer, H.; Lauche, R.; Dobos, G. Characteristics of randomized controlled trials of yoga: A bibliometric analysis. *BMC Complement. Altern. Med.* **2014**, *14*, 328. [CrossRef] [PubMed]
122. Kaley-Isley, L.C.; Peterson, J.; Fischer, C.; Peterson, E. Yoga as a Complementary Therapy for Children and Adolescents: A Guide for Clinicians. *Psychiatry* **2010**, *7*, 20–32. [PubMed]
123. Balasubramaniam, M.; Telles, S.; Doraiswamy, P.M. Yoga on Our Minds: A Systematic Review of Yoga for Neuropsychiatric Disorders. *Front. Psychiatry* **2012**, *3*, 117. [CrossRef] [PubMed]
124. Jensen, P.S.; Kenny, D.T. The effects of yoga on the attention and behavior of boys with Attention-Deficit/hyperactivity Disorder (ADHD). *J. Atten. Disord.* **2004**, *7*, 205–216. [CrossRef] [PubMed]
125. Haffner, J.; Roos, J.; Goldstein, N.; Parzer, P.; Resch, F. The effectiveness of body-oriented methods of therapy in the treatment of attention-deficit hyperactivity disorder (ADHD): Results of a controlled pilot study. *Z. Kinder Jugendpsychiatr. Psychother.* **2006**, *34*, 37–47. [CrossRef] [PubMed]
126. Khalsa, S.B.; Hickey-Schultz, L.; Cohen, D.; Steiner, N.; Cope, S. Evaluation of the mental health benefits of yoga in a secondary school: A preliminary randomized controlled trial. *J. Behav. Health Serv. Res.* **2012**, *39*, 80–90. [CrossRef] [PubMed]
127. Mendelson, T.; Greenberg, M.; Dariotis, J.; Feagans Gould, L.; Rhoades, B.; Leaf, P. Feasibility and Preliminary Outcomes of a School-Based Mindfulness Intervention for Urban Youth. *J. Abnorm. Child Psychol.* **2010**, *38*, 985–994. [CrossRef] [PubMed]
128. Sibinga, E.; Webb, L.; Ghazarian, S.; Ellen, J. School-Based Mindfulness Instruction: An RCT. *Pediatrics* **2016**, *137*. [CrossRef] [PubMed]

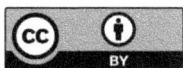

![children logo] *children*

MDPI

Article

Do Mothers Benefit from a Child-Focused Cognitive Behavioral Treatment (CBT) for Childhood Functional Abdominal Pain? A Randomized Controlled Pilot Trial

Claudia Calvano [1], Martina Groß [2] and Petra Warschburger [1,*]

[1]   Counseling Psychology, University of Potsdam, Potsdam 14469, Germany; calvano@uni-potsdam.de
[2]   Deutsche Morbus Crohn/Colitis ulcerosa Vereinigung (DCCV e.V.), Berlin 10179, Germany; mgross@dccv.de
*   Correspondence: warschb@uni-potsdam.de; Tel.: +49-331-977-2988

Academic Editor: Hilary McClafferty
Received: 13 December 2016; Accepted: 6 February 2017; Published: 15 February 2017

Abstract: While the efficacy of cognitive-behavioral treatment (CBT) approaches for childhood functional abdominal pain (FAP) is well-established for child outcomes, only a few studies have reported on parent-specific outcomes. This randomized controlled pilot trial analyzed effects of a group CBT on maternal variables (i.e., pain-related behavior, worries and self-efficacy, as well as general psychosocial strain). *Methods*: The sample constituted of 15 mothers in the intervention group (IG) and 14 mothers in the waitlist control group (WLC). Outcome measures were assessed pre-treatment, post-treatment and at three months follow-up. *Results*: Analyses revealed significant, large changes in maladaptive maternal reactions related to the child's abdominal pain in the IG compared to the WLC—i.e., reduced attention ($d = 0.95$), medical help-seeking ($d = 0.92$), worries ($d = 1.03$), as well as a significant increase in behaviors that encourage the child's self-management ($d = 1.03$). In addition, maternal self-efficacy in dealing with a child's pain significantly increased in the IG as well ($d = 0.92$). Treatment effects emerged post-treatment and could be maintained until three months follow-up. There were no effects on general self-efficacy and maternal quality of life. *Conclusion*: While these results are promising, and underline the efficacy of the CBT approach for both the child and mothers, further studies, including long-term follow-ups, are warranted.

Keywords: functional abdominal pain; parents; CBT; behavior; self-efficacy; RCT; waitlist control

1. Introduction

Functional abdominal pain (FAP) is very prevalent in childhood [1], highly impairing [2] and persistent when untreated [3]. Not only do the children suffer from increased psychological distress [4,5] and a poor health-related quality of life [6,7], childhood FAP also affects the family functioning and is commonly associated with parental stress [8]. Furthermore, literature suggests that parents often influence a child's coping and course of abdominal pain [8,9] therefore a parent's reaction when the child experiences pain can be pivotal. This is especially true for parental protective behaviors, such as excusing the child from school or household chores and increased attention when their child is in pain—which are often seen as maladaptive behaviors—and can be associated with a child's impairment [10–12] and increased healthcare use due to abdominal pain [13].

Current literature reports that a significant number of parents experience high psychological strain and a poor quality of life [14–16]. Taking this into account, analyses of treatment effects on parents' psychosocial well-being should be of interest to researchers as well. The efficacy of cognitive behavioral treatment (CBT) approaches for FAP, in reducing a child's pain and disability, is well-established [17–20]. Despite the critical role parents play in pediatric pain, comparatively few data exist focusing on parent-specific outcomes in relation to these approaches [21,22]. Results from controlled trials have suggested that significant effects on parental protective behavior and threat beliefs can be seen up to 12 months post-intervention [23–25]. A short-term improvement of maladaptive parental responses was also reported [25]. However, thus far, there is no data analyzing the effects on parents' self-efficacy, which can be an important mediating mechanism underlying behavioral changes [26,27]. In pediatric pain research, self-efficacy refers to the perceived competence in dealing with pain in everyday life [28]. Analyzing this construct may extend current knowledge on parent-specific treatment effects [22] and could identify possible mediators for long-term sustenance of change.

This report aims to fill these gaps by analyzing the effects of an outpatient, manualized CBT group for children suffering from FAP (described in [29]), on the mothers' behavior, worries, self-efficacy and quality of life. Data are derived from a randomized controlled trial (RCT) that included a waitlist control group (WLC) and three months follow-up. Positive, large-sized effects on self-reported pain, coping and health-related quality of life were observed in the children's outcomes [30,31]. In line with these favorable effects on the affected children, we hypothesize that the mothers in the intervention group (IG) compared to the WLC, will report a more pronounced reduction of child's pain and gastrointestinal (GI) symptoms.

Additionally, we hypothesize that mothers in the IG compared to the WLC will show a more pronounced reduction in: (1) attention, protective behavior, medical help-seeking; in (2) pain-related worries; and a more pronounced increase in (3) behavior encouraging child's self-management; and in (4) their self-efficacy in dealing with the child's pain. In an exploratory manner, we will analyze whether positive changes will also be observed in the mothers' general self-efficacy and quality of life.

2. Materials and Methods

2.1. Study Design and Procedure

The study is a prospective RCT with a parallel waitlist design for the evaluation of a group cognitive behavioral program for children aged 6–12 years suffering from FAP (Current Controlled Trials registration ISRCTN 69830258). Figure 1 displays the RCT flow chart, which follows CONSORT guidelines. The complete CONSORT checklist is provided (Table S1) as an online supplementary document. Eligible families were recruited from an epidemiological study on the psychological well-being of primary school children over a 15-month period (recruitment: April 2008–July 2009). Eligibility criteria for further medical and psychological examination referred to the children, and were defined as the occurrence of chronic abdominal pain at least once a week and lack of organic findings which could account for the symptoms. The 144 eligible cases were invited for further examination to confirm self-reported questionnaire data. This included referring the child for a medical examination for the diagnosis of pediatric FAP and a psychological examination by a standardized diagnostic parent interview [32] to eliminate the possibility that the child fulfills criteria for a psychiatric disorder, according to ICD-10. For pain symptomatology, Rome-III diagnosis of Functional Abdominal Pain Syndrome (FAPS) [33] had to be fulfilled. Diagnosis of FAPS, according to Rome III, requires abdominal pain at least once per week for at least two months, along with associated impairment in everyday life or occurrence of other bodily complaints. A detailed description of the study design can be found in previous publications by the authors [30,31].

In total, 29 families were included and randomized to either the IG ($n = 15$) or the WLC ($n = 14$), applying a 1:1 allocation ratio. A computer-assisted randomization sequence was generated, with no restriction, and conducted by a person not involved in the study, and one of the authors enrolled the participants and assigned them to interventions based on the randomization results. Due to the waitlist control design, blinding was not possible. Data were collected at diagnostic examination (T0), two weeks pre-treatment (T1), 2 weeks post-treatment (T2) and 3 months post-treatment (T3). Data collection, as well as the intervention, took place in the outpatient Patient Training Center (PTC) for chronically ill children and their parents, associated with the Counseling Psychology Department of the University of Potsdam, over a 20-month period (interventions: April 2008–December 2009). In the IG, four groups were conducted consecutively. One child in the IG dropped out after the second child session due to an injury (broken leg) and the family did not participate any longer in the training program (the parents did not take part in the parent session, which was scheduled after the third child session) [29]. The participants in the WLC were offered a participation in the training program, only after completion of T3 assessments, which was approximately five months after inclusion. The study was approved by the Ethics Committee of the University of Potsdam.

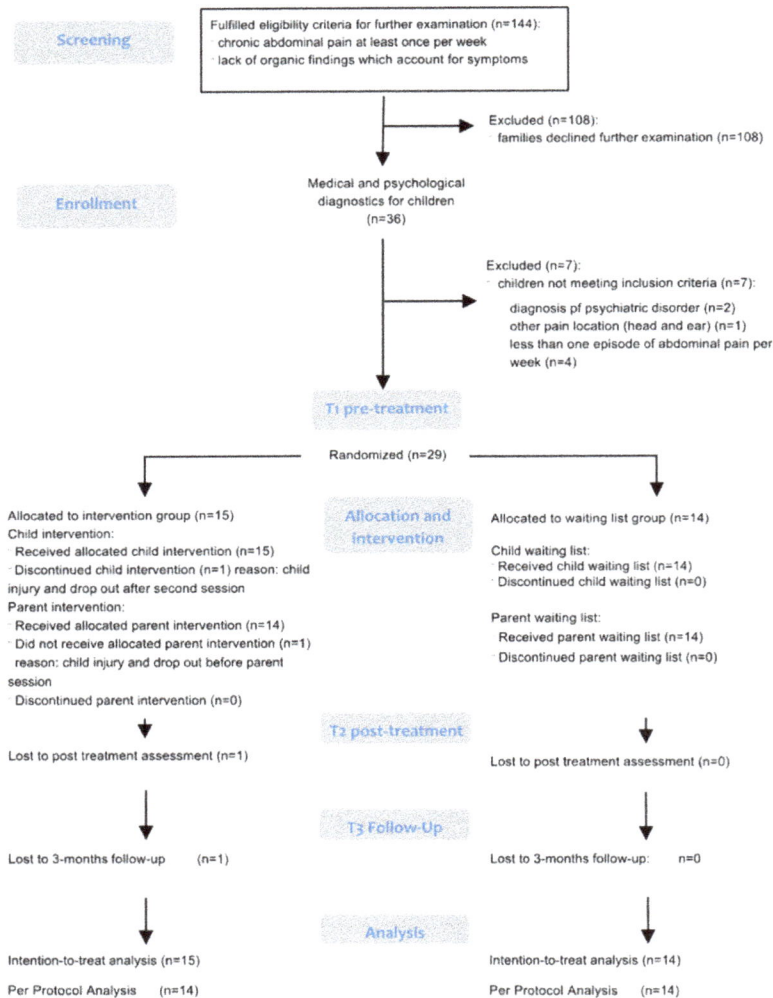

Figure 1. Trial flow chart. Adapted and extended for parent analysis from [31].

2.2. Intervention

Families assigned to the IG received the manualized, cognitive-behavioral, child-centered group intervention entitled "Stop the pain with Happy Pingu" [29], including six group sessions for the children (weekly; each 90 min) and one parent group session (90 min). The primary aim of the training was to enhance the children's self-management skills to cope with their pain. In order to attain this goal, children participated alone in the sessions without their parents, learned different skills to cope with their pain and were encouraged to do their regular homework (relaxation and practice of coping skills) on their own. In particular, children were instructed to apply cognitive-behavioral techniques, such as progressive muscle relaxation, distraction, cognitive restructuring and stopping negative thoughts [29,31].

The main goal of the parent session was to foster trust in the new competencies that the child had acquired. Parents received detailed information about the contents of the preceding sessions with the children and the biopsychosocial disease model underlying the intervention. Thereby, parents were asked to reflect on their own role in maintaining the disorder. The group training allowed the mutual exchange of personal experiences and the discussion of potential maladaptive reactions. In particular, parents were encouraged to rely on the competencies the child had learned and to support their child to implement these skills in their pain-coping activities. This was based on a mutual exchange led by the trainer, not on practices of behavioral responses. In addition, parents were informed how to recognize clinical alarm signals, according to the recommendations of the Subcommittee on Chronic Abdominal Pain in Children [34]. Since carbohydrate malabsorptions are common concerns in children suffering from FAP, nutritional guidelines were discussed, with the focus on a balanced diet [29]. This part of the parent session was conducted by a nutrition scientist, with the remaining contents, as well as the child sessions, conducted by one of the authors.

2.3. Measures

For this study, primary outcomes refer to pain-related measures (i.e., parental perception of pain and GI symptoms, parent's behavior, worries and self-efficacy). Secondary outcomes refer to general self-efficacy and the parent's quality of life. In addition, treatment satisfaction in the IG was also assessed. Except for the demographic and socioeconomic measures (T0), primary and secondary outcome data were assessed pre-treatment (T1), post-treatment (T2) and at 3 months follow-up (T3). Parents of the intervention group reported on treatment satisfaction for the intervention at post-treatment (T2).

2.3.1. Demographic and Socioeconomic Measures

Child age, gender and number of siblings were reported by the mothers. In addition, child psychological distress was assessed in the parent report of the validated German version of the Strengths and Difficulties Questionnaire (SDQ) [35]. To evaluate its clinical impact, the total problem score was compared with German normative values; scores were classified as normal, borderline and abnormal psychological distress. Socioeconomic status (SES) was assessed according to the procedure defined by Blossfeld [36], which was a validated and broadly used measure to include the parent's educational level and current work situation.

2.3.2. Treatment Satisfaction

To assess treatment satisfaction, we adapted the parent version of the Therapy Evaluation Questionnaire [37], a validated questionnaire originally developed for the psychotherapy setting. In our study, 15 of the 21 items were adapted to properly fit to our context (i.e., "therapy"/"therapist" was replaced by "training"/"trainer" and "problem" was replaced by "pain"). The 21 items were split into two scales: treatment success (7 items, e.g., "I got a better understanding of child's pain"; "I was able to positively change my behavior in the course of training") and treatment process (14 items, e.g., "The trainer understood our situation"; "I was able to openly talk to the trainer about the problems which made us come here"). Answer format was on a 5-point scale: (1) not at all/never; (2) hardly/seldom; (3) partly/sometimes; (4) predominantly/mostly; (5) exactly/always. According to the manual, we also calculated the total score as the mean of all items. The questionnaire was administered to the mothers of the IG at the T2 session post-treatment ($n = 14$). The raw scores and total score had good internal consistencies (treatment success: $\alpha = 0.83$; treatment process: $\alpha = 0.81$; total score: $\alpha = 0.89$). Scale scores and the total score were compared with normative data.

2.3.3. Parental Perceptions of Changes in Abdominal Pain

Mothers were asked about changes in their child's abdominal pain symptoms (i.e., intensity, duration and frequency) in short, standardized interviews conducted by a psychologist at T1, T2 and T3. Answers were recorded on graded scales for a standardized recording of answers. Data from pre-intervention assessment (T1) referred to the last seven days and included pain location, intensity, frequency and duration. T1 data were then analyzed for a sample description. At post-intervention (T2) and follow-up (T3), parents were asked to rate the change of pain since the end of the intervention ("How did the abdominal pain change since the end of the intervention?") with respect to the overall change of pain (very much improved; somewhat improved; not changed; somewhat worsened; very much worsened), perceived changes in pain intensity (intensity decreased; not changed; intensity increased), perceived changes in pain frequency (frequency decreased; not changed; frequency increased), and perceived changes in duration of pain (duration decreased; not changed; duration increased). These T2 and T3 data were analyzed descriptively and presented in the results section.

2.3.4. Parent-Reported Outcome Measures

The following parent-reported outcome measures were assessed at all three points of measurement (T1–T3).

(1) Gastrointestinal Symptoms: Mothers were asked to report on their child's GI symptoms in accordance with the current Rome-III classification ("My child was suffering during the last month from . . . "; six items: abdominal pain, diarrhea, constipation, nausea, vomiting, bloating; [33]). Items of this symptom list were answered on a five-point frequency scale (never, almost never, sometimes, often, almost always). We calculated a mean score as an indicator of GI symptom severity, which yielded an acceptable internal consistency (Cronbach's alpha = 0.72).

(2) Parental pain-related behavior: A self-developed 24-item questionnaire was administered, covering different adaptive and maladaptive aspects of parental behavior and worries related to their child's abdominal pain. Following the introductory sentence, "When my child has abdominal pain, . . . " mothers rated their reactions on a five-point Likert scale (never, seldom, sometimes, often, always). The inventory comprises the following six subscales: "protection" (five items, e.g., "let him/her stay home from school"; "allow things which are usually forbidden"; $\alpha = 0.77$, "attention" (6 items, e.g., "I comfort my child"; $\alpha = 0.77$), "medical help-seeking and home remedies" (4 items, e.g., "I consult a doctor"; "I give him a hot water bottle"; $\alpha = 0.72$), "support child's coping" (3 items, e.g., "I support my child to distract on his own"; "I support my child to relax on his own"; $\alpha = 0.86$) , and "worries" (6 items, e.g., "I am worried"; "I am concerned about my child's future"; $\alpha = 0.83$). Compilation of the items was based on literature of parent behavior [38,39] and pre-tested in another pilot-study [40]. Psychometric properties were sufficient with internal consistencies >0.70 for all scales and sufficient selectivity for all items (part-whole-correlations >0.30). As hypothesized, the scale "protection" showed significant positive correlations to attention ($r_{T1} = 0.406$, $p = 0.029$), medical help-seeking ($r_{T1} = 0.404$, $p = 0.030$) and worries ($r_{T1} = 0.436$, $p = 0.018$). The negative correlation to the scale "support child's coping" was not statistically significant ($r_{T1} = -0.189, p = 0.327$).

(3) Parental pain-related self-efficacy: We adapted a validated, illness-specific self-efficacy scale for parents with children suffering from atopic dermatitis or asthma [41,42] to measure pain-specific self-efficacy expectations. The pain-specific self-efficacy scale was preceded by a short introduction ("Dealing with abdominal pain challenges you. We would like to know how confident you are about dealing with those challenges."). The nine-item scale covers self-efficacy

expectations with respect to preventive actions (two items; e.g., "My child spontaneously wants to do something that could worsen the pain. I am able to refuse his/her wish."), being consequent (two items; e.g., "My child is in pain in the morning and doesn't want to go to school. I am able to encourage my child to go to school."), as well as intervening actions when the child is in acute pain (Five items; e.g., "My child is in hard pain. I am able to distract my child."). The items were answered on a six-point Likert scale ("very unsure"–"very sure"). Internal consistency of the total score for parental pain-specific self-efficacy was acceptable (Cronbach's alpha = 0.72).

(4) General self-efficacy: Self-efficacy was measured by the validated and broadly used General Self-Efficacy Scale (GSES; [43]). Schwarzer and Jerusalem [44] report internal consistencies from 0.82–0.93 and a 2-year retest-reliability of 0.47 (men) and 0.63 (women). The GSES total score is positively associated with self-esteem and optimism, and negatively correlated with anxiety and depression [43]. The GSES covers 10 items, enquiring about the subjective evaluation of one's ability to cope with new or difficult demands in life (e.g., "When there are obstacles, I find my way to assert myself"; "I can find a solution for every problem"). Answer format was four-point ("not true", "hardly true", "somewhat true", "exactly true"). Higher raw scores are associated with higher perceived self-efficacy. Internal consistency in our sample was excellent (Cronbach's alpha = 0.92).

(5) Parental quality of life: We used the "Ulm Quality of Life Inventory for Parents of Chronically Ill Children" (ULQUIE) [45] to assess mothers' self-reported quality of life. The questionnaire was developed for parents of chronically ill children and has been shown to discriminate between clinical and non-clinical groups, as well as different stages of illness [45]. The authors had reported acceptable to good internal consistency for the total score in the validation study on 244 parents of chronically ill children [45]. The 29 items have a five-point answer format (never, seldom, sometimes, often, always) and refer to the last seven days. The wording was adapted to our study and "chronic illness" was replaced by "abdominal pain". We used the total score as a global measure for mothers quality of life, which yielded excellent internal consistency in our sample (Cronbach's α = 0.91).

2.4. Data Analysis

Statistical analyses were carried out using SPSS Statistics (Version 22). All scale scores were transformed to the range of 0–100 to enhance comparability of measures within the study. Effects for primary and secondary outcomes were analyzed by two-factorial analysis of variance for repeated measures, using group (IG × WLC) and the factor time (T1 × T2 × T3) as a repeated measurement factor. Hypotheses refer to a significant group × time interaction (i.e., an increase or decrease of measures in mothers of the IG compared to the WLC over the three measurement points). In case of significant overall effects, changes from T1–T2, T1–T3 and T2–T3 in the outcome measure will be analyzed by post hoc tests, applying Bonferroni correction of alpha-level. Main effects for group and time will be reported as well. In case the assumption of sphericity is violated (Mauchly-Test), the Greenhouse–Geisser correction of degrees of freedom and significance level will be applied [46]. In an exploratory fashion, changes in child pain will be correlated with changes in maternal outcomes. For this, results with at least a statistical trend ($p < 0.100$) will be reported. Change will be measured by the mean difference in the outcomes between T1–T2 and T1–T3.

As previously mentioned, one child dropped out from the IG due to a physical injury after the second of six sessions. No other adverse events occurred. For this one case, the mother did not participate in the parent session and the parent report of the post-intervention and their 3 month follow-up is consequently missing. We replaced the missing data of this case for T2 and T3 according to the last observation carried forward (LOCF) method for an intention to treat (ITT) analysis (Figure 1). Besides the ITT analysis, data were also analyzed by per protocol analysis (PPA). Besides this one dropout, we were able to report a full retention rate. There was no a priori power calculation for this study, as power calculation was performed for child's self-reported abdominal pain, which was our main outcome of the trial [31]. For the current analysis on maternal effects, we performed a post hoc power calculation and defined a power of 1-β >0.80 as sufficient. For each effect, Cohen's *d* was used as a measure for effect size. Cohen's *d* represents the treatment effect in units of standard deviations (*SDs*), with interpretation of Cohen's *d* = 0.20 as a low, *d* = 0.50 as a moderate and *d* = 0.80 as a high effect. Significance level was set at alpha = 0.05.

3. Results

3.1. Sample and Baseline Pain Characteristics

The 29 randomized children were between 6.6 and 11.9 years old (*M* = 9.59, *SD* = 1.54), and predominantly girls (*n* = 25; 86.2%). All 29 children were suffering from abdominal pain for three months or longer. For the parents in the IG, all mothers participated in the parent sessions and in two cases, the fathers participated as well. With respect to the data analysis, only the mothers of the IG and WLC participated in the assessment sessions T1–T3. There were no missing data, except for the one dropout, and therefore 14/15 randomized mothers in the IG participated in the parent session. A summary of demographic and baseline pain characteristics can be found in Table 1.

Table 1. Demographic data and baseline pain characteristics of the sample (*n* = 29).

Variables	IG (*n* = 15)	WLC (*n* = 14)	*p*-Value
Single parent			
yes	14	11	0.280
no	1	3	
Educational level mother			
≤10 years	5	7	0.362
>10 years	10	7	
Educational level father			
≤10 years	4	4	0.909
>10 years	11	10	
Job situation mother			
not employed	1	1	0.960
(self-) employed	14	13	
Job situation father			
not employed	0	0	NA
(self-) employed	15	14	
Number of siblings			
M (*SD*)	1.79 (1.67)	1.50 (0.76)	0.566
range	0–7	1–3	
Psychological distress of the child [1]			
Total problem score			
Normal	8	11	
Borderline	5	2	0.415
Abnormal	1	1	
Abdominal pain intensity (last 7 days)			
M (*SD*)	3.00 (1.00)	2.64 (1.28)	0.407
range	1–4	1–5	
Abdominal pain frequency *			
M	9.13	11.61	0.396
SD	(4.91)	(9.55)	
range	2–20	3–30	
Abdominal pain duration **			
M (*SD*)	57.13 (34.41)	61.79 (73.00)	0.826
range	15–120	10–300	

All variables were collected from the mother's report. All frequencies are depicted for the number of cases *n*; for metric variables, mean (*M*), standard deviation (*SD*) and range are depicted. *p*-value refers to the significance value according to χ^2/*t*-test when *p* < 0.05. NA, not applicable (as there were no cases of unemployed fathers, group comparisons were not conducted); IG, intervention group; WLC, wait list control group. [1] data on psychological distress (*n* = 14 in the IG due to missing item) are based on German normative values [35] and are published for the total sample in [30]; * number of days last month; ** minutes on average.

3.2. Initial Analyses

All outcome measures were tested for a priori baseline differences between groups. There was a significantly higher baseline value in the IG only for the total score of quality of life ($t(27) = 2.187$, $p = 0.038$), which is included as a covariate in the repeated measures analysis for this outcome. Between mothers in the IG versus WLC, there were no baseline differences at T1 in the sum score of GI symptoms ($t(27) = 1.111$, $p = 0.276$), pain-related self-efficacy ($t(27) = -1.725$, $p = 0.096$) and general self-efficacy ($t(27) = 0.297$, $p = 0.789$). Mothers did also not differ on the baseline measures of pain-related behavior and worries (attention $t(27) = -0.938$, $p = 0.357$; protection $t(27) = -1.678$, $p = 0.105$; support child's coping $t(27) = -1.427$, $p = 0.165$; medical help-seeking $t(27) = -0.346$, $p = 0.732$; worries $t(27) = 0.683$, $p = 0.500$).

Treatment Satisfaction

For the IG, the mothers' evaluation of the intervention yielded high scores on the different scales of treatment success ($M = 74.75$, $SD = 13.54$, range 53.57–92.86) and treatment process ($M = 96.05$, $SD = 4.49$, range 87.50–100). The total score for treatment satisfaction was therefore high ($M = 88.95$, $SD = 7.16$, range 76.19–97.62). Taking the German cutoff values (percentile ranks: 0–10 clearly under average; 11–25 under average; 26–75 average; 76–90 over average; 91–100 clearly over average; [37]), treatment success was rated under average in 21.4% of participants; as average in 7.1%; as over average in 14.3% and as clearly over average in 57.1%. For the scale treatment process, 100% of ratings were over average. Taking the total score, 100% of ratings were categorized as clearly over average.

3.3. Primary Outcomes

3.3.1. Maternal Perceptions of Changes in Pain

Analysis of the mother's evaluation of changes in pain revealed highly significant differences between the groups, both for post-intervention T2 and for the follow-up assessment T3. As items were not assessed at T1, the dropout data could not be replaced in this analysis, resulting in 14 participants analyzed in the IG. For the overall change of pain at T2, 13/14 mothers in the IG reported that pain had very much improved ($n = 1$ reported somewhat improved), whereas in the WLC, 10/14 reported no change ($n = 3$ reported somewhat improved and $n = 1$ worsened; $\chi^2(3) = 25.00$, $p < 0.001$). Results at T3 were comparable. For the overall change at T3, 13/14 mothers in the IG reported that pain had very much improved ($n = 1$ reported somewhat improved), whereas in the WLC, 12/14 reported no change ($n = 1$ reported very much improved and $n = 1$ very much worsened; $\chi^2(3) = 24.29$, $p < 0.001$). A similar pattern was found when analyzing the data for pain intensity, frequency and duration (data not shown).

Table 2 summarizes the results of repeated measures ANOVA for the outcomes GI symptoms, pain-related self-efficacy, general self-efficacy and maternal quality of life. Results for maternal pain-related behavior and worries are summarized in Table 3.

Table 2. Outcome measures (means, *SDs*) with results of repeated measures ANOVA (main effects for group, time, and group × time interaction).

	IG *n* = 15		WLC *n* = 14		Main Effect Time	Main Effect Group	Group × Time Interaction			
								Post Hoc Test [b]		
	M	SD	*M*	SD	*p/d*	*p/d*	*p* [a]/*d* [a]	*F*	*p*	*d*
Gastrointestinal Symptoms										
Baseline	32.22	11.72	26.49	15.90	<0.001/1.36	0.492/0.27	0.003/0.97	1.722 (1–2)	0.201 (1–2)	0.51 (1–2)
Post	18.61	11.12	20.24	12.43				5.390 (2–3)	0.028 (2–3)	0.89 (2–3)
Follow-up	11.67	9.61	23.81	16.24				13.128 (1–3)	0.001 (1–3)	1.39 (1–3)
Pain-related self-efficacy										
Baseline	65.33	12.79	72.22	7.98	0.059/0.70	0.730/0.13	0.011/0.92	5.483 (1–2)	0.027 (1–2)	0.90 (1–2)
Post	73.63	11.93	70.00	9.58				1.101 (2–3)	0.303 (2–3)	0.40 (2–3)
Follow-up	77.63	13.92	70.79	10.38				7.496 (1–3)	0.011 (1–3)	1.05 (1–3)
General self-efficacy										
Baseline	70.44	15.78	69.74	13.84	0.030/0.76	0.705/0.16	0.818/0.18	NA	-	-
Post	73.33	12.60	70.25	13.43				-	-	-
Follow-up	76.22	15.47	74.10	16.79				-	-	-
Quality of life										
Baseline	76.03	6.73	67.86	12.70	0.278/0.43	0.886/0.06	0.487/0.28	-	-	-
Post	71.55	11.40	65.70	10.96				-	-	-
Follow-up	77.87	11.25	72.29	14.78				-	-	-

p, significance level; *d*, effect size. All scores were transformed to a range of 0–100. [a] for group × time interaction; when violated sphericity, df and *p*-value correction (Greenhouse-Geisser); [b] test of within-subject contrasts for interaction, with 1 = T1; 2 = T2; 3 = T3. NA, post-hoc analyses not applicable due to non-significant group × time interaction.

Table 3. Mothers' pain-related behavior and worries (means, SDs) with results of repeated measures ANOVA (main effects for group, time, and group × time interaction).

	IG n = 15		WLC n = 14		Main Effect Time	Main Effect Group	Group × Time Interaction			
							p^a/d^a	Post Hoc Test [b]		
	M	SD	M	SD	p/d	p/d		F	p	d
Attention						0.001/1.04	<0.001/1.59	0.004/0.95			
Baseline	51.39	19.71	57.14	12.17				9.746 (1–2)	0.004 (1–2)	1.20 (1–2)
Post	34.72	12.27	58.93	16.00				0.044 (2–3)	0.835 (2–3)	0.09 (2–3)
Follow-up	31.39	13.81	54.46	12.71				7.320 (1–3)	0.012 (1–3)	1.04 (1–3)
Protection					0.109/0.59	0.0004/1.21	0.466/0.34			
Baseline	17.67	17.61	28.93	18.52				NA	–	–
Post	12.33	15.34	29.29	17.41				–	–	–
Follow-up	8.00	9.60	26.07	16.66				–	–	–
Support coping					<0.001/1.17	0.0342/0.37	0.002/1.03			
Baseline	51.67	19.21	60.12	11.40				8.147 (1–2)	0.008 (1–2)	1.10 (1–2)
Post	69.44	17.16	59.52	15.28				0.276 (2–3)	0.603 (2–3)	0.20 (2–3)
Follow-up	75.56	17.10	62.50	17.30				11.994 (1–3)	0.002 (1–3)	1.33 (1–3)
Help-seeking					<0.001/1.46	0.032/0.87	0.005/0.92			
Baseline	28.75	15.99	30.80	15.97				5.891 (1–2)	0.022 (1–2)	0.93 (1–2)
Post	12.08	10.94	25.00	13.31				1.100 (2–3)	0.304 (2–3)	0.40 (2–3)
Follow-up	11.67	11.54	28.57	16.39				8.108 (1–3)	0.008 (1–3)	1.10 (1–3)
Worries					<0.001/1.69	0.222/0.48	0.002/1.03			
Baseline	41.11	19.79	36.01	20.39				7.133 (1–2)	0.013 (1–2)	1.03 (1–2)
Post	21.11	17.21	32.44	16.19				0.444 (2–3)	0.511 (2–3)	0.26 (2–3)
Follow-up	14.72	13.90	28.87	13.02				10.120 (1–3)	0.004 (1–3)	1.23 (1–3)

p, significance level; *d*, effect size. All scores were transformed to a range of 0–100. "support coping" refers to the scale "support child's coping"; "help-seeking" refers to the scale "medical help-seeking and home remedies"; [a] for group × time interaction; when violated sphericity, df and *p*-value correction (Greenhouse–Geisser); [b] test of within-subject contrasts for interaction, with 1 = T1; 2 = T2; 3 = T3. NA, post-hoc analyses not applicable due to non-significant group × time interaction.

3.3.2. Gastrointestinal (GI) Symptoms

In line with our hypothesis, we found a significant decrease in the occurrence of child's GI symptoms overtime, as perceived by the mothers, in the IG compared to the WLC (interaction $F(2, 54) = 6.345, p = 0.003, d = 0.97$). Of note, there was also an overall main time-effect (Table 2) and both groups showed a decrease from study inclusion to the T2 assessment (time effect $F_{1-2}(1, 27) = 12.871$, $p_{1-2} = 0.001, d_{1-2} = 1.38$).

However, there was a significant decrease of GI symptoms in the IG during the follow-up time span between T2–T3 (interaction $F_{2-3}(1, 27) = 5.390, p_{2-3} = 0.028, d_{2-3} = 0.89$) and overall from T1 to T3 (interaction F_{1-3} (1, 27) = 13.128, $p_{1-3} = 0.001, d_{1-3} = 1.39$), with large effect sizes.

3.3.3. Pain-Related Self-Efficacy

In line with our hypothesis, we found a significant and large-sized increase in maternal pain-related self-efficacy in dealing with child's abdominal pain in the IG over time (group $\times$ time interaction $F(1.58, 42.78) = 5.660, p = 0.011, d = 0.92$). Post hoc analyses for the interaction term revealed significant changes with large effect sizes from T1 to T2 and overall from T1 to T3 (Table 2). While from T2 to T3 the scores further increased in the IG, the interaction term was not significant ($F_{2-3}(1, 27) = 1.101, p_{2-3} = 0.303, d_{2-3} = 0.40$).

3.3.4. Maternal Pain-Related Behavior

We found significant, large treatment effects ($d = 0.92–d = 1.03$) consistent with all hypotheses for attention, medical help-seeking, support child's coping and worries. Post hoc analyses revealed that all changes were significant from T1 to T2 as well as overall from T1 to T3, with large effect sizes from $d = 0.93–d = 1.33$. Detailed results for the main effects (time, group) and treatment effect (group $\times$ time interaction, including post-hoc analyses for interaction) are summarized in Table 3. For the follow-up time span, the changes in the IG could be maintained and significant group differences with large effect sizes emerged, consistent with the direction of hypotheses ($d_{2-3} = 2.10$ for significant less attention in the IG, $d_{2-3} = 1.22$ for less medical help-seeking and home remedies, $d_{2-3} = 0.94$ for less worries and $d_{2-3} = 0.80$ for more support of child's coping).

The scale "protection" was the only one for which results were not consistent with hypotheses, as the interaction term was not significant ($F(2, 54) = 0.775, p = 0.466, d = 0.34$). On a descriptive level, scores were reduced in the IG by on average 9.67 points, however, there were also large-sized differences on group level overall and at all time points ($F_{1-2}(1, 27) = 6.437, p_{1-2} = 0.017, d_{1-2} = 0.98$; $F_{2-3}(1, 27) = 12.494, p_{2-3} = 0.001, d_{2-3} = 1.37$; F_{1-3} (1, 27) = 8.331, $p_{1-3} = 0.008, d_{1-3} = 1.11$).

3.4. Secondary Outcomes

3.4.1. General Self-Efficacy

Analysis of variance revealed a significant increase of general self-efficacy in both groups over time (main effect time $F(2, 52) = 3.747, p = 0.030, d = 0.76$). Scores increased from T1 to T3 on average by 5.78 (IG) respectively 4.36 (WLC) points. Changes in time were significant from T2 to T3 ($F_{2-3}(1, 26) = 5.078, p_{2-3} = 0.033, d_{2-3} = 0.88$) and T1–T3 ($F_{1-3}(1, 26) = 5.438, p_{1-3} = 0.028, d_{1-3} = 0.92$). There was no significant main effect for group ($F(1, 26) = 0.146, p = 0.705$), nor group $\times$ time interaction ($F(2, 52) = 0.201, p = 0.818$; Table 2).

3.4.2. Maternal Quality of Life

Analysis of covariance controlling for the baseline T1 value did not show significant effects for time ($F(1, 26) = 1.228, p = 0.278$), group ($F(1, 26) = 0.021, p = 0.886$) or for group $\times$ time interaction ($F(1, 26) = 0.497, p = 0.478$). However, statistical power was insufficient, ranging from $1\text{-}\beta = 0.05–0.37$ for the ULQUIE analyses (Table 2).

All presented results were derived from an ITT analysis. Result patterns of the PPA were similar, with increased effect sizes.

In an exploratory manner, we analyzed whether changes in the child's pain corresponded with changes in maternal outcomes. Only results with $p < 0.100$ were reported. For the child's pain, we used both the GI symptom score as perceived by the mother, as well as the child's self-reported pain as a mean score covering pain intensity, frequency and duration per day. Data for the pain diary were derived from a previous publication [31] and are based on a 14 day pain diary. Bivariate correlations within the IG showed that for changes between T1 and T2, a pronounced decrease of self-reported abdominal pain was positively correlated with a pronounced decrease of maternal attention ($r = 0.519$, $p = 0.047$). A pronounced decrease of mother-reported GI symptoms corresponded with a higher increase in the support of child's coping ($r = -0.509$, $p = 0.052$) and higher decrease in help-seeking ($r = 0.464$, $p = 0.082$), although not statistically significant. For the overall change between T1 and T3, a pronounced decrease in GI symptoms was significantly correlated with a pronounced decrease in help-seeking ($r = 0.596$, $p = 0.088$).

4. Discussion

While the efficacy of CBT on a child's pain has been confirmed in several studies [17,18,20,47,48], only a few studies have reported on changes in parent outcomes [23–25]. This paper aimed to analyze whether any effects on the mothers of children suffering from FAP were noticeable, after participation in a group CBT focusing on their child's self-management. We observed significant, large-sized effects, even though only one parent session was included. We first analyzed changes in the mother's perception of her child's symptom load. Mothers in the IG reported a clear improvement of abdominal pain and GI symptoms, which is in line with results for proxy reported pain in other treatment trials for FAP [23,24,49,50] and also corresponds to previously reported positive effects reported by the children [31].

We also assessed a broad range of pain-related maternal behaviors. According to the cognitive-behavioral pain model, hypotheses differentially referred to an increase of adaptive behavior, defined as supporting the child's coping skills (i.e., distraction and relaxation), and a decrease of maladaptive behavior, defined as attention to pain, protective behavior and medical help-seeking. With the exception of protective reactions, all treatment effects on maternal behavior were significant, with large effect sizes and even maintained over the follow-up span. These results suggest that a broad range of maternal behavior can be influenced by even a short intervention. Palermo et al. [25] also reported similar significant, medium sized effects on parent's encouragement of their child's activities. In addition, in an uncontrolled study, Frerker et al. [51] observed long-term reductions in solicitous behavior and short-term increases in distraction after treatment. Contrary to hypotheses and other trials [23–25], no significant decrease of protective reactions in the IG compared to the WLC was observed. A floor effect might explain this result, since despite the fact that scores halved from pre-intervention to follow-up in the IG, the IG displayed very low scores already at pre-treatment, impeding further improvement.

Consistent with our hypothesis, the mothers in the IG also reported significantly less worries concerning their child's abdominal pain at follow-up, which might imply that psychoeducation was successful ("pain is real, but not dangerous"). These results are promising, as there is evidence that the parent's conceptual pain model is critical for their child's prognosis [52]. Other CBT trials also report effects on parental cognitive-affective variables, like the reduction of perceived threats [24] and reduction of self-blame [25]. Participation in the training program also led to significant improvements in the mother's pain-related self-efficacy, which is in line with research on other chronic diseases [41,42]. Thus far, no trial in childhood FAP research has included parent's pain-specific self-efficacy as an outcome measure. As perceived self-efficacy constitutes an important variable in the context of chronic illness, explaining and predicting the implementation of treatment [28,42] and behavior change [27], further investigations of the parent's pain-specific self-efficacy might give additional insight into other mechanisms of change.

Taking recent systematic reviews into account [21,22,53], evidence for treatment efficacy on parent and child outcomes, may also depend on the degree to which the parents are involved. Recent studies have reported that parental involvement varies between 25%–50% of total therapy time [53] and also varies with respect to the setting. In our intervention, parental involvement was comparably low, with a 6:1 ratio of child to parent therapy time (14% of total therapy time)—despite the young age of the children in our sample. Of note, trials can differ greatly with respect to the age range of participants. While we focused on younger children aged 6–12 years, others included a broader age range (e.g., aged 7–17 years [23] or only older children and adolescents aged 11–17 years [25]). However, the specific contents of these parent interventions are quite similar, covering, for instance, psychoeducation on FAP, the cognitive-behavioral model and discussions of parental behavior [23,49]. Since all other interventions have included more comprehensive parent sessions [22,53], the large-sized effects on parent outcomes are especially of interest. Perhaps parent involvement in FAP treatment does not need to be very extensive, as our results indicate that the approach of one accompanying parent session is still very effective.

In accordance with integrative views on childhood chronic pain [8,54], the effects of our intervention effect the child as well as the parent—which probably interact with one another in a self-reinforcing circle of positive effects. The improvement of maternal behavior might positively influence changes on the child level, while the reduction of child's pain and impairment may be a motor for change in the mother's behavior and worries. Levy et al. [55] found that changes in a parent's threat perception significantly mediates changes in the child's pain. Although these conclusions are limited due to the small sample size, exploratory correlation analyses provided promising first results on the mutual benefits of a child's pain and maternal behavior. Future trials should systematically analyze both the child and parent effects of CBT interventions and mediational pathways, in order to gain further insight into possible reciprocal effects of treatment.

One further conclusion of this trial is that while we observed large-sized treatment effects on almost all abdominal pain-related measures, the constructs conceptualized on an unspecific, general level were not affected by treatment.

With respect to general self-efficacy, we did not observe an intervention effect. To put this in context with the level of self-efficacy, we compared the score of our total sample ($n = 29$) at baseline ($M = 30.90$, $SD = 4.38$; range 19–40) with the score of the normative sample derived from the validation study [56]. Paired t-test revealed that our sample reported even significantly higher general self-efficacy than the normative population-based score for adult women ($M = 28.8$, $SD = 4.9$; $p = 0.015$). Based on these results, the non-significant effects on general self-efficacy could be attributed to a ceiling effect. We can only speculate that the comparatively high level of self-efficacy might have catalyzed the significant changes found in pain-specific measures of self-efficacy and behavior in the IG. However, the potentially positive effects of general self-efficacy pointed out by other studies [57] needs to be analyzed in larger samples. In general, the different treatment responses of pain-specific versus general self-efficacy, as found in this study, are in line with the current literature. Since for chronic conditions, disease-specific measures are more sensitive to change [58,59] and accordingly, treatment effects for parents in the context of other pediatric chronic conditions have also been reported [60].

We also did not observe significant changes in the mother's quality of life in our sample. This might be attributable to the fact that treatment content of the parent session was focused on pain-specific issues like the disease model and the child's coping with pain, and therefore changes in the parent's general well-being were not primarily focused on. One other reason might also be that for the mother's quality of life, we already observed high levels at baseline. Exploratory comparisons to other ULQUIE data show that our sample, with $M = 72.09$ and $SD = 10.72$ for the total score in both groups at baseline, not only showed significantly higher scores than reported for parents of children with other chronic pediatric conditions [61,62], but also that values did not significantly differ from a healthy control sample ($M = 74.0$, $SD = 28.6$, $p = 0.345$; [61]). These data might suggest that parents in our trial were not severely strained to begin with. This is in line with results from a study on parental quality of life in a sample of parents with children suffering from inflammatory bowel disease who also reported higher quality of life scores in most of the domains [63]. On the other side, this observation contradicts other evidence on increased maternal psychosocial strain in FAP samples (e.g., [14–16]). It can be assumed that the relatively high scores on maternal quality of life in our study are attributable to the fact that recruitment for this trial took place in the general population, not in a clinical setting. To the best of our knowledge, there are few data on the quality of life of parents with children with FAP; therefore further studies with more representative samples are warranted.

This trial also has to be reviewed in the context of methodological strengths and limitations. We included various dimensions of parental experience and behavior as outcome measures and we were consequently able to draw differentiated conclusions, not only regarding maladaptive maternal reactions, but also regarding adaptive reactions and pain-specific self-efficacy. While the measure for parent behavior was a self-developed questionnaire based on clinical experience and literature, psychometric properties were satisfactory. Assessment of changes in child pain was conducted by an interview, which was standardized, but did not include established measures for pain assessment like a Numeral Rating Scale. Of note, the data on changes in pain are the mother's subjective perception of her child's pain level and not meant to be a validated proxy marker for the child's pain experience. However, maternal perceptions of child's pain are considered as important pathways for change and pain-related outcomes like healthcare seeking [23,64]. Additionally, this RCT was conducted according to CONSORT guidelines. The retention rate over the follow-up time span was excellent (96.6%) and there were no missing data on the questionnaires. The intervention was standardized and is available as manualized treatment program [29]. However, one should mention the comparably low sample size, with <20 individuals in each treatment arm, which can be traced back to the calculation of the sample size for the primary study outcome [31]; however, statistical power was sufficient for the main analyses in this paper ($1-\beta > 0.80$). As a common problem in pediatric pain research, only mothers participated in the assessment sessions and therefore we unfortunately do not have data of the fathers. However, Frerker et al. [51] did not find different changes in parental behavior after treatment in mothers versus fathers. Nonetheless, RCTs including a sufficient number of fathers are warranted to enable conclusions with respect to gender-related treatment effects. In addition, interpretation and generalizability of results may be constrained due to the selectivity of the non-treatment-seeking sample with a high rate of decliners for further examination and single-site conduction of this trial. Replication of results, including a multi-site approach with a one-year follow-up and active control group, is currently ongoing [65].

The evaluations of our CBT program gave not only promising evidence for its efficacy, but it also identified possible decisive catalysts for improvement, which should be targeted in further clinical practice. Of note, we cannot imply the degree of parent involvement which is needed, or whether we need a child or a parent focus. Nonetheless, child's self-management, together with parent interventions such as psychoeducation on FAP, and taking parental concerns seriously, such as discussing everyday demands and working on adaptive alternatives, seem to constitute promising strategies for improvement of the psychosocial situation of both children and parents. Identification of the mechanisms at work in the circle of positive effects can deliver valuable implications for management of FAP in pediatric practice and also amend integrative parent-child approaches in childhood FAP [8].

5. Conclusions

Functional abdominal pain in children is a common and impairing condition, affecting not only the children themselves but also the parents. Taking into account the growing evidence on parent-specific changes in pediatric pain management, as well as the positive effects of our CBT program on the child level that have recently been published, this study aimed to analyze whether the mothers randomized to the CBT IG for their child's FAP, may benefit from participation in the program as well. Despite a strong focus on child's self-management, large-sized effects on mother's behavior, worries and self-efficacy in dealing with child's pain were observed in the IG, whereas for the mothers in the waitlist control group, no changes were observed. Of note, despite these pain-specific effects, the mother's perception of their self-efficacy in everyday life and their quality of life was not significantly affected.

These results add to the current knowledge on treatment changes experienced by mothers of children suffering from FAP. The fact that, in our sample, the mothers strongly benefited from the training program, together with previously reported child benefits, implies that the circle many families find themselves in can be broken with these interventions. Extending this line of research and taking a broader family perspective [8,9], a thorough investigation of treatment effects on the family level are also warranted. Therefore, additional studies are needed to gain a better understanding of mechanisms of FAP treatment.

Supplementary Materials: The following is available online at www.mdpi.com/2227-9067/4/2/13/s1, Table S1: CONSORT Checklist.

Acknowledgments: C.C. is supported by a grant of the German Research Foundation (DFG; WA 1143/9-1). M.G. was supported by a grant of Potsdam Graduate School.

Author Contributions: M.G. and P.W. conceived the study and the study design; M.G. recruited patients and collected data; C.C. was responsible for data analysis and together with P.W. for interpretation of data; C.C. drafted the article; and C.C., M.G. and P.W. critically revised the article. All authors were given the opportunity to discuss the results and comment on the manuscript. C.C. and P.W. take responsibility for the work as whole. All authors approved the final manuscript.

Conflicts of Interest: The authors declare no conflict of interest. The founding sponsors had no role in the design of the study; in the collection, analyses, or interpretation of data; in the writing of the manuscript, and in the decision to publish the results.

References

1. Korterink, J.J.; Diederen, K.; Benninga, M.A.; Tabbers, M.M. Epidemiology of pediatric functional abdominal pain disorders: A meta-analysis. *PLoS ONE* **2015**, *10*, e0126982. [CrossRef] [PubMed]
2. Warschburger, P.; Hänig, J.; Friedt, M.; Posovszky, C.; Schier, M.; Calvano, C. Health-related quality of life in children with abdominal pain due to functional or organic gastrointestinal disorders. *J. Pediatr. Psychol.* **2014**, *39*, 45–54. [CrossRef] [PubMed]
3. Lisman-van Leeuwen, Y.; Spee, L.A.A.; Benninga, M.A.; Bierma-Zeinstra, S.M.A.; Berger, M.Y. Prognosis of abdominal pain in children in primary care—A prospective cohort study. *Ann. Fam. Med.* **2013**, *11*, 238–244. [CrossRef] [PubMed]
4. Gulewitsch, M.D.; Enck, P.; Schwille-Kiuntke, J.; Weimer, K.; Schlarb, A.A. Rome III criteria in parents' hands: Pain-related functional gastrointestinal disorders in community children and associations with somatic complaints and mental health. *Eur. J. Gastroenterol. Hepatol.* **2013**, *25*, 1223–1229. [CrossRef] [PubMed]
5. Campo, J.V.; Bridge, J.; Ehmann, M.; Altman, S.; Lucas, A.; Birmaher, B.; Di Lorenzo, C.; Iyengar, S.; Brent, D.A. Recurrent abdominal pain, anxiety, and depression in primary care. *Pediatrics* **2004**, *113*, 817–824. [CrossRef] [PubMed]
6. Petersen, S.; Hägglöf, B.L.; Bergström, E.I. Impaired health-related quality of life in children with recurrent pain. *Pediatrics* **2009**, *124*, e759–e767. [CrossRef] [PubMed]
7. Varni, J.W.; Bendo, C.B.; Nurko, S.; Shulman, R.J.; Self, M.M.; Franciosi, J.P.; Saps, M.; Pohl, J.F. Health-related quality of life in pediatric patients with functional and organic gastrointestinal diseases. *J. Pediatr.* **2015**, *166*, 85–90. [CrossRef] [PubMed]
8. Palermo, T.M.; Chambers, C.T. Parent and family factors in pediatric chronic pain and disability: An integrative approach. *Pain* **2005**, *119*, 1–4. [CrossRef] [PubMed]
9. Palermo, T.M.; Valrie, C.R.; Karlson, C.W. Family and parent influences on pediatric chronic pain: A developmental perspective. *Am. Psychol.* **2014**, *69*, 142–152. [CrossRef] [PubMed]
10. Walker, L.; Claar, R.; Garber, J. Social consequences of children's pain: When do they encourage symptom maintenance? *J. Pediatr. Psychol.* **2002**, *27*, 689–698. [CrossRef] [PubMed]

11. Levy, R.L.; Whitehead, W.E.; Walker, L.S.; von Korff, M.; Feld, A.D.; Garner, M.; Christie, D. Increased somatic complaints and health-care utilization in children: Effects of parent IBS status and parent response to gastrointestinal symptoms. *Am. J. Gastroenterol.* **2004**, *99*, 2442–2451. [CrossRef] [PubMed]
12. Peterson, C.C.; Palermo, T.M. Parental reinforcement of recurrent pain: The moderating impact of child depression and anxiety on functional disability. *J. Pediatr. Psychol.* **2004**, *29*, 331–341. [CrossRef] [PubMed]
13. Walker, L.S.; Levy, R.L.; Whitehead, W.E. Validation of a measure of protective parent responses to children's pain. *Clin. J. Pain* **2006**, *22*, 712–716. [CrossRef] [PubMed]
14. Campo, J.V.; Bridge, J.; Lucas, A.; Savorelli, S.; Walker, L.; Di Lorenzo, C.; Iyengar, S.; Brent, D.A. Physical and emotional health of mothers of youth with functional abdominal pain. *Arch. Pediatr. Adolesc. Med.* **2007**, *161*, 131–137. [CrossRef] [PubMed]
15. Eccleston, C.; Crombez, G.; Scotford, A.; Clinch, J.; Connell, H. Adolescent chronic pain: Patterns and predictors of emotional distress in adolescents with chronic pain and their parents. *Pain* **2004**, *108*, 221–229. [CrossRef] [PubMed]
16. Lipani, T.A.; Walker, L.S. Children's appraisal and coping with pain: relation to maternal ratings of worry and restrictions in family activities. *J. Pediatr. Psychol.* **2006**, *31*, 667–673. [CrossRef] [PubMed]
17. Palermo, T.M.; Eccleston, C.; Lewandowski, A.S.; Williams, A.C.; Morley, S. Randomized controlled trials of psychological therapies for management of chronic pain in children and adolescents: An updated meta-analytic review. *Pain* **2010**, *148*, 387–397. [CrossRef] [PubMed]
18. Sprenger, L.; Gerhards, F.; Goldbeck, L. Effects of psychological treatment on recurrent abdominal pain in children—A meta-analysis. *Clin. Psychol. Rev.* **2001**, *31*, 1192–1197. [CrossRef] [PubMed]
19. Eccleston, C.; Palermo, T.M.; Williams, A.C.; Lewandowski Holley, A.; Morley, S.; Fisher, E.; Law, E. Psychological therapies for the management of chronic and recurrent pain in children and adolescents. *Cochrane Database Syst. Rev.* **2012**, *12*, CD003968. [CrossRef] [PubMed]
20. Eccleston, C.; Palermo, T.M.; Williams, A.C.; Lewandowski Holley, A.; Morley, S.; Fisher, E.; Law, E. Psychological therapies for the management of chronic and recurrent pain in children and adolescents. *Cochrane Database Syst. Rev.* **2014**, *5*, CD003968. [CrossRef]
21. Eccleston, C.; Palermo, T.M.; Fisher, E.; Law, E. Psychological interventions for parents of children and adolescents with chronic illness. *Cochrane Database Syst. Rev.* **2012**, *8*, CD009660. [CrossRef]
22. Eccleston, C.; Fisher, E.; Law, E.; Bartlett, J.; Palermo, T.M. Psychological interventions for parents of children and adolescents with chronic illness. *Cochrane Database Syst. Rev.* **2015**, *4*. [CrossRef]
23. Levy, R.L.; Langer, S.L.; Walker, L.S.; Romano, J.M.; Christie, D.L.; Youssef, N.; DuPen, M.M.; Feld, A.D.; Ballard, S.A.; Welsh, E.M.; et al. Cognitive-behavioral therapy for children with functional abdominal pain and their parents decreases pain and other symptoms. *Am. J. Gastroenterol.* **2010**, *105*, 946–956. [CrossRef]
24. Levy, R.L.; Langer, S.L.; Walker, L.S.; Romano, J.M.; Christie, D.L.; Youssef, N.; DuPen, M.M.; Ballard, S.A.; Labus, J.; Welsh, E.; et al. Twelve-month follow-up of cognitive behavioral therapy for children with functional abdominal pain. *JAMA Pediatr.* **2013**, *167*, 178–184. [CrossRef] [PubMed]
25. Palermo, T.M.; Law, E.F.; Fales, J.; Bromberg, M.H.; Jessen-Fiddick, T.; Tai, G. Internet-delivered cognitive-behavioral treatment for adolescents with chronic pain and their parents: A randomized controlled multicenter trial. *Pain* **2016**, *157*, 174–185. [CrossRef] [PubMed]
26. Bandura, A. *Self-Efficacy: The Exercise of Self-Control*; W.H. Freeman: New York, NY, USA, 1997.
27. Jones, V.; Whitehead, L.; Crowe, M.T. Self-efficacy in managing chronic respiratory disease: Parents' experiences. *Contemp. Nurse* **2016**, *52*, 341–351. [CrossRef] [PubMed]
28. Bursch, B.; Tsao, J.C.I.; Meldrum, M.; Zeltzer, L.K. Preliminary validation of a self-efficacy scale for child functioning despite chronic pain (child and parent versions). *Pain* **2006**, *125*, 35–42. [CrossRef] [PubMed]
29. Groß, M.; Warschburger, P. *Chronische Bauchschmerzen im Kindesalter: Das "Stopp-den-Schmerz-mit-Happy-Pingu"-Programm*; Hogrefe: Göttingen, Germany, 2011.
30. Groß, M.; Warschburger, P. Chronic abdominal pain: Psychosocial strain and treatment-associated changes in coping. *Verhaltenstherapie* **2013**, *23*, 80–89. [CrossRef]
31. Groß, M.; Warschburger, P. Evaluation of a cognitive-behavioral pain management program for children with chronic abdominal pain: A randomized controlled study. *Int. J. Behav. Med.* **2013**, *20*, 434–443. [CrossRef] [PubMed]
32. Schneider, S. *Kinder-DIPS: Diagnostisches Interview bei psychischen Störungen im Kindes- und Jugendalter*, 2nd ed.; Springer: Heidelberg, Germany, 2009.

33. Rasquin, A.; Di Lorenzo, C.; Forbes, D.; Guiraldes, E.; Hyams, J.S.; Staiano, A.; Walker, L.S. Childhood functional gastrointestinal disorders: Child/adolescent. *Gastroenterology* **2006**, *130*, 1527–1537. [CrossRef] [PubMed]
34. SCAP. Chronic abdominal pain in children: Clinical Report. *Pediatrics* **2005**, *115*, 812–815.
35. Woerner, W.; Becker, A.; Rothenberger, A. Normative data and scale properties of the German parent SDQ. *Eur. Child. Adolesc. Psychiatry* **2004**, *13* (Suppl. 2), ii3–ii10. [CrossRef] [PubMed]
36. Blossfeld, H.-P. Berufseintritt und Berufsverlauf: Eine Kohortenanalyse über die Bedeutung des ersten Berufs in der Erwerbsbiographie. *Mitt. Arb.- Berufsforsch.* **1985**, *18*, 177–197.
37. Mattejat, F.; Remschmidt, H. *Fragebögen zur Beurteilung der Behandlung (FBB)*; Hogrefe: Göttingen, Germany, 1999.
38. Lohaus, A.; Klein-Heßling, J. Problemlösungen sind erlernbar. Zur Evaluation von Stressbewältigungs- und Entspannungstrainings für Kinder im Grundschulalter. *Rep. Psychol.* **2003**, *28*, 96–102.
39. Sharrer, V.W.; Ryan-Wenger, N.M. Measurements of stress and coping among school-aged children with and without recurrent abdominal pain. *J. Sch. Health* **1991**, *61*, 86–91. [CrossRef] [PubMed]
40. Groß, M. *Recurrent Abdominal Pain in Childhood. Development and Evaluation of Cognitive-Behavioral Pain Management Program—A Pilot Study*; Diploma Psychology, University of Potsdam: Potsdam, Germany, May 2007.
41. Buchholz, H.T.; Warschburger, P.; von Schwerin, A.-D.; Petermann, F. SEND: Eine Skala zur Erhebung der spezifischen Selbstwirksamkeit für Eltern neurodermitiskranker Vorschulkinder. *Z. Med. Psychol.* **2003**, *12*, 63–68.
42. Warschburger, P.; von Schwerin, A.-D.; Buchholz, T.; Petermann, F. Eine Skala zur Erfassung von elterlichen Selbstwirksamkeitserwartungen im Umgang mit dem Asthma ihres Kindes. *Z. Klin. Psychol. Psychother.* **2003**, *32*, 184–190. [CrossRef]
43. Schwarzer, R.; Jerusalem, M. *Skalen zur Erfassung von Lehrer- und Schülermerkmalen: Dokumentation der Psychometrischen Verfahren im Rahmen der Wissenschaftlichen Begleitung des Modellversuchs Selbstwirksame Schulen*; Freie Universität Berlin: Berlin, Germany, 1999.
44. Schwarzer, R.; Jerusalem, M. Generalized Self-Efficacy scale. In *Measures in Health Psychology: A User's Portfolio*; Weinman, J., Wright, S., Johnston, M., Eds.; NFER-NELSON: Windsor, UK, 1995; pp. 35–37.
45. Goldbeck, L.; Storck, M. ULQIE: A quality-of-life inventory for parents of chronically ill children. *Z. Klin. Psychol. Psychother.* **2002**, *31*, 31–39. [CrossRef]
46. Field, A.P. *Discovering Statistics Using SPSS (and Sex and Drugs and Rock 'n' Roll)*, 3rd ed.; SAGE Publications: Los Angeles, SC, USA, 2009.
47. Fisher, E.; Heathcote, L.; Palermo, T.M.; Williams, A.C.; Lau, J.; Ellert, U.; Neuhauser, H.; Roth-Isigkeit, A. Systematic review and meta-analysis of psychological therapies for children with chronic pain. *J. Pediatr. Psychol.* **2014**, *39*, 763–782. [CrossRef] [PubMed]
48. Huertas-Ceballos, A.A.; Logan, S.; Bennett, C.; Macarthur, C. Psychosocial interventions for recurrent abdominal pain (RAP) and irritable bowel syndrome (IBS) in childhood. *Cochrane Database Syst. Rev.* **2008**, CD003014. [CrossRef]
49. Sanders, M.R.; Shepherd, R.W.; Cleghorn, G.; Woolford, H. The treatment of recurrent abdominal pain in children: A controlled comparison of cognitive-behavioral family intervention and standard pediatric care. *J. Consult. Clin. Psychol.* **1994**, *62*, 306–314. [CrossRef] [PubMed]
50. Robins, P.M.; Smith, S.M.; Glutting, J.J.; Bishop, C.T. A randomized controlled trial of a cognitive-behavioral family intervention for pediatric recurrent abdominal pain. *J. Pediatr. Psychol.* **2005**, *30*, 397–408. [CrossRef] [PubMed]
51. Frerker, M.; Hechler, T.; Schmidt, P.; Zernikow, B. [Pain-related parental behavior: Maternal and paternal responses to chronic pain of their child and modifications following inpatient interdisciplinary pain treatment]. *Schmerz* **2016**, *30*, 241–247. [CrossRef] [PubMed]
52. Crushell, E.; Rowland, M.; Doherty, M.; Gormally, S.; Harty, S.; Bourke, B.; Drumm, B. Importance of parental conceptual model of illness in severe recurrent abdominal pain. *Pediatrics* **2003**, *112*, 1368–1372. [CrossRef] [PubMed]
53. Law, E.F.; Fisher, E.; Fales, J.; Noel, M.; Eccleston, C. Systematic review and meta-analysis of parent and family-based interventions for children and adolescents with chronic medical conditions. *J. Pediatr. Psychol.* **2014**, *39*, 866–886. [CrossRef] [PubMed]
54. Palermo, T.M.; Lewandowski Holley, A. The importance of the family environment in pediatric chronic pain. *JAMA Pediatr.* **2013**, *167*, 93–94. [CrossRef]

55. Levy, R.L.; Langer, S.L.; Romano, J.M.; Labus, J.; Walker, L.S.; Murphy, T.B.; van Tilburg, M.A.L.; Feld, L.D.; Christie, D.L.; Whitehead, W.E. Cognitive mediators of treatment outcomes in pediatric functional abdominal pain. *Clin. J. Pain* **2014**, *30*, 1033–1043. [CrossRef] [PubMed]

56. Hinz, A.; Schumacher, J.; Albani, C.; Schmid, G.; Brähler, E. Bevölkerungsrepräsentative Normierung der Skala zur Allgemeinen Selbstwirksamkeit. *Diagnostica* **2006**, *52*, 26–32. [CrossRef]

57. Romppel, M.; Herrmann-Lingen, C.; Wachter, R.; Edelmann, F.; Düngen, H.D.; Pieske, B.; Grande, G.A. Short form of the General Self-Efficacy Scale (GSE-6): Development, psychometric properties and validity in an intercultural non-clinical sample and a sample of patients at risk for heart failure. *GMS Psychosoc. Med.* **2013**, *10*, Doc01. [PubMed]

58. Lacasse, A.; Bourgault, P.; Tousignant-Laflamme, Y.; Courtemanche-Harel, R.; Choiniere, M. Development and validation of the French-Canadian Chronic Pain Self-efficacy Scale. *Pain Res. Manag.* **2015**, *20*, 75–83. [CrossRef] [PubMed]

59. McWilliams, L.A.; Kowal, J.; Wilson, K.G. Development and evaluation of short forms of the Pain Catastrophizing Scale and the Pain Self-efficacy Questionnaire. *Eur. J. Pain* **2015**, *19*, 1342–1349. [CrossRef] [PubMed]

60. Warschburger, P.; von Schwerin, A.D.; Buchholz, H.T.; Petermann, F. An educational program for parents of asthmatic preschool children: Short- and medium-term effects. *Patient Educ. Couns.* **2003**, *51*, 83–91. [CrossRef]

61. Goldbeck, L. The impact of newly diagnosed chronic paediatric conditions on parental quality of life. *Qual. Life Res.* **2006**, *15*, 1121–1131. [CrossRef] [PubMed]

62. West, C.A.; Besier, T.; Borth-Bruhns, T.; Goldbeck, L. Effectiveness of a family-oriented rehabilitation program on the quality of life of parents of chronically ill children. *Klin. Padiatr.* **2009**, *221*, 241–246. [CrossRef] [PubMed]

63. Greenley, R.N.; Cunningham, C. Parent quality of life in the context of pediatric inflammatory bowel disease. *J. Pediatr. Psychol.* **2009**, *34*, 129–136. [CrossRef] [PubMed]

64. Calvano, C.; Warschburger, P. Chronic abdominal pain in children and adolescents: Parental threat perception plays a major role in seeking medical consultations. *Pain Res. Manag.* **2016**, *2016*, 3183562. [CrossRef] [PubMed]

65. Warschburger, P.; Calvano, C.; Becker, S.; Friedt, M.; Hudert, C.; Posovszky, C.; Schier, M.; Wegscheider, K. Stop the pain: Study protocol for a randomized-controlled trial. *Trials* **2014**, *15*, 357. [CrossRef]

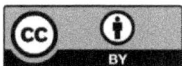

children

Review

Clinical Hypnosis, an Effective Mind–Body Modality for Adolescents with Behavioral and Physical Complaints

Anju Sawni [1,*] and Cora Collette Breuner [2]

[1] Department of Pediatrics, Hurley Children's Hospital/Hurley Medical Center, Michigan State University College of Human Medicine, Flint, MI 48503, USA
[2] Department of Pediatrics, Adolescent Medicine Division and Department of Orthopedics and Sports Medicine, Seattle Children's Hospital, University of Washington, Seattle, WA 98105, USA; Cora.Breuner@seattlechildrens.org
* Correspondence: Asawni1@hurleymc.com; Tel.: +1-810-262-9283 (ext. 5); Fax: +1-810-810-262-9736

Academic Editor: Hilary McClafferty
Received: 2 February 2017; Accepted: 20 March 2017; Published: 24 March 2017

Abstract: Mind–body medicine is a system of health practices that includes meditation/relaxation training, guided imagery, hypnosis, biofeedback, yoga, art/music therapy, prayer, t'ai chi, and psychological therapies such as cognitive behavioral therapy. Clinical hypnosis is an important mind–body tool that serves as an adjunct to conventional medical care for the adolescent patient. Clinical hypnosis specifically uses self-directed therapeutic suggestions to cultivate the imagination and facilitate the mind–body connection, leading to positive emotional and physical well-being. There are many similarities between clinical hypnosis and other mind–body/self-regulatory modalities such as visual imagery, mindfulness meditation, yoga, and biofeedback that incorporate experiential learning and mechanisms for change. They may be viewed as subtypes of the hypnotic experience and share the common experience of trance as the entrée into self-empowered change in physiologic and psychological states. Clinical hypnosis can be used by health care providers to teach adolescents coping skills to deal with a wide variety of conditions such as chronic headaches, recurrent abdominal pain, anxiety, depression, grief and bereavement, phobias, anger, family stressors, sleep disorders, or enuresis. Clinical vignettes are given to help illustrate the effectiveness of hypnosis in adolescents.

Keywords: mind–body therapies; adolescents; pain; headache; stress; anxiety; depression; hypnosis; guided imagery; mindfulness; emotional regulation

1. Introduction

Mind–body medicine is a philosophy and a system of health practices that enlist the mind in improving emotional well-being and physical health. These practices include meditation/relaxation training, guided imagery, hypnosis, biofeedback, yoga, art/music therapy, prayer, t'ai chi, and psychological therapies such as cognitive behavioral therapy.

Mind–body therapies focus on balancing the autonomic nervous system (ANS) by activating the parasympathetic branch of the ANS to reduce the sympathetic physiological response to stress and by regulating the hypothalamic pituitary adrenal axis, both of which are indicators of stress. This reduction of stress on the mind and body may help control or reverse certain underlying disease processes. Evidence suggests that the mind and body have constant bidirectional communication through neuro-endocrine, neuro-chemical, immunological, and energetic pathways.

Higher cognitive centers and limbic emotional centers are capable of regulating virtually all aspects of the immune system and therefore have a profound effect on health and illness-termed psychoneuroimmunology [1–3].

These therapies may improve the quality of life and reduce the physical symptoms for adolescents with various chronic diseases.

Data from the 2012 National Health Interview Survey show that mind–body therapies were used in adolescents aged 13 to 17 years, and more often among females versus males (5.7% vs. 1.7%). Children and youth were more likely to use mind–body therapies for pain-related conditions or emotional, behavioral, or mental conditions and if they received specialty or mental health care. The most common reasons for the use of mind–body therapies were to improve overall health/general wellness, to reduce stress levels or relax, and to feel better emotionally [4,5].

Mind–body therapies such as clinical hypnosis are considered safe and can be effective for adolescents with medical conditions such as tension or migraine headaches, enuresis, recurrent abdominal pain, constipation, sleep difficulties, acute or chronic pain, anxiety, and other emotional and stress-related symptoms [6,7].

2. Stress and the Developing Adolescent Brain

Adolescence is a period of rapid physical growth, intellectual and cognitive development, as well as a time for creating autonomy, and promoting both self-esteem and strong peer relationships. During adolescence, teens experience the ebb and flow of emotions between self-confidence, insecurity, invincibility, anxiety, worry, doubt, and self-worth as a result of rapid changes occurring in the brain and neuro-biological and neuro-endocrine systems.

The rapidly developing adolescent brain is sensitive to stress and adverse events due to changes in hormones and the plasticity in the structure and function of the brain [8].

Brain development during adolescence involves changes in the frontal and parietal cortices, the site of higher-order cognitive and socioemotional processes (i.e., executive function). The cortex is fine-tuned through synaptic pruning in areas that play a role in judgment, impulse control, planning, and emotion regulation [9–11].

Glucocorticoid receptors are found in the amygdala, hippocampus, and prefrontal cortex (PFC); exposure to stressful experiences (leading to increase in glucocorticoids) has been shown to alter the size and neuronal architecture of these areas as well as lead to functional differences in learning, memory, and other aspects of executive functioning. Specifically, chronic stress is associated with hypertrophy and over-activity in the amygdala and orbitofrontal cortex, and can lead to loss of neurons and neural connections in the hippocampus and medial PFC. The PFC turns off the cortisol response and regulates the autonomic balance (i.e., sympathetic versus parasympathetic effects), it also plays an important role in the development of executive functions, such as decision-making, working memory, behavioral self-regulation, and mood and impulse control [12]. The consequences of structural changes in the brain include more anxiety related to both hyper activation of the amygdala and less control as a result of PFC atrophy, as well as impaired memory and mood control due to hippocampal reduction [13].

The adolescent brain is particularly vulnerable to stressors in the youth's social and emotional environment. Executive functions, such as the ability to direct attention and solve problems efficiently, the awareness of threat, and effective fear processing are diminished when there are significant emotional stimuli during adolescence [14–17]. Rapid neurobiological changes during times of emotional stress may predispose adolescents to difficulties with emotion regulation [8]. Difficulties in emotion regulation are a feature of many emotional and behavioral problems seen in adolescents, including anxiety, depression, conduct problems, cutting, disordered eating, and substance abuse [18–20].

The prevalence of mental health disorders is 22% in adolescents 13 to 18 years old. Anxiety disorders are the most common condition (31.9%), followed by behavior disorders (19.1%), mood disorders (14.3%), and substance use disorders (11.4%). Approximately 40% of those with one class of disorder also meet criteria for another class of lifetime disorder [21,22].

With increasing exposure to technology and screen time (on smart phones, computers, television, and social media sites), more mental health concerns, and persistent economic, racial, and ethnic disparities in health status, we now have new morbidities in adolescents called the 'millennial morbidities'. These morbidities may lead to stress-related problems such as chronic headaches, abdominal pain, anxiety, depression, and other emotional problems [23].

Adolescents who experience emotional stress often complain of chronic physical symptoms that respond poorly to standard medications. Cognitive and emotion regulation, including the ability to modulate responses to stress, is increasingly found to contribute to overall adjustment, including social emotional development (e.g., peer relations). Mind–body/self-regulation therapies such as clinical hypnosis operate at the physiological, attentional, emotional, cognitive, and behavioral levels and teach adolescents' coping skills to control their inner wellbeing with respects to thoughts, emotions, attention, and performance [24,25]. Research shows that mind–body/self-regulation therapies can help develop appropriate connections between the relevant prefrontal structures in adolescents, thereby stabilizing arousal and reducing harmful risk-taking behaviors [26]. They may reduce the impact of stress-related conditions, lessen depression and anxiety, alleviate pain, improve quality of life, and increase emotion regulation and subjective well-being [27–34].

3. Clinical Hypnosis: An Effective Mind–body Modality for Adolescents

There are many similarities between clinical hypnosis and other mind–body/self-regulatory modalities such as visual imagery, mindfulness mediation, yoga, and biofeedback that incorporate experiential learning and mechanisms for change. They all have some overlap and may be viewed as subtypes of the hypnotic experience and share the common experience of trance (what happens when we engage in changing our mind) as the entrée into self-empowered change in physiological and psychological states. However, clinical hypnosis specifically uses self-directed therapeutic suggestions to cultivate the imagination and facilitate the mind–body connection, leading to positive physical, emotional, and behavioral change. Using brain imaging, cognitive neuroscientists have identified the power that therapeutic suggestions have on attention functions and associated brain networks and their impact on physical and mental experience [29,35].

Clinical hypnosis is a teachable coping skill that most adolescents (except those with moderate to severe mental retardation) are able to learn with minor effort, and it is safe, effective, and has no adverse side effects in trained hands.

Although there is no universally agreed-upon definition of hypnosis, it can be best described as the cultivation of the imagination in an altered state of consciousness (awareness and alertness) within a focused state (with or without physical relaxation), in which an individual is selectively focused, absorbed, and concentrating upon a particular idea or image aimed at improving mental or physical health. In adolescents, visual imagery/progressive muscle relaxation is often used to get into this altered state of awareness. It is an internal, imaginative process (similar in feeling to daydreaming and/or using the imagination to see, hear, touch, smell, and taste things) that is used to focus attention and become absorbed so that a hypnotic state/trance is entered into. In this state, perceptions and sensations can be enhanced, modified, or changed to inhibit and control reflexive actions, delay gratification, use problem-solving strategies, increase self-esteem, and decrease anxiety, stress, or discomfort. Hypnosis is a natural state and most adolescents move in and out of spontaneous hypnotic-like states as they focus their concentration, for example, while playing video games, "text-messaging", watching favorite movies, listening to music/stories, or otherwise engaging in fantasy/daydreaming [7].

Hypnosis in adolescents is more permissive and less directive than in adults, as it utilizes the natural hypnotic abilities that teens bring to the clinical encounter. Adolescents can enter into the hypnotic state easily and rapidly and, while in this state of deep concentration, are highly responsive to therapeutic suggestions/goals ("hypnotherapy"). Examples of therapeutic suggestions include decreasing or eliminating undesirable symptoms, reframing and rethinking distorted thoughts about situations and stressors, building positive expectations, re-enforcing control over reaction to problems/situations, and strengthening the concept/belief in the ability of the mind and body to work together to create desirable changes in behavior/outcome. Hypnotherapy allows the adolescent to gain a sense of control, increase self-esteem and competence, and reduce stress.

Clinical hypnosis is indicated when (1) an adolescent is responsive to hypnotic suggestions; (2) a problem is treatable with hypnosis; (3) good rapport exists between the adolescent and provider; (4) the adolescent is motivated to remedy the problem; and (5) no iatrogenic harm is anticipated by use. Caution is indicated in adolescents with a history of physical, sexual, or emotional abuse and those with post-traumatic stress disorder (PTSD), in which case coordination of care with a qualified mental health expert is strongly advisable.

Clinical hypnosis is an effective and powerful tool and with appropriate clinical pediatric hypnosis training (skills-based pediatric hypnosis workshops, www.nphti.org). Pediatric/adolescent health care providers' can help adolescents cope and deal with a wide variety of conditions such as chronic headaches/recurrent abdominal pain, anxiety, depression, grief and bereavement, phobias, anger, family stressors, sleep disorders, or enuresis [36–47].

Hypnosis can also be effective for managing procedure pain [48] and chronic pain related to disease—i.e., malignancy, sickle cell, chronic headaches, and abdominal pain (recurrent abdominal pain, inflammatory bowel disease) [49–54].

Clinical hypnosis/self-regulation therapies also can be helpful when integrated into a multimodal treatment plan for adolescents with Attention deficit hyperactivity disorder (ADHD). Hypnosis can be beneficial in teaching them to quiet their mind, slowing and focusing, so that they can sort out frustration or anger produced when the mind works faster than the ability to communicate, and direct them in a positive manner [55–58].

For more detailed descriptions and references of the wide range of clinical conditions for which hypnosis is applicable and effective in adolescents, readers can consult the two standard textbooks on clinical hypnosis by Kohen and Olness, Sugarman and Wester [59,60], as well as an excellent review article by Kohen and Kaiser [61].

4. Application of Clinical Hypnosis—Clinical Vignettes

Through clinical vignettes, this article illustrates common applications of clinical hypnosis in adolescent health care. These vignettes demonstrate the ease, value, and benefit of having pediatric/adolescent health care providers empower and teach clinical hypnosis strategies to adolescents.

The success of clinical hypnosis depends on establishing a strong rapport with the adolescent and individualizing the therapy to the specific goals and characteristics of the adolescent. During the initial visit, the clinician learns the adolescent's personal and family history, and assesses motivation, expectations, strengths, and other internal resources—such as capacity to self-regulate their emotions—the clinician should emphasize that the adolescent is in control. They should offer choices and options and teach the adolescent that they can use the skill (clinical hypnosis) when he/she chooses. The clinician should offer to be the teacher or coach, emphasize the adolescent's ability for control and mastery, and utilize the teen's language and imagery. They should reinforce whatever happens, get feedback from the teen, and address anxiety as well as pain. It is important to have a follow-up plan, such as emphasizing the importance of clinical-hypnosis practice and keeping a calendar of the practice and symptoms (this can easily be done on the teen's smart-phone; the majority of teens have a one). The provider should schedule a follow up appointment in a few weeks to reassess/reinforce progress. The use of other cognitive and behavioral strategies should be incorporated as well to address the symptom.

4.1. Clinical Vignette 1: Chronic Daily Headaches

A 16-year-old female was referred by her neurologist for chronic headaches. Her neurological work up for headaches was negative, with no anatomical or pathological etiology. She had a history of daily headaches, that did not wake her up from sleep but did cause her to miss school and not socialize with her friends. She took over-the-counter ibuprofen/acetaminophen with little relief. She would sleep to help her headaches.

Past medical history and social history were non-contributory. No history of depression, anxiety, or school problems. Family/home life was stable with no acute/chronic toxic stressors.

Mental status evaluation revealed normal cognition and no apparent psychiatric disorder such as a conversion disorder, psychosis, or thought disorder.

The initial session with her and her parents focused on obtaining a thorough history, performing a physical exam, and reviewing labs/imagery. Pain assessment scale using range of 0–10 was used (10 = worst imaginable headache, 0 = no headache, her average score was 8). When asked at which number she would be able to go to school/function so that the headache did not bother her, she replied ≤3.

The clinician then educated the patient and parents on the mind–body connection, with a more formalized introduction/discussion and demystification of hypnosis, emphasizing that learning strategies such as clinical hypnosis can be very effective in managing headache pain.

It was explained that clinical hypnosis could help her take control of her pain/headaches and she could do something so that her headaches would not bother her anymore. The patient and parents were receptive to learning clinical hypnosis. The patient was motivated to get rid of her headaches and resume her normal life.

A second visit was scheduled to teach the patient clinical hypnosis techniques. When designing a hypnotic or hypnosis/trance experience, the clinician utilizes the adolescent's imagination and perception of the symptom and how it affects them as well as probes into the adolescent's interests, strengths, and goals. The adolescent is taught to use techniques such as progressive muscle relaxation, focused breathing, and visual imagery to help them get into a relaxed and focused state (with or without physical relaxation). In this relaxed state, the brain is more focused and receptive to learning techniques to feel better and ultimately make the headache pain dissipate. Prior to incorporating visual imagery and giving a therapeutic suggestion to alleviate the symptom or problem, the clinician asks the adolescent what they would like to imagine that is fun and makes them happy (i.e., a favorite place or favorite things) and if they would like to imagine doing that to help them get into a deeper relaxed state (this reinforces that the teen is in control and empowers them). In this deeper relaxed state, the mind is open and receptive to ideas to help them with their symptoms. In this case the clinician asked the patient to draw a picture of what her headache felt like to her. She drew a picture of a hammer pounding her head. Then both the clinician and the patient devised a method to stop the hammer from pounding her head. The patient used her imagination to visualize having a stop sign come up before the hammer hit her head which would stop the hammer and thus would stop the headache. She then practiced visualizing the stop sign coming up and saying stop to the hammer before it hit her head (the therapeutic suggestion). The clinician then developed a concrete plan with the teen to help practice her clinical hypnosis techniques. Some clinicians ask their patients to keep a calendar of their practice (easy to do on their smartphone). The focus is on practicing clinical hypnosis, not on the symptoms. At the follow up visit a month later, she was practicing her clinical hypnosis, she had kept a calendar of when she practiced hypnosis and pain scale of the headaches. Her headaches were infrequent and not interfering with her daily activities or school.

4.2. Clinical Vignette 2: Needle Phobia

This was a 14-year-old male was referred by his primary care doctor to learn clinical hypnosis for needle phobia. He became very anxious and hysterical prior to obtaining any immunizations or blood draws and was therefore behind on immunizations and screening lab tests.

Past medical history was significant for attention deficit hyperactivity disorder, treated with methylphenidate. There was no history of other psychiatric diagnosis.

He was motivated to learn clinical hypnosis. He recognized that he needed immunizations to stay healthy but was afraid of shots. He was motivated and willing to overcome his "fear of shots". The clinician discussed mind–body/clinical hypnosis techniques with him and used a distraction technique (listening to his music on his iPod) and the hypnotic concept of disassociation i.e., dissociate body and mind, to encourage him to give his arm to the nurse to let her give him the shot so that he could stay healthy, and while she did what she needed to do, he could focus on something else like listening to his music. Also, exposure therapy with desensitization is the treatment of choice for phobias. He was exposed to the equipment (e.g., cleaning swab, syringe, needle) and procedure for injections, so those items no longer created panic symptoms. A "pretend needle" was used to do practice session. After rehearsing this for one session he then "practiced getting the shot" (exposure therapy), while listening to his music (distraction), "gave his arm to the nurse" (disassociation). He did well in the practice session. The patient came back two days later and went through the clinical hypnosis technique of distraction and disassociation and successfully received his immunizations.

4.3. Clinical Vignette #3: Primary Nocturnal Enuresis

A 14-year-old male was referred by his pediatrician for management of primary nocturnal enuresis. History revealed that he had nocturnal enuresis six/seven nights/week and never had a period of complete dryness. He was in the ninth grade and played hockey with practices late at night and quite a few games away from home. He was very embarrassed about his bedwetting and thus very motivated to stop.

Family history was positive for nocturnal enuresis in father until age 16.

He reported drinking a lot of fluids after each hockey practice and game. He had a difficult time unwinding and falling asleep and was a deep sleeper.

He denied drugs, alcohol, or tobacco use and did well in school. There were no other stressors at home or school.

He was motivated to learn clinical hypnosis and stop bedwetting. The clinician discussed the mind–body connection—i.e., the brain and bladder were communicating with each other. He was told that his brain and bladder talked to each other very well, and cooperated and worked well because during the day he never wet his pants even if he had to go really badly, he could hold his pee. He was shown a drawing of genitourinary anatomy and physiology, and was engaged in building curiosity about how the body works, thus helping him be in a spontaneous hypnotic state. The drawing showed how urine was sent from the kidneys to the bladder. The bladder was shown as a container with a muscle at the tip that has a gate that is closed and keeps the urine in the bladder until he goes to the bathroom and the mother computer (i.e., the brain) gives a signal to open the gate when it is full so he can pee. The drawing showed the brain and bladder connection, with bi-directional arrows communicating between the full bladder and the brain, keeping the gate closed until he gets the message from the brain to open it.

The clinician explained, that because he was a deep sleeper, his brain and bladder did not talk well/forgot at night so he had to remind them to talk to each other like they did during the day before he went to sleep.

Then the clinician had him imagine having this conversation in his head to practice how he would have the brain and bladder talk to each other. For example, the clinician coached the patient to say "bladder, tonight let the brain know when you are full. Brain, you have a choice. When the bladder says its full, tell me to wake up, walk to the bathroom, open the gate, pee in the toilet, close the gate, and go back to my comfortable dry bed, or, instead tell the bladder gate to stay closed and locked all night until morning, when I get up from my nice, warm, dry bed and go to the bathroom".

With either choice, the bed is dry in the morning. The patient then wanted to sleep through the night and decided to send a message to brain to keep the gate closed to his bladder till he woke up in the morning. Other behavior modification techniques such as no fluids 1 hour before bed, and bladder

Kegel strengthening exercises during the day were taught. The patient kept a calendar of his clinical hypnosis practice and of dry nights.

He focused on dry nights, positive behaviors, feeling proud and good when his bed was dry, which gave him positive messages of success. He went through two sessions and at a two-month follow up his enuresis had resolved completely.

4.4. Clinical Vignette 4: Anxiety with Sleep Disturbance

A 13-year-old female was referred by her pediatrician for concerns regarding palpitations/panic attacks and sleep problems that started a few months earlier. The patient reported symptoms of shortness of breath, sharp chest pain, and hyperventilation. Extensive medical evaluation by a pediatrician and a cardiologist were negative for physical/anatomical abnormalities.

Patient continued experiencing palpitations and felt as if she "could not catch her breath, and her throat was closing".

She also reported having trouble sleeping, and frequently watched scary movies on her iPad at night to help her sleep. She occasionally took melatonin to help her sleep.

Her mom reported that she was a "worrier" thought often about her safety, as well as her parents' safety, and was concerned that something was wrong with her.

There were no recent illness/stressors in the family and no acute life changes. Family history was positive for anxiety in the father. She lived at home with parents, was an only child and got along well with both parents. She was in the eighth grade, doing virtual home schooling for past two years and was doing well. She did not like crowds and school, so parents decided to do home/virtual school. She had one close friend and cousins with whom she socialized. She liked to play the piano and do arts and crafts. She was referred to a psychologist and also saw a psychiatrist once. She was diagnosed with "social anxiety" by psychiatrist after one visit and told to take sertraline but she never started as her mother did not want to give her medications.

The clinician educated the patient and mom on the benefits of learning mind–body techniques such as focused breathing/visual imagery/clinical hypnosis, to help her cope with her panic attacks/anxiety/worried thoughts.

The patient was open and motivated to learning clinical hypnosis/relaxation techniques. She was taught focused breathing, progressive muscle relaxation, and visual imagery techniques to help her relax and get into a state of focused concentration. The clinician discussed imagining something that made her happy or feel good; her favorite imagery was being up at a lake on the boat. While in this relaxed state the clinician gave her therapeutic suggestions to notice that her breathing was calm, strong, and comfortable; her heart was beating normally and was strong and well; and she was healthy. Her parents were fine and she did not have to worry about her health or her parents' health.

The clinician also discussed other behavioral modification techniques when she felt anxious such as coloring and journaling to help her worry less and distract her when her worry thoughts were taking over her mind. She was shown smart phone e apps (e.g., calm, breathe & relax, mind shift, stop, breathe & think) that helped her practice her breathing.

The patient was told to schedule regular practice time and instructed to keep a calendar of her clinical hypnosis exercise breathing practice and to note the days she felt good/less worried. It was recommended that she continue therapy with a psychologist. She was also advised on proper sleep hygiene techniques (i.e., no screen time one hour before bed, no TV). At a one-month follow-up she was doing better. She was practicing her clinical hypnosis/breathing/visual imagery exercises before bed, two to three times a week. Her mom noticed her overall mood was better and she had fewer panic attacks although she still got anxious, especially when she had to go to new places or places with crowds. She practiced her focused breathing when she would get anxious and she reported sleeping better. At the two month follow up, she had no more panic attacks or excessive worrying.

4.5. Clinical Vignette 5: Substance Abuse

A 17-year-old male was referred by his primary care doctor for management of substance abuse, anxiety, and panic attacks. The patient experienced his first acute panic attack one week prior to his visit which resulted in an emergency room (ED) visit. He was started on short acting alprazolam for acute panic attacks in ED. Was prescribed escitalopram but did not take it because he "(did not) want to take medication". The patient had a history of smoking marijuana (MJ) daily for past four months and weekly for the past year and more recently admitted to smoking a more potent form of MJ oil called "wax/butane hash oil". He denied any other illicit drug use or any prescription drug abuse except for an occasional beer.

He had a past history of mild depressive symptoms/anxiety which was progressively getting worse the past year. For the past several months, he was more socially isolated and stayed in his room and smoked marijuana. He denied self-harm or suicidal thoughts.

He had a lot of worry/concerns/anxiety about his physical health especially the negative effects of marijuana on his health.

He had a lot of psychosomatic complaints, chest pain, numbness and tingling in hands/arms, nonspecific abdominal pain, back pain, and musculoskeletal pain. Since the acute panic episode, he was motivated to stop marijuana and any illicit drug use. He recognized that when he smoked the more potent marijuana "wax", he would be more anxious, feel panicky, heart beating fast, chest hurting, nausea, abdominal pain, and numbness.

Past medical history was significant for attention deficit disorder for which he was prescribed methylphenidate for a few months but stopped two years prior. He currently reported having difficulty focusing at school and declining grades. Family history was positive for anxiety in sister.

He was a senior in high school. His hobbies included making music on his computer and playing in a band. He admitted to peer pressure to smoke marijuana. He denied being sexually active. He worked part time at a fast food restaurant.

A complete physical and neurological exam was normal. Vital signs were all normal.

He needed a lot of reassurance that physically he was fine.

He was open to learning clinical hypnosis/focused breathing/to help with panic attacks/anxiety. He was taught progressive muscle relaxation/focused breathing/visual imagery to help him get into a relaxed alter state of focused consciousness. He visualized himself playing his electronic music/making music. While in this relaxed state, he was given therapeutic suggestions of noting that his body was healthy, that his heart, lungs, hands, and chest were all fine.

He was told he did not need drugs to make good music. He was reminded that when he smoked marijuana he did not feel good. Smoking MJ made him anxious and it was not good for his health, it made his heart beat fast, chest hurt, and nauseous. The clinician discussed the importance of regular practice of clinical hypnosis/breathing exercises. At three week follow up, he was practicing his clinical hypnosis daily and had no further panic attacks or ED visits.

He was followed monthly and for several months he continued to be pre-occupied about his physical health and have vague physical complaints. At each visit he was reassured that physically he was healthy.

He did admit to occasionally smoking marijuana on weekends with his friends but only a few hits as he noted that when he smoked too much he would feel his heart beat fast and get anxious. He was also started on Concerta for his ADHD.

4.6. Clinical Vignette 6: Crohn's Disease with Abdominal Pain

A 17-year-old female with Crohn's disease was referred by her gastroenterologist with severe abdominal pain after multiple hospitalizations for relapse. It was hoped that clinical hypnosis would help her as she was going away to college in the fall and prior to going away was scheduled for small bowel resection/with colostomy.

Mom and patient were interested in "holistic therapies" to help her with the surgery as well as with management of her abdominal discomfort/Crohn's disease while away at college. Mom took herbs/nutritional supplements. Clinician discussed nutrition/healthy eating with patient and mother and added probiotics and omega-3 essential fatty acid supplements to her daily medication regimen.

Patient was very motivated to feel better and manage her Crohn's disease. The clinician taught her clinical hypnosis prior to surgery using progressive muscle relaxation/visual imagery (going to her favorite place in her imagination), then gave her therapeutic suggestions to notice how well the surgery went and how well she was healing, how healthy her gut was, and she could eat healthy foods.

She chose the suggestion "that she wanted to send a message (via text messaging) from her brain to her gut that it was healing well. The clinician reinforced that if her stomach bothered her she could breathe and go to her favorite place and imagine herself feeling good. The surgery was successful and she recovered without complications and was having less abdominal pain. She left for college feeling more confident that she could manage her distress/pain and Crohn's disease.

The above case studies are an example of the benefits of using clinical hypnosis to help adolescents manage common medical conditions. However, it is important to keep in mind that not every adolescent will respond so quickly and positively and that proper certification is essential when applying pediatric hypnosis. Certified pediatric hypnosis training is provided by National Pediatric Hypnosis Training Institute-Inaugural Annual Skill Development Workshops in Pediatric Clinical Hypnosis (Introductory, Intermediate, and Advanced; www.nphti.org).

Not only is a trained clinical provider important for success but so is building a positive rapport with the teen and family with ongoing re-assessment, flexibility, and brainstorming for problem resolution, good outcomes, and healing. As with any skill, regular practice of clinical hypnosis by the teen enhances competence, confidence, and positive outcomes, whereas absence of regular practice is more likely to result in slower and/or less positive results. Homework assignments for the adolescent and their parents involves practice of clinical hypnosis—i.e., keeping a calendar of practice and specifying when they will practice—counseling parents about their level of involvement, and encouraging/motivating adolescents to take charge and control of their symptoms and life in order to have a positive outcome.

5. Conclusions

Clinical hypnosis is a natural state that can be cultivated, with permission from the adolescent and builds on the adolescent's existing strengths and interests. It is an altered state of consciousness (awareness and alertness) within a focused state (with or without physical relaxation), in which an individual is selectively focused, absorbed, and concentrating upon a particular idea or image aimed at improving mental or physical health. Clinical hypnosis is a teachable skill that most adolescent patients are able to learn with minor effort, and is safe, effective, and free of adverse side effects in trained hands. Hypnosis promotes the cultivation of imagination and patients' positive expectations and motivation for success.

Hypnosis in adolescents is more permissive and less directive than in adults, as it utilizes the natural hypnotic abilities that teens bring to the clinical encounter. As a result, adolescents can enter into the hypnotic state quicker and easier than adults and are highly responsive to therapeutic suggestions/goals (hypnotherapy).

Examples of therapeutic suggestions include decreasing or eliminating undesirable symptoms, reframing and rethinking distorted thoughts about situations and stressors, building positive expectations, and re-enforcing control over reaction to problems/situations, and strengthening the concept/belief in the ability of the mind and body to work together to create desirable changes in behavior/outcome. Clinical hypnosis allows the adolescent to gain a sense of control, increase self-esteem and competence, and reduce stress, therefore helping them to manage their physical and emotional well-being. For some problems, hypnosis may be the treatment of choice (e.g., enuresis, headaches, abdominal pain, procedural pain/anxiety, and adjustment reaction to stress).

For more complex problems/conditions, hypnosis may be more adjunctive but a highly effective and important modality in the overall management.

6. Suggested Training

(1)   American Society for Clinical Hypnosis. http://www.asch.net.
(2)   National Pediatric Hypnosis Training Institute. http://www.nphti.org.

Author Contributions: Anju Sawni was the lead author of this review article. She provided contributions to this article through organizing, writing, literature review, case presentations and editing of the major sections. Cora Collette Breuner provided contributions to the article through, literature review, editing, writing and advising of the article.

Conflicts of Interest: The authors declare no conflict of interest.

References

1.   Pert, C. *Molecules of Emotion*; Simon and Schuster: New York, NY, USA, 1997.
2.   Chiarmonte, D.R. Mind–body therapies for primary care physicians. *Prim. Care* **1997**, *24*, 787–807. [CrossRef]
3.   *Psychoneuroimmunolgy*, 4th ed.; Ader, R. (Ed.) Academic Press: Cambridge, MA, USA, 2007.
4.   Clarke, T.C.; Black, L.I.; Stussman, B.J.; Barnes, P.M.; Nahin, R.L. *Trends in the Use of Complementary Health Approaches among Adults: United States, 2002–2012*; National health Statistics Reports, no 79; National Center for Health Statistics: Hyattsville, MD, USA, 2015.
5.   Child and Adolescent Health Measurement Initiative. *What's New in the 2012 NHIS Child Complementary and Alternative Medicine Supplemen?* Data Resource Center for Child & Adolescent Health: Washinton, DC, USA, 2013; Available online: www.childhealthdata.org (accessed on 25 January 2017).
6.   Sussman, D.; Culbert, T. Pediatric Self-regulation. In *Developmental-Behavioral Pediatrics*, 3rd ed.; Levine, M.D., Carey, W.B., Crocker, A.C., Eds.; W.B. Saunders: Philadelphia, PA, USA, 1999; pp. 843–850.
7.   Kohen, D.P. A pediatric perspective on mind–body medicine. In *Integrative Pediatrics*; Culbert, T., Olness, K., Eds.; Oxford University Press: New York, NY, USA, 2009; pp. 267–301.
8.   Romeo, R.D. Adolescence: A central event in shaping stress reactivity. *Dev. Psychobiol.* **2010**, *52*, 244–253. [CrossRef] [PubMed]
9.   Giedd, J.N.; Blumenthal, J.; Jeffrie, N.O.; Castellanos, F.X.; Liu, H.; Zijdenbos, A.; Rapoport, J.L. Brain development during childhood and adolescence: A longitudinal MRI study. *Nat. Neurosci.* **1999**, *2*, 861–863. [CrossRef] [PubMed]
10.   Stroud, L.; Foster, E.; Handwerger, K.; Papandonatos, G.D.; Granger, D.; Kivilighan, K.T.; Niaura, R. Stress response and the adolescent transition: Performance versus peer rejection stress. *Dev. Psychobiol.* **2009**, *21*, 47–68. [CrossRef] [PubMed]
11.   Sumter, S.R.; Bokhorsta, C.L.; Miersa, A.C.; Van Pelt, J.; Westenberg, P.M. Age and puberty differences in stress responses during a public speaking task: Do adolescents grow more sensitive to social evaluation? *Psychoneuroendocrinology* **2010**, *35*, 1510–1516. [CrossRef] [PubMed]
12.   Shonkoff, J.P.; Garner, A.S. Committee on psychosocial aspect of child and family health, Committee on early childhood adoption and dependent care and Section on Developmental and Behavioral Pediatrics. The Lifelong Effects of Early Childhood Adversity and Toxic Stress. *Pediatrics* **2011**, *29*, e232–e246.
13.   McEwen, B.S.; Gianaros, P.J. Stress- and allostasis-induced brain plasticity. *Ann. Rev. Med.* **2011**, *62*, 431–445. [CrossRef] [PubMed]
14.   Silk, J.S.; Siegel, G.J.; Whalen, D.J.; Ostapenko, L.J.; Ladoucer, C.D.; Dahl, R.E. Pubertal changes in emotional information processing: Pupillary, behavioral, and subjective evidence during emotional work identification. *Dev. Psychopathol.* **2009**, *21*, 7–26. [CrossRef] [PubMed]
15.   Blakemore, S.J. Development of the social brain during adolescence. *Q. J. Exp. Psychol.* **2008**, *61*, 40–49. [CrossRef] [PubMed]
16.   Arnsten, A.F.T.; Shansky, R.M. Adolescent vulnerable period for stress-induced prefrontal cortical function? Introduction to Part IV. *Ann. N. Y. Acad. Sci.* **2004**, *1021*, 143–147. [CrossRef] [PubMed]
17.   Andersen, S.L.; Teicher, M.H. Stress, sensitive periods and maturational events in adolescent depression. *Trends Neurosci.* **2008**, *31*, 183–191. [CrossRef] [PubMed]

18. Beato-Fernández, L.; Rodríguez-Cano, T.; Pelayo-Delgado, E.; Calaf, M. Are there gender-specific pathways from early adolescence psychological distress symptoms toward the development of substance use and abnormal eating behavior? *Child Psychiatry Hum. Dev.* **2007**, *37*, 193–203. [CrossRef] [PubMed]
19. Cisler, J.M.; Olatunji, B.O.; Felder, M.T.; Forsyth, J.P. Emotion regulation and the anxiety disorders: An Integrative Review. *J. Psychopathol. Behav. Assess.* **2010**, *32*, 68–82. [CrossRef] [PubMed]
20. Andersen, S.L.; Teicher, M.H. Desperately driven and no brakes: Developmental stress exposure and subsequent risk for substance abuse. *Neurosci. Biobehav. Rev.* **2009**, *33*, 516–524. [CrossRef] [PubMed]
21. U.S. Department of Health and Human Services; Centers for Disease Control and Prevention. *Mental Health Surveillance among Children—United States, 2005–2011*; MMWR: Atlanta, GA, USA, 2013; Volume 62, pp. 1–35. Available online: http://www.cdc.gov/mmwr/preview/mmwrhtml/su6202a1.htm (accessed on 25 January 2017).
22. Merikangas, R.; He, J.P.; Burstein, M.; Swanson, S.A.; Avenevoli, S.; Cui, L.; Benjet, C.; Georgiades, K.; Swendsen, J. Lifetime prevalence of mental disorders in U.S. adolescents: Results from the National Comorbidity Survey Replication–Adolescent Supplement (NCS-A). *J. Am. Acad. Child Adolesc. Psychiatry* **2010**, *49*, 980–989. [CrossRef] [PubMed]
23. Palfrey, J.S.; Tonniges, T.F.; Green, M.; Richmond, J. Introduction: Addressing the millennial morbidity—The context of community pediatrics. *Pediatrics* **2005**, *115*, 1121–1123. [CrossRef] [PubMed]
24. Bell, M.A.; Deater-Deckard, K. Biological systems and the development of self-regulation: Integrating behavior, genetics, and psychophysiology. *J. Dev. Behav. Pediatr.* **2007**, *28*, 409–420. [CrossRef] [PubMed]
25. Greenberg, M.T. Promoting resilience in children and youth: Preventive interventions and their interface with neuroscience. *Ann. N. Y. Acad. Sci.* **2006**, *1094*, 139–150. [CrossRef] [PubMed]
26. Atkins, S.M.; Bunting, M.F.; Bolger, D.J.; Dougherty, M.R. Training the adolescent brain: Neural plasticity and the acquisition of cognitive abilities. In *The Adolescent Brain: Learning, Reasoning, and Decision Making*; Reyna, V.F., Chapman, S.B., Dougherty, M.R., Confrey, J., Eds.; American Psychological Association: Washington, DC, USA, 2012; pp. 211–242.
27. Pascoea, M.C.; Bauerb, I.E. A systematic review of randomized control trials on the effects of yoga on stress measures and mood. *J. Psychiatr. Res.* **2015**, *68*, 270–282. [CrossRef] [PubMed]
28. Hölzel, B.K.; Lazar, S.W.; Gard, T.; Schuman-Olivier, Z.; Vago, D.R.; Ott, U. How Does Mindfulness Meditation Work? Proposing Mechanisms of Action from a Conceptual and Neural Perspective. *Perspect. Psychol. Sci.* **2011**, *6*, 537–559. [CrossRef] [PubMed]
29. Baijal, S.; Jha, A.P.; Kiyonaga, A.; Singh, R.; Srinivasan, N. The influence of concentrative meditation training on the development of attention networks during early adolescence. *Front. Psychol.* **2011**, *12*, 153. [CrossRef] [PubMed]
30. Cahn, B.R.; Polich, J. Meditation states and traits: EEG, ERP, and neuroimaging studies. *Psychol. Bull.* **2006**, *132*, 180–211. [CrossRef] [PubMed]
31. Britton, W.B.; Bootzin, R.R.; Cousins, J.C.; Hasle, B.P.; Peck, T.; Shapiro, S.L. The contribution of mindfulness practice to a multicomponent behavioral sleep intervention following substance abuse treatment in adolescents: A treatment-development study. *Subst. Abus.* **2010**, *31*, 86–97. [CrossRef] [PubMed]
32. Tang, Y.Y.; Holzel, B.K.; Posner, M.I. The neuroscience of mindfulness meditation. *Nat. Rev. Neurosci.* **2015**, *16*, 213–225. [CrossRef] [PubMed]
33. Sibinga, E.M.; Kerrigan, D.; Stewart, M.; Johnson, K.; Magyari, T.; Ellen, J.M. Mindfulness-based stress reduction for urban youth. *J. Altern. Complement. Med.* **2011**, *17*, 213–218. [CrossRef] [PubMed]
34. Sibinga, E.M.; Webb, L.; Ghazarian, S.R.; Ellen, J.M. School-based mindfulness instruction: An RCT. *Pediatrics* **2016**, *137*, 1–8. [CrossRef] [PubMed]
35. Raz, A. Does neuroimaging of suggestion elucidate hypnotic trance? *Int. J. Clin. Exp. Hypn.* **2011**, *59*, 363–377. [CrossRef] [PubMed]
36. Kaiser, P. Chlldhood Anxiety, Worry, and Fear: Individualizing Hypnosis Goals and Suggestions for Self-Regulation. *Am. J. Clin. Hypn.* **2011**, *54*, 16–31. [CrossRef] [PubMed]
37. Cyr, L.R.; Culbert, T.; Kaiser, P. Helping children with stress and anxiety: An integrative medicine approach. *Biofeedback* **2003**, *31*, 12–17.
38. Yapko, M. *Mindfulness and Hypnosis: The Power of Suggestion to Transform Experience*; W.W. Norton & Co.: New York, NY, USA, 2011.
39. Kaiser, P. Childhood anxiety and psychophysiological reactivity: Hypnosis to build discrimination and self-regulation skills. *Am. J. Clin. Hypn.* **2014**, *56*, 343–367. [CrossRef] [PubMed]

40. Kuttner, L.; Friedrichsdorf, S.J. Hypnosis and palliative care. In *Therapeutic Hypnosis with Children and Adolescents*, 2nd ed.; Sugarman, L.I., Wester, W.C., Eds.; Crown House Publishing: Carmarthen, UK, 2014; pp. 491–509.

41. Golden, W. Cognitive Hypnotherapy for Anxiety Disorders. *Am. J. Clin. Hypn.* **2012**, *54*, 263–274. [CrossRef] [PubMed]

42. Kerns, C.M.; Read, K.L.; Klugman, J.; Kendall, P.C. Cognitive-behavioral therapy for youth with social anxiety: Differential short and long-term treatment outcomes. *J. Anxiety Disord.* **2013**, *27*, 210–215. [CrossRef] [PubMed]

43. Yapko, M.D. *Applying Hypnosis in Treating Depression: Innovations in Clinical Practice*; Routledge Press: New York, NY, USA, 2006.

44. Kohen, D.P.; Murray, K. Depression in Children and Youth: Applications of Hypnosis to Help Young People Help Themselves. In *Applying Hypnosis in Treating Depression: Innovations in Clinical Practice*; Yapko, M.D., Ed.; Routledge Press: New York, NY, USA, 2006; pp. 189–216.

45. Kohen, D.P. Depression. In *Therapeutic Hypnosis with Children and Adolescents*; Sugarman, L.I., Wester, W.C., II, Eds.; Crown House Publishing: Carmarthen, UK, 2014; Chapter 9; pp. 187–208.

46. Kuttner, L. Treating pain, anxiety and sleep disorders with children and adolescents. In *Advances in the Use of Hypnosis in Medicine, Dentistry, Pain Prevention and Management*; Brown, D.C., Ed.; Crown House Publishers: Bethel, CT, USA, 2009; Chapter 11; pp. 177–194.

47. Schlarb, A.A.; Liddle, C.C.; Hautzinger, M. JuST—A multimodal treatment program for treatment of insomnia in adolescents: A pilot study. *Nat. Sci. Sleep* **2011**, *3*, 13–20. [PubMed]

48. Curtis, S.; Wingert, A.; Ali, S. The Cochrane Library and Procedural Pain in Children: An Overview of Reviews. *Evid. Based Child Heal. A Cochrane Rev. J.* **2012**, *7*, 1363–1399. [CrossRef]

49. Eccleston, C.; Palermo, T.M.; Williams, A.C.; Lewandowski, A.; Morley, S. Psychological therapies for the management of chronic and recurrent pain in children and adolescents. *Cochrane Database Syst. Rev.* **2009**. [CrossRef]

50. Hammond, D.C. Review of the efficacy of clinical hypnosis with headaches and migraines. *Int. J. Clin. Exp. Hypn.* **2007**, *55*, 207–219. [CrossRef] [PubMed]

51. Kohen, D.P.; Zajac, R. Self-hypnosis training for headaches in children and adolescents. *J. Pediatr.* **2007**, *150*, 635–639. [CrossRef] [PubMed]

52. Shaoul, R.; Sukhotnik, I.; Mogilner, J. Hypnosis as an adjuvant treatment for children with inflammatory bowel disease. *J. Dev. Behav. Pediatr.* **2009**, *30*, 268. [CrossRef] [PubMed]

53. Anbar, R.D. Self-hypnosis for the treatment of functional abdominal pain in childhood. *Clin. Pediatr.* **2001**, *40*, 447–451. [CrossRef] [PubMed]

54. Vlieger, A.M.; Rutten, J.M.; Govers, A.M.; Frankenhuis, C.; Benninga, M.A. Long-term follow-up of gut-directed hypnotherapy vs. standard care in children with functional abdominal pain or irritable bowel syndrome. *Am. J. Gastroenterol.* **2012**, *107*, 627–631. [CrossRef] [PubMed]

55. Bogels, S.; Hopgstad, B.; van Dun, L.; de Schutter, S. Mindfulness training for adolescents with externalizing disorders and their parents. *Behav. Cogn. Psychother.* **2008**, *36*, 193–209. [CrossRef]

56. Van der Oord, S.; Bögels, S.M.; Peijnenburg, D. The Effectiveness of Mindfulness Training for Children with ADHD and Mindful Parenting for their Parents. *J. Child Fam. Stud.* **2012**, *21*, 139–147. [CrossRef] [PubMed]

57. Zylowska, L.; Ackermann, D.L.; Yang, M.H.; Futrell, J.L.; Horton, N.L.; Hale, S.T.; Pataki, C.; Smalley, S.L. Mindfulness meditation training in adults and adolescents with ADHD. A feasibility study. *J. Attent. Disord.* **2007**, *11*, 737–746. [CrossRef] [PubMed]

58. Culbert, T.; Banez, G.; Reiff, M. Children who have Attentional disorders: Interventions. *Pediatr. Rev.* **1994**, *15*, 5–15. [CrossRef] [PubMed]

59. Kohen, D.P.; Olness, K.N. *Hypnosis and Hypnotherapy with Children*, 4th ed.; Routledge Publications, Taylor'& Francis: New York, NY, USA, 2011.

60. Sugarman, L.I.; Wester, W.C. *Therapeutic Hypnosis with Children and Adolescents*, 2nd ed.; Crown House Publishing: Carmarthen, UK, 2014.

61. Kohen, D.P.; Kaiser, P. Clinical hypnosis with children and adolescents—What? Why? How? Origins, applications, and efficacy. *Children* **2014**, *1*, 74–98. [CrossRef] [PubMed]

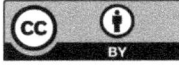

Article

A Pilot Study of Mindfulness Meditation for Pediatric Chronic Pain

Lynn C. Waelde [1,2], Amanda B. Feinstein [3], Rashmi Bhandari [3], Anya Griffin [3], Isabel A. Yoon [3] and Brenda Golianu [3,*]

1   Pacific Graduate School of Psychology, Palo Alto University, Palo Alto, CA 94304, USA; lwaelde@paloaltou.edu
2   Department of Psychiatry and Behavioral Sciences, Stanford University School of Medicine, Stanford, CA 94305, USA
3   Department of Anesthesia, Stanford University School of Medicine, Stanford, CA 94305, USA; abfein@stanford.edu (A.B.F.); rbhandar@stanford.edu (R.B.); anyag@stanford.edu (A.G.); iayoon@stanford.edu (I.A.Y.)
*   Correspondence: bgolianu@stanford.edu; Tel.: +1-650-724-5338

Academic Editor: Hilary McClafferty
Received: 28 February 2017; Accepted: 18 April 2017; Published: 26 April 2017

Abstract: Despite advances in psychological interventions for pediatric chronic pain, there has been little research examining mindfulness meditation for these conditions. This study presents data from a pilot clinical trial of a six-week manualized mindfulness meditation intervention offered to 20 adolescents aged 13–17 years. Measures of pain intensity, functional disability, depression and parent worry about their child's pain were obtained at baseline and post-treatment. Results indicated no significant changes in pain or depression, however functional disability and frequency of pain functioning complaints improved with small effect sizes. Parents' worry about child's pain significantly decreased with a large effect size. Participants rated intervention components positively and most teens suggested that the number of sessions be increased. Three case examples illustrate mindfulness meditation effects and precautions. Mindfulness meditation shows promise as a feasible and acceptable intervention for youth with chronic pain. Future research should optimize intervention components and determine treatment efficacy.

Keywords: mindfulness; meditation; pediatric; chronic pain; adolescent; group therapy

1. Introduction

Pediatric chronic pain is a significant problem in the United States, with prevalence rates across pain subtypes ranging from 11% to 38% [1]. Children with chronic pain experience impairments in emotional [2], social [3], and school functioning [4,5]. Chronic pain in childhood not only pervasively impacts quality of life [6], but also leaves youth at risk for progression of pain into adulthood [7].

Psychological approaches to pain management are known to be an important part of interdisciplinary treatment for pediatric chronic pain [8]. Such approaches typically include cognitive behavioral therapy [9,10], biofeedback [11], and hypnosis [12]. Research suggests that psychological therapies may improve pain and functioning [13].

Mindfulness, often defined as paying attention on purpose and nonjudgmentally in the present moment [14], is a strategy that has received little attention in the field of pediatric pain, despite the growing application of mindfulness-based interventions to address chronic pain in adults [15]. Mindfulness-based interventions for youth have ranged from delivering mindfulness strategies within broader cognitive behavioral packages [16] to developmentally modifying the Mindfulness-Based Stress Reduction (MBSR) program [17]. Jastrowski-Mano et al. [18] published the first small ($n = 6$)

randomized controlled pilot study on MBSR for pediatric pain. Due to high attrition and difficulties with recruitment, they were unable to draw conclusions about the efficacy or feasibility of MBSR for this population. Ruskin and colleagues [19] reported on the development of an MBSR group for adolescents with chronic pain and cited challenges as well, including insufficient post-test data which affected their ability to draw conclusions about outcomes. Two more recent studies examining mindfulness-based programs for adolescents with chronic pain indicated that such interventions were feasible and acceptable [20,21]. Chadi et al. [20] utilized a combination of MBSR and Mindfulness-Based Cognitive Therapy adapted to adolescents and reported no improvements in psychological or pain symptoms, though they did report pre/post-reductions in salivary cortisol levels. Ali et al. [21] utilized a developmentally modified MBSR protocol in a pilot cohort study and reported significant pre/post-improvements in fibromyalgia symptoms, anxiety, and functional disability. Given that previous studies utilizing mindfulness for pediatric chronic pain have reported feasibility and some positive outcomes, more research is needed to further explore the acceptability and efficacy of therapeutic modalities that incorporate mindfulness for this challenging patient population.

The current study was designed to pilot a mindfulness meditation program using a manualized intervention entitled Inner Resources for Teens (IRT) [22], a six-week protocol developed and adapted for teenagers from a similar course utilized for adults named Inner Resources for Stress [23]. Like MBSR, the IRT program teaches mindfulness in daily life and mindfulness meditation, but also includes techniques such as breath-focused imagery and repetition of cue words that are intended to provide additional cognitive structure. Unlike MBSR, IRT does not include hatha yoga or movement-based practices. Previous randomized controlled trials (RCT) of the Inner Resources for Stress intervention for adults have demonstrated pre/post-improvements relative to control groups in diurnal cortisol slope, life satisfaction, and remission from chronic depression [24,25].

The aims of this study were to examine the feasibility, acceptability, and usefulness of the mindfulness meditation intervention, as well as the acceptability of specific treatment components of the IRT program. A secondary aim of this study was to document qualitative case descriptions from three participants to highlight benefits and challenges of using mindfulness meditation with this population.

2. Methods

2.1. Participants and Setting

Twenty patients diagnosed with chronic pain were recruited from a university-based pediatric pain management clinic. All participants had a history of chronic pain for more than 12 months. They continued to receive multidisciplinary pain management standard of care throughout the intervention. The mean age of participations was 15.1 (standard deviation (SD) = 1.36) and ages ranged from 13 to 17. Two participants (10%) were male. Types of pain included abdominal pain, headaches, fibromyalgia, musculoskeletal pain, complex regional pain syndrome, and joint pain (see Table 1). The mean duration of chronic pain was 2.8 years (range 2.2 to 7).

Table 1. Types of Pain Experienced by Participants.

Pain Type	n (%)
Headache	7 (35)
Abdominal pain	6 (30)
Joint pain, rheumatologic	2 (10)
Musculoskeletal pain	2 (10)
Flank pain, polycystic kidney disease	1 (5)
Complex regional pain syndrome	1 (5)
Erythromelalgia	1 (5)

2.2. Procedures

This study was conducted at a tertiary pediatric pain clinic within a children's hospital setting on the West Coast in the United States. The study was approved by the university's Institutional Review Board. Consent and assent procedures took place at the clinic visit. Participants completed baseline questionnaires on the day of the first mindfulness session, including demographics, pain intensity ratings, and domains of physical and psychological functioning. Following the final session, they also completed ratings of pain and function and responded to open-ended questions evaluating the feasibility and acceptability of the intervention.

2.3. Intervention

The mindfulness intervention consisted of a six-session group-based intervention to teach and practice skills for maintaining sustained nonjudgmental present moment awareness. Three groups were held four months apart, containing nine, three and eight participants, respectively. The intervention was led by a clinical psychologist (author L.W.) and a clinical psychology doctoral student who was trained and supervised in the intervention. The techniques were adapted specifically for adolescents and included a guided body tour, tension release, mindfulness meditation, breath-focused imagery, and repetition of cue words. The Guided Body Tour consisted of noticing and then visualizing breath flow to parts of the body. Complete Breath involved noticing every part of the breath from the inhalation through the exhalation. Repetition of secular cue words consisted of repeating the sounds "Hum Sah," meant to represent the sound of breathing in synchrony with the breath, repeating "Hum" with every inhalation and "Sah" with the exhalation. Tension Release was a breath-focused visualization exercise designed to enhance participants' ability to let go of any "tension or holding",

Sessions were 60 min in length, and began and ended with a 20-min period of therapist-led teaching and practice of mindfulness meditation. The middle 20 min of each session included therapist presentations of didactic material, including the discussion of ways to apply the practice to presenting problems. A major focus of the didactic/discussion sessions was to encourage use of mindfulness skills and techniques in daily life, particularly in response to dealing with pain. Participants were asked to practice these techniques at home for at least 15 min per day for six weeks and to practice them as much as possible in daily life. Participants were provided with a manual, entitled *Inner Resources for Teens* [22] which contained age-appropriate readings and suggestions for the daily practice of the techniques. The manual included four 15-min audio recordings of guided mindfulness meditations that participants used for home practice. The audio recordings were provided on compact disc (CD) and participants were encouraged to convert the recordings to other listening devices.

2.4. Measures

Demographic information collected from participants included age, sex, and duration of chronic pain problem. Qualitative information was obtained from written surveys.

Pain Intensity: Adolescents rated their usual pain intensity and worst pain intensity in the past seven days on the 11-point Numeric Rating Scale (NRS-11) from 0 = "No pain" to 10 = "Worst pain possible" at baseline and post-treatment [26]. The NRS-11 has evidenced validity in the assessment of pain intensity in children and adolescents [26].

Depression: The Children's Depression Inventory (CDI) is a self-report assessment of symptoms of depression that includes 27 items that are scored on a 3-point scale [27]. Total scores range from 0 to 54. Psychometric evidence supporting its use in youth are described by other authors [28,29].

Functional Disability: The 15-item Functional Disability Inventory (FDI) [30] evaluates the physical impact of chronic condition as reported by youth and their caregivers (proxy report) on activities of daily living (e.g., walking, school, sleep) on a Likert scale ranging from 0 = "No trouble" to 4 = "Impossible", where higher scores signify greater functional impairment. The measure has shown sound reliability and validity when used with youth who experience chronic medical challenges [31].

The Stanford Pediatric Pain Functioning Inventory (SPPFI): The SPPFI is a clinical tool which evaluates the frequency of pain functioning complaints during the past week. The survey consisted of 24 questions designed for teenagers (aged 13–18) and a similar version for their parents (proxy report). The item stem for the first five items states: "Due to my pain in the past week, it was hard for me to . . . ." Some of the items for this stem include "Walk more than a block," and "Do physical education (PE), sports, or exercise." The next 15 items have the stem "Because of my pain in the past week, I . . . ." Some of the items following this stem include "Spent time on my bed or couch," "Had low energy," "Had trouble paying attention," and "Worried about making my pain worse." The last four items had the stem "In the past week my pain . . . ." Some of the items for this stem included "Interrupted family activities," "Made my parents worry," and "Made my parents miss work." Parent items had the stem "This past week, my child's pain . . . " which included items such as "Caused me to worry," "Affected our family's activities," "Caused me/my spouse to miss work." Participants rated items on a 5-point response scale with 0 = "Never," 1 = "Almost never," 2 = "Sometimes," 3 = "Often," 4 = "Always",

The Project Evaluation questionnaire was administered at post-treatment and included open-ended questions assessing the feasibility and acceptability of the treatment. Participants and parents indicated the desired length and number of sessions the intervention should include. Participants also rated the components of the intervention on a scale 6-point scale, with 0 = "Not sure," 1 = "Not at all useful," 2 = "A little bit useful," 3 = "Moderately useful," 4 = "Quite a bit useful," and 5 = "Extremely useful." Ratings of 0 and 1 were reported as "Not useful," and ratings of 2–5 were reported as "Useful."

3. Results

Of the 20 participants enrolled the study, four did not meet the attendance criteria of four out of six sessions (attrition rate = 20%). Attrition was due to transportation difficulties ($n = 1$), a new medical condition that precluded group participation ($n = 1$), and participant concerns that the sessions were not adequately reducing pain ($n = 2$). Two additional participants were lost to follow-up because they were not able to attend the last session and scheduling difficulties prevented them from scheduling an in-person post-treatment assessment; therefore, follow-up assessment data were available for 14 participants.

Paired *t*-tests examined changes from baseline to post-treatment (see Table 2). Participant ratings of pain intensity (usual pain and worst pain) did not change from baseline to post-treatment. Likewise, participant ratings of depression were unchanged. Although improvements in ratings of functional disability frequency of pain functioning complaints were not statistically significant, there were numerical pre/post-decreases equivalent to a small Cohen's *d* effect size [32]. Parents' ratings of the worry caused by their child's pain significantly decreased from baseline to post-treatment, with a large effect size.

Table 2. Means, Standard Deviations, and Effects Sizes of Change from Baseline to Post-treatment.

Variable	Baseline $n = 20$		Post-Treatment $n = 14$			
	M	*SD*	*M*	*SD*	*t*	*d*
NRS-usual pain	5.6	1.9	5.6	2.0	−0.4	0
NRS-most severe pain	8.6	1.6	8.8	1.4	−0.8	0
CDI	38.7	7.1	38.9	6.9	−0.1	0
FDI	13.8	6.6	12.5	9.9	0.6	0.20
Teen SPPFI	31.8	14.9	27.4	17.5	0.83	0.30
Parent SPPFI-child's pain caused me to worry [a]	2.7	1.2	1.8	1.2	3.3 *	0.75

Note: NRS = Numerical Rating Scale; SPPFI = Stanford Pediatric Pain Functioning Inventory; CDI = Children's Depression Inventory; FDI = Functional Disability Inventory. [a] Parent SPPFI were available for 11 parents. * $p < 0.01$. M = Mean; SD = standard deviation; *t* = paired *t*-test; *d* = Cohen's *d* effect size

The program evaluation questionnaire assessed the acceptability of aspects of the intervention. Participants and parents also provided data on the acceptability of the number of sessions the intervention should include (see Table 3). None of the participants indicated that they thought the intervention should be shorter. Less than one-third ($n = 4$; 28.6%) of participants indicated that six weeks was the ideal length for the mindfulness meditation program, and the remaining participants ($n = 10$; 71.4%) endorsed that the intervention should include more than 8 or 10 sessions. None of the participants indicated that the intervention should be shorter than 60 min. The majority of the participants ($n = 10$; 71.4%) indicated that 60 min was the ideal session length and less than a third ($n = 4$; 28.6%) indicated that it should be longer. Only one parent thought the intervention should be shorter in terms of number and length of sessions, and around half of parents agreed that the current format of six 60 min sessions was preferred. Results indicated that the majority of participants rated the intervention components as useful (see Table 4). Practice in daily life and the group sessions were the most highly rated components, with 12 participants (85.7%) rating them as useful. Meditation and repetition of cue words, unguided by an audio recording, was rated as useful by 11 participants (78.6%). Of the four audio recordings of guided practice, Complete Breath and "Hum Sah" were the most highly rated, followed by the Guided Body Tour and Tension Release.

Table 3. Participant and Parent Recommendations for Intervention Duration from Project Evaluation.

	Teen Participants n (%)	Parents n (%)
Number of weekly sessions		
4	0	1 (9.1)
6 (number of pilot sessions)	4 (28.6)	5 (45.5)
8	4 (28.6)	1 (9.1)
10	6 (42.9)	4 (36.4)
Length of weekly session in minutes		
30	0	1 (9.1)
60 (length of pilot sessions)	10 (71.4)	7 (63.6)
90	4 (28.6)	3 (27.3)

Table 4. Number and Proportion of Participants Rating Intervention Components as Useful.

Intervention Component	n (%)
Inner Resources for Teens manual	10 (71.4)
Guided Body Tour CD	9 (64.3)
Complete Breath CD	10 (71.4)
Hum Sah CD	10 (71.4)
Tension Release CD	8 (57.1)
Meditation practice without CD	11 (78.6)
Hum Sah practice without CD	11 (78.6)
Practice in daily life	12 (85.7)
Group sessions	12 (85.7)

Note: CD = audio recording on compact disc used for guided practice.

Case Illustrations

Case #1. A 15-year-old male participant with multiple pain complaints, including headaches and myofascial pain, was able to learn and practice the meditation techniques and use them to cope with stressors associated with his medical conditions. Although his awareness of pain was slightly increased during the initial sessions, after approximately three weeks of practicing the techniques he became aware that the pain increased his distress and that he could use mindful awareness to reduce his experience of stress, feel more relaxed, and attenuate his experience of pain. He attended all six sessions. He continued to improve after the conclusion of the intervention, by self-report and clinical assessment in follow-up medical visits.

Case #2. A 14-year-old female with fibromyalgia and depression reported improvements in both physical and emotional symptoms after participating in the full six-week program. She reported that this intervention was helpful and described through the program evaluation questionnaires that she learned a new method for coping with her symptoms. Peer support seemed to be of particular benefit to this participant, as she was able to normalize the experience of chronic pain. She especially liked the practice of cue word repetition during periods of sitting meditation and in her daily life, as she reportedly found that it decreased her worry and rumination and reduced her experience of pain. At the midpoint of the intervention, she reported that mindfulness allowed her to address the emotional impact of chronic pain, particularly anxiety, resulting in self-reported reduction in usual pain level. This improvement increased her ability to begin and maintain a daily exercise program and led to full symptom resolution three months after completion of the intervention.

Case #3. A 16-year-old female participant with functional abdominal pain and a longstanding history of participation in pain management treatments (e.g., interventional blocks, multiple medication trials and psychological interventions) reported that she utilized distraction as her primary method of coping with chronic pain. Although she reported successful use of the techniques for coping with anxiety, such as when trying to fall asleep or prior to a music competition, she found the concurrent use of mindfulness and distraction to cope with pain to be confusing and ineffective, resulting in exacerbation of pain symptoms. Due to the focus on body awareness with mindfulness practice, she reported that she became more aware of pain sensations and increasingly distressed. With support of the study team, she was withdrawn from the mindfulness program after two sessions. She continued to participate in outpatient pain management, including psychological services. There were no long-term sequelae and her pain level returned to baseline upon termination of the intervention.

4. Discussion

The current study examined a novel intervention for training in mindfulness meditation, Inner Resources for Teens, which combined mindfulness in daily life, meditation practices, breath-focused cue word repetition, and visualization for adolescents with chronic pain. The intervention was reported as feasible, acceptable, and useful for the majority of participants by adolescent- and parent-report (as well as case study description). There were small quantitative improvements in functioning and reduced disability, suggesting a small effect size; however, due to the small number of patients these were not found to be statistically significant. Parent's concern and worry about their child demonstrated a statistically significant decrease with a large effect size. The adolescents in our pilot study demonstrated acceptable adherence to the intervention, with 80% attending at least four of the six sessions. The majority of participants reported satisfaction with the intervention and expressed the desire for additional sessions after the six weekly sessions were completed. The 60-min session length used in the current study was preferred by most participants and parents.

The group format of the intervention was a highly rated component, consistent with previous work indicating that social support is a valued component of mindfulness interventions for pediatric chronic pain [21]. Practice in daily life was also highly rated, similar to work with adults showing that integrating mindfulness practice in daily life was more commonly practiced than sitting meditation [25]. At the end of the six-week program, participants preferred the unguided meditation and cue word repetition over practice using audio recordings. It is possible that the guided practices were more important at an earlier stage, when participants were first learning the practices. Of the four audio recordings of guided practice, Complete Breath and "Hum Sah" were the most highly rated, followed by the Guided Body Tour and Tension Release. Both the Guided Body Tour and Tension Release may serve to focus attention on bodily sensations to a greater degree than breath-focused meditations and may be less tolerable for adolescents with chronic pain.

As illustrated in Case #3, increased body awareness may be difficult for adolescents with chronic pain, particularly if they primarily rely upon distraction as a pain coping strategy. It is notable that all of the intervention components were rated as useful by a majority of participants, suggesting that the combination of mindfulness, cue word repetition, and meditation exercises was acceptable within the scope of a single intervention. This combination of components differs from interventions such as MBSR, which do not include visualization and cue word repetition [17]. However, as illustrated in Cases #1 and #2, these practices were useful for stress and anxiety. Case #1 noted that his pain initially increased as he brought awareness to his breathing and body, but he was able to tolerate the minor exacerbation in pain intensity until he experienced reduced stress and anxiety about the pain, which in turn reduced his perception of pain. Case #2 reported that the use of breath-focused cue word repetition was helpful in redirecting her attention from worry and rumination and provided useful structure during the initial phases of learning the techniques.

There were no significant changes post-intervention in pain intensity or depression quantitative measures, which is not a surprising finding. Previous studies of mindfulness [20,21] have not reported reductions in pain as an outcome of the intervention, so it may be that these practices are more specific to the distress and dysregulation that accompany the pain experience [33]. Alternatively, it may be that the timing of teaching intervention components is the critical factor. Previous work shows that initial instructions to observe and accept experience—a defining feature of most mindfulness approaches—reduces pain tolerance relative to a control condition and may tax self-regulatory capacity [34]. Longer training may be required to use mindfulness techniques to control or down-regulate the pain experience [35]. Focused practices, such as visualization or cue word repetition, may provide useful structure for teens who are unable to tolerate increased present moment awareness during the initial phase of training.

Parents demonstrated reduced worry about their child's chronic pain over the six-week intervention period. It may be that parents had increased confidence in their child's ability to implement self-management skills, and this confidence decreased parental worry and catastrophizing. Increased parental catastrophizing has been associated with increased child disability in pediatric patients with chronic pain [36], therefore this parent outcome is a promising target for future implementations of mindfulness training.

Limitations of the study include reliance on self-report measures with only limited inclusion of parent-reported data. In addition, the measure of parent worry was based on an item from an assessment tool (i.e., SPPFI), limiting the interpretation of this construct. Although the heterogeneity of pain complaints may be a limitation that restricts recommending this intervention to specific pain populations, it is also a strength with regard to generalizability across pain conditions in terms of the usefulness of this intervention. Not providing intervention components to family members was an additional limitation that was expressly desired by families and should be addressed in future research.

Future Directions

Given that most of the teen participants indicated that the number of sessions should be increased, future implementations should consider a longer format (8 to 10 weekly sessions). The 60-min session length used in the current study seemed optimal to most participants. The impact of the intervention on parents' worry about their child's pain appears indicative of benefits that parents, themselves, may receive through their child's knowledge and implementation of pain coping skills. With additional parent-proxy report measures utilized in future studies, it may be possible to further delineate parental perspectives on functional improvements gained via mindfulness interventions, in the context of other parental self-reported outcomes. Future work is recommended to explore how parents may directly benefit from their own mindfulness training within the context of concurrent adolescent and parent groups. Given that previous research and the results of this pilot study indicate that pain experience may initially fluctuate with mindfulness training, introducing more structured practice, such as cue word repetition, during the first session of the intervention may provide the necessary support for patients as they gain skills to reduce anxiety and increase self-regulatory capacity.

Likewise, future studies should consider the coping style of individual participants as well as their developmental needs, as the focus of mindfulness practice on present moment awareness and physical sensations may seem overwhelming for some adolescents at first. It may be that initially distraction techniques may provide some much-needed relief from the painful sensations, whereas at a later stage, the use of mindfulness techniques may help to decrease anxiety and amplification of the pain experience. The gradual incorporation of mindfulness techniques into the therapy process may produce optimal results. Additional work is also needed to study the method of delivery as a group intervention compared to individual instruction. The group intervention may allow for much-needed social interaction as well as peer validation, whereas the individualized approach may allow for further personalization of the techniques. Future research may explore the relative merits of both distraction and mindfulness techniques to determine the most beneficial use of these strategies for different pain contexts and strategies. Moreover, improved clarification about the aim and rationale for mindfulness treatment may align participant expectancies with the aims of the intervention during each phase of the training. Because the current brief intervention did not demonstrate decreases in pain or increases in functioning, future studies are needed to explore dose and duration of treatment to optimize pain and symptom management.

5. Conclusions

In conclusion, a mindfulness program such as the IRT shows promise as an intervention for helping adolescents with chronic pain and appears to be a feasible tool in the armamentarium of non-pharmacological treatments. The results of this pilot study demonstrate the continued need to further develop pediatric chronic pain mindfulness interventions, exploring a variety of treatment components to determine the most feasible, acceptable and efficacious interventions for this population within the context of a multidisciplinary approach to pediatric chronic pain management.

Author Contributions: L.C.W., B.G., and R.B. conceived and designed the study. B.G., L.C.W., and R.B. recruited and tested subjects. L.C.W. analyzed data. All authors were involved in data interpretation and writing of the manuscript. Aaron Fett and Jason Thompson served as co-interventionists. David Spiegel, M.D. provided invaluable consultation regarding study design.

Conflicts of Interest: The authors declare no conflict of interest.

References

1. King, S.; Chambers, C.T.; Huguet, A.; MacNevin, R.C.; McGrath, P.J.; Parker, L.; MacDonald, A.J. The epidemiology of chronic pain in children and adolescents revisited: a systematic review. *Pain* **2011**, *152*, 2729–2738. [CrossRef] [PubMed]
2. Pinquart, M.; Shen, Y. Depressive symptoms in children and adolescents with chronic physical illness: An updated meta-analysis. *J. Pediatr. Psychol.* **2011**, *36*, 375–384. [CrossRef] [PubMed]
3. Forgeron, P.A.; King, S.; Stinson, J.N.; McGrath, P.J.; MacDonald, A.J.; Chambers, C.T. Social functioning and peer relationships in children and adolescents with chronic pain: A systematic review. *Pain Res. Manag.* **2010**, *15*, 27–41. [CrossRef] [PubMed]
4. Chan, E.; Piira, T.; Betts, G. The school functioning of children with chronic and recurrent pain. *Pediatr. Pain Lett.* **2005**, *7*, 11–16.
5. Simons, L.E.; Logan, D.E.; Chastain, L.; Stein, M. The relation of social functioning to school impairment among adolescents with chronic pain. *Clin. J. Pain* **2010**, *26*, 16–22. [CrossRef] [PubMed]
6. Gold, J.I.; Yetwin, A.K.; Mahrer, N.E.; Carson, M.C.; Griffin, A.T.; Palmer, S.N.; Joseph, M.H. Pediatric chronic pain and health-related quality of life. *J. Pediatr. Nurs.* **2009**, *24*, 141–150. [CrossRef] [PubMed]
7. Walker, L.S.; Dengler-Crish, C.M.; Rippel, S.; Bruehl, S. Functional abdominal pain in childhood and adolescence increases risk for chronic pain in adulthood. *Pain* **2010**, *150*, 568–572. [CrossRef] [PubMed]
8. Eccleston, C.; Palermo, T.M.; Williams, A.C.d.C.; Lewandowski Holley, A.; Morley, S.; Fisher, E.; Law, E. Psychological therapies for the management of chronic and recurrent pain in children and adolescents. *Cochrane Libr.* **2014**.

9. Robins, P.M.; Smith, S.M.; Glutting, J.J.; Bishop, C.T. A randomized controlled trial of a cognitive-behavioral family intervention for pediatric recurrent abdominal pain. *J. Pediatr. Psychol.* **2005**, *30*, 397–408. [CrossRef] [PubMed]
10. Kashikar-Zuck, S.; Ting, T.V.; Arnold, L.M.; Bean, J.; Powers, S.W.; Graham, T.B.; Passo, M.H.; Schikler, K.N.; Hashkes, P.J.; Spalding, S. Cognitive behavioral therapy for the treatment of juvenile fibromyalgia: A multisite, single-blind, randomized, controlled clinical trial. *Arthritis Rheumatol.* **2012**, *64*, 297–305. [CrossRef] [PubMed]
11. Labbé, É.L.; Williamson, D.A. Treatment of childhood migraine using autogenic feedback training. *J. Consult. Clin. Psychol.* **1984**, *52*, 968–976. [CrossRef] [PubMed]
12. Vlieger, A.M.; Menko–Frankenhuis, C.; Wolfkamp, S.C.; Tromp, E.; Benninga, M.A. Hypnotherapy for children with functional abdominal pain or irritable bowel syndrome: A randomized controlled trial. *Gastroenterology* **2007**, *133*, 1430–1436. [CrossRef] [PubMed]
13. Fisher, E.; Heathcote, L.; Palermo, T.M.; de C Williams, A.C.; Lau, J.; Eccleston, C. Systematic review and meta-analysis of psychological therapies for children with chronic pain. *J. Pediatr. Psychol.* **2014**, *39*, 763–782. [CrossRef] [PubMed]
14. Kabat-Zinn, J. *Full catastrophe living: The program of the stress reduction clinic at the University of Massachusetts Medical Center*; Delta: New York, NY, USA, 1990.
15. Cherkin, D.C.; Sherman, K.J.; Balderson, B.H.; Cook, A.J.; Anderson, M.L.; Hawkes, R.J.; Hansen, K.E.; Turner, J.A. Effect of mindfulness-based stress reduction vs cognitive behavioral therapy or usual care on back pain and functional limitations in adults with chronic low back pain: A randomized clinical trial. *JAMA* **2016**, *315*, 1240–1249. [CrossRef] [PubMed]
16. Pielech, M.; Vowles, K.E.; Wicksell, R. Acceptance and Commitment Therapy for Pediatric Chronic Pain: Theory and Application. *Children* **2017**, *4*, 10. [CrossRef] [PubMed]
17. Kabat-Zinn, J.; Lipworth, L.; Burney, R. The clinical use of mindfulness meditation for the self-regulation of chronic pain. *J. Behav. Med.* **1985**, *8*, 163–190. [CrossRef] [PubMed]
18. Jastrowski Mano, K.E.; Salamon, K.S.; Hainsworth, K.R.; Anderson Khan, K.J.; Ladwig, R.J.; Davies, W.H.; Weisman, S.J. A randomized, controlled pilot study of mindfulness-based stress reduction for pediatric chronic pain. *Altern. Ther. Health Med.* **2013**, *19*, 8–14. [PubMed]
19. Ruskin, D.; Kohut, S.A.; Stinson, J. The development of a mindfulness-based stress reduction group for adolescents with chronic pain. *J. Pain Manag.* **2014**, *7*, 301.
20. Chadi, N.; McMahon, A.; Vadnais, M.; Malboeuf-Hurtubise, C.; Djemli, A.; Dobkin, P.L.; Lacroix, J.; Luu, T.M.; Haley, N. Mindfulness-based Intervention for Female Adolescents with Chronic Pain: A Pilot Randomized Trial. *J. Can. Acad. Child Adolesc. Psychiatry* **2016**, *25*, 159. [PubMed]
21. Ali, A.; Weiss, T.R.; Dutton, A.; McKee, D.; Jones, K.D.; Kashikar-Zuck, S.; Silverman, W.K.; Shapiro, E.D. Mindfulness-Based Stress Reduction for Adolescents with Functional Somatic Syndromes: A Pilot Cohort Study. *J. Pediatr.* **2017**, *183*, 184–190. [CrossRef] [PubMed]
22. Waelde, L.C. *Inner Resources for Teens: Treatment Manual and Materials*; Inner Resources Center, Pacific Graduate School of Psychology, Palo Alto University: Palo Alto, CA, USA, 2011.
23. Waelde, L.C. *Inner Resources for Stress: Treatment Manual and Materials*; Inner Resources Center, Pacific Graduate School of Psychology, Palo Alto University: Palo Alto, CA, USA, 2005.
24. Butler, L.D.; Waelde, L.C.; Hastings, T.A.; Chen, X.H.; Symons, B.; Marshall, J.; Kaufman, A.; Nagy, T.F.; Blasey, C.M.; Seibert, E.O.; et al. Meditation with yoga, group therapy with hypnosis, and psychoeducation for long-term depressed mood: A randomized pilot trial. *J. Clin. Psychol.* **2008**, *64*, 806–820. [CrossRef] [PubMed]
25. Waelde, L.C.; Meyer, H.; Thompson, J.T.; Thompson, L.; Gallagher-Thompson, D. Randomized controlled trial of Inner Resources meditation for family dementia caregivers. *J. Clin. Psychol.* **2017**, (in press). [CrossRef] [PubMed]
26. Miró, J.; Castarlenas, E.; Huguet, A. Evidence for the use of a numerical rating scale to assess the intensity of pediatric pain. *Eur. J. Pain* **2009**, *13*, 1089–1095. [CrossRef] [PubMed]
27. Rush, A.J.; Beck, A.T.; Kovacs, M.; Hollon, S. Comparative efficacy of cognitive therapy and pharmacotherapy in the treatment of depressed outpatients. *Cognit. Ther. Res.* **1977**, *1*, 17–37. [CrossRef]
28. Saylor, C.F.; Finch, A.; Spirito, A.; Bennett, B. The Children's Depression Inventory: A systematic evaluation of psychometric properties. *J. Consult. Clin. Psychol.* **1984**, *52*, 955. [CrossRef] [PubMed]

29. Strauss, C.C.; Forehand, R.; Frame, C.; Smith, K. Characteristics of children with extreme scores on the Children's Depression Inventory. *J. Clin. Child Adolesc. Psychol.* **1984**, *13*, 227–231. [CrossRef]

30. Walker, L.S.; Greene, J.W. The functional disability inventory: measuring a neglected dimension of child health status. *J. Pediatr. Psychol.* **1991**, *16*, 39–58. [CrossRef] [PubMed]

31. Claar, R.L.; Walker, L.S. Functional assessment of pediatric pain patients: psychometric properties of the functional disability inventory. *Pain* **2006**, *121*, 77–84. [CrossRef] [PubMed]

32. Cohen, J. *Statistical Power Analysis for the Behavioral Sciences*, 2nd ed.; Lawrence Erlbaum Associates, Inc: Hillsdale, NJ, USA, 1988.

33. Chapman, C.R.; Tuckett, R.P.; Song, C.W. Pain and stress in a systems perspective: reciprocal neural, endocrine, and immune interactions. *J. Pain* **2008**, *9*, 122–145. [CrossRef] [PubMed]

34. Evans, D.R.; Eisenlohr-Moul, T.A.; Button, D.F.; Baer, R.A.; Segerstrom, S.C. Self-regulatory deficits associated with unpracticed mindfulness strategies for coping with acute pain. *J. Appl. Soc. Psychol.* **2014**, *44*, 23–30. [CrossRef] [PubMed]

35. Kingston, J.; Chadwick, P.; Meron, D.; Skinner, T.C. A pilot randomized control trial investigating the effect of mindfulness practice on pain tolerance, psychological well-being, and physiological activity. *J. Psychosom. Res.* **2007**, *62*, 297–300. [CrossRef] [PubMed]

36. Palermo, T.M.; Law, E.F.; Essner, B.; Jessen-Fiddick, T.; Eccleston, C. Adaptation of Problem-Solving Skills Training (PSST) for Parent Caregivers of Youth with Chronic Pain. *Clin. Pract. Pediatr. Psychol.* **2014**, *2*, 212–223. [CrossRef] [PubMed]

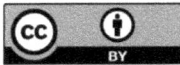

Review

Mind–Body Therapy for Children with Attention-Deficit/Hyperactivity Disorder

Anne Herbert [1] and Anna Esparham [2,*]

[1]   Gottlieb Memorial Hospital, Loyola University Health System, 701 North Ave, Melrose Park, IL 60160, USA; anne.herbert@luhs.org
[2]   Division of Integrative Medicine, University of Kansas Medical Center, 3901 Rainbow Blvd, Mailstop 1017, Kansas City, KS 66160, USA
*   Correspondence: aesparham@kumc.edu; Tel.: +1-913-588-6208

Academic Editor: Hilary McClafferty
Received: 30 November 2016; Accepted: 18 April 2017; Published: 25 April 2017

Abstract: Attention-deficit/hyperactivity disorder (ADHD) is pervasive among the pediatric population and new treatments with minimal adverse effects are necessary to be studied. The purpose of this article is to review current research studying mind–body therapies for treatment of children diagnosed with ADHD. Literature was reviewed pertaining to the effectiveness of movement-based therapies and mindfulness/meditation-based therapies for ADHD. Many positive effects of yoga, Tai Chi, physical activity, and meditation may significantly improve symptoms of ADHD among children.

Keywords: attention-deficit/hyperactivity disorder (ADHD); mind–body; pediatric; children; mindfulness; meditation; yoga; integrative medicine; alternative; complementary

---

1. Introduction

Attention-deficit/hyperactivity disorder (ADHD) is a widespread chronic disorder affecting children's well-being and success in life. The historical understanding of ADHD has changed over the years [1]. ADHD was defined in the Diagnostic and Statistical Manual of Mental Disorders (DSM)-III-R in 1987 as a disorder with a specific diagnostic checklist and three subtypes: primarily inattentive, primarily hyperactive, and combined. According to the American Psychiatric Association in the DSM-V, to be considered ADHD, a child must have symptoms before the age of 12, for at least six months, and affecting two domains of life. The prevalence of the three subtypes of ADHD are: primarily inattentive (20–30% of diagnosed population), primarily hyperactive-impulsive (less than 15%), and combined subtype (50–75%) [2]. The prevalence of ADHD in the US among children is estimated at 11% [3]. ADHD is very common among children and adolescents, consisting of about 50% of child psychiatric diagnoses [1].

2. Attention-Deficit/Hyperactivity Disorder

2.1. Etiology

A landmark theory about the primary dysfunction of ADHD was developed by Russel Barkley called the Hybrid Neuropsychological Model of Executive (Self-Regulatory) Function [4]. This theory explains ADHD as primarily a disorder of maladaptive behavioral inhibition and impairment of four executive functions. According to Barkley, behavioral inhibition has three functions: inhibiting a prepotent response, stopping an ongoing response, and controlling interference. Behavioral inhibition creates an opportunity for the executive functions to take place leading to a response. The four executive functions Barkley identified are (a) working memory, (b) self-regulation of affect, motivation and arousal, (c) internalization of speech, and (d) reconstitution. In individuals with ADHD, behavioral inhibition is dysfunctional, thereby impairing the four executive functions. In turn, motor response in the forms of motor control, fluency and syntax are affected because these actions are controlled directly by the four executive functions. Therefore, individuals with ADHD have a cascade of dysfunction, beginning with a deficit in behavioral inhibition, leading to an impairment of the four executive functions, resulting in altered motor responses [4]. Barkley's theory must be considered in the present literature review regarding how mind–body therapy has the potential to affect executive functioning in ADHD.

ADHD has been correlated with many different genetic and environmental influences. It has been identified that genetic factors, environment, brain structure, neural pathways, and neurotransmitter levels influence ADHD and its symptoms [2,5,6]. In-utero influences such as alcohol and tobacco exposure during pregnancy, low birth weight, toxemia, eclampsia, poor maternal health, maternal age, and certain complications during labor can predispose a child to ADHD. Furthermore, psychosocial adversity in a child's life such as marital discord, low socioeconomic level, paternal criminality, maternal mental disorders, large family size, or foster care placement have been correlated with an increased risk for ADHD [5]. Further areas of study may be necessary to include the mechanism of action on how these predisposing risks affect executive function in children with ADHD.

ADHD has been identified as a *complex trait* disorder meaning that it is affected by many susceptibility genes. Each gene affects the risk of developing the disorder on a small scale (p. 51) [6]. Research on genetic associations with ADHD exhibit significant amounts of inconsistent results most likely due to its complexity. Twin and adoption studies show that genetic factors may account for over 70% of the of ADHD symptom variance. Mean heritability for ADHD has been shown to be 77% in twin studies [5]. An extensive meta-analysis by Gizer et al. reviewed the candidate genes associated with ADHD. Their analysis showed significant associations for several genes that influence neurotransmitter function including serotonin, dopamine and norepinephrine regulation. These were found to include *DAT1*, *DRD4*, *DRD5*, *5HTT*, *HTR1B*, and *SNAP25* [6]. One of the most extensively studied was the candidate gene *DAT1*, which codes for a carrier protein that allows for the reuptake of dopamine into the presynaptic neuron [6]. Studies also show genetic differences for the norepinephrine transporter (*NET*) that affects ADHD functioning [7,8]. Dysregulation of dopamine and norepinephrine is thought to play a role in ADHD symptoms [5,7]. The genetic variations associated with ADHD decrease norepinephrine and dopamine activity in the synapses. Stimulant medications, such as methylphenidate and amphetamine, may help overcome this by increasing the availability of norepinephrine and dopamine by inhibiting transporter functions [7].

A longitudinal study among children showed that children homozygous for the major A allele for *NET* were more likely to have a lifetime diagnosis of ADHD [7]. The major A allele may also be associated with higher ADHD symptoms scores. Sigurdardottir et al. found that individuals with the major A allele showed higher *NET* binding potential than controls. Higher *NET* availability was found to be associated with higher symptom scores on the Conners' Adult ADHD Rating Scale: The Self-Report Screening Version (CAARS-S:SV) and Observer-Screen Version (CAARS-O:SV) [8]. Specific brain regions and neurotransmitters have been identified as playing a role in ADHD symptoms. Previous theories explain that the prefrontal cortex of the brain has the overall function of forming "cross-temporal structures of behavior that have a unifying purpose or goal" (p. 71) [4]. The prefrontal cortex is hypothesized to have a role in self-regulation of drive and motivational states that precede goal-directed actions. Because of this, the prefrontal cortex and its executive functions have an influence over motor control in the form of response, anticipatory setting to respond, or inhibition of response. Persons with damage to the prefrontal cortex present with similar symptoms to those with ADHD, having deficient inhibition and executive functioning [4]. Decreased volume of total cerebral brain matter in the frontal cortex, cerebellum and subcortical structures are also associated with ADHD. Hypofunction of anterior cingulate cortex may be associated with disinhibition in ADHD. Furthermore, frontosubcortical pathways that operate with catecholamines are affected in

ADHD. Stimulant medications act on these pathways to increase inhibition of frontal cortical activity on subcortical regions. In addition, the corpus callosum and cerebellum play a role in cognitive functioning. Communication between the two regions may be degraded in ADHD [2].

Certain brain wave activity and patterns have been found among individuals with ADHD that set them apart from their counterparts. Electroencephalography (EEG) is used to analyze brain activity in individuals with ADHD. EEG studies can be analyzed both quantitatively and qualitatively. Certain studies investigate waveform amplitude, absolute and relative power, dominant and subordinate frequency analysis, wave percentage time, and coherence between regions. EEG provides a measure of the "background state" of the brain. Since the 1930s, EEG studies have identified that a subgroup of children with ADHD tend to have an increase in theta and delta slow wave activity, mostly in the frontal region [1]. During inattentive or unfocused states, the slow theta waves (3.5–8.0 Hz) dominate the prefrontal and frontal cortices, as well as other midline loci of the brain. During relaxed, wakeful states, alpha waves (9.0–11 Hz) take over these areas of the brain. Increasing awareness, planning, and purposeful actions cause the sensorimotor rhythm (12–15 Hz) to appear in the motor cortex [9]. Training the sensorimotor rhythm through neurofeedback has been hypothesized to improve inhibitory responses and control of attention in children with ADHD [10,11]. Focused attention or sustained mental effort causes beta-1 (13–21 Hz) and beta-2 activity (22–30 Hz) to be active in the prefrontal, frontal and central midline areas (p. 434) [9]. As the brain moves from a sleeping to attentive state, the wave frequency in central, midline and frontal regions increases and the amplitude decreases. Many individuals with ADHD have been shown to exhibit increased theta/beta wave ratios. Individuals with ADHD also exhibit differences in Event-Related Potential (ERP) tests. The ERP tests evaluate the brain's electrical response to stimuli directly after the stimulus. It is conducted by presenting two types of stimuli, "Go" and "No-Go." When presented with the "Go" stimulus, the participant must respond, while when the "No-Go" stimulus is presented, the participant is supposed to inhibit a response. According to the review by Monastra et al., participants with ADHD perform significantly poorer on "Go," "No-Go" tests. Slow Cortical Potentials (SCPs) are event-related current shifts in the brain that originate from the upper cortical layer and last 300 msec to a few seconds. Negative electrical shifts have been linked to reduced activation of regions related to orientation and attention, which is of interest to ADHD research. SCP biofeedback training is currently being studied where participants in this treatment receive "feedback" related to their regulation of positive or negative current shifts. Reduced ADHD symptoms were reported in two studies of SCP biofeedback training, but there is not enough controlled research to be able to consider it as an effective treatment at this time [9]. However, it is not yet universal that EEG-neurofeedback can diagnose ADHD based on brainwaves as it may only differentiate a relatively small group of these children.

Lazzaro et al. investigated brain wave activity of adolescents with ADHD compared to age- and sex-matched counterparts [12]. The study recruited 54 male adolescents 11–17 years of age, 34 were unmedicated, and the rest were taken off of medication two weeks prior to the study. They were age-matched with 54 male adolescents without ADHD as a control group. The participants underwent a baseline resting, open-eye EEG and then the experimental EEG where they were asked to focus their sight on a black dot 60 cm away to limit eye movement. Brain activity was then measured for two minutes. There was significantly increased theta and alpha-1 activity across anterior, midline, posterior, left and right hemisphere brain regions among ADHD participants. Delta and alpha-2 activity was not significantly increased among ADHD participants compared to control [12]. In summary, the majority of individuals with ADHD presented with excess theta activity and decreased beta in the frontal and central midline regions, also known as cortical hypoarousal. However, there is a minority of individuals with ADHD who exhibit cortical hyperarousal or no changes in quantitative electroencephalography (QEEG) compared to healthy controls. As far as diagnostic value of QEEG, the reported sensitivity and specificity of the theta/beta power ratio has been shown to be comparably accurate in differentiating ADHD from healthy counterparts when compared with behavioral rating scale measures [9].

Heart rate variability (HRV) may be a useful marker for therapeutic changes in ADHD and illustrates the relationship between ADHD and the autonomic nervous system. Abnormal catecholaminergic function has been linked to ADHD, resulting in "underarousal of the sympathetic system in children with ADHD" (p. 1366) [13]. Stimulants increase the dopamine and norepinephrine activity. In turn, studies have shown increases in blood pressure and heart rate due to these medications. One study consisting of 37 children with ADHD, ages 6–12 years, showed a significant change in HRV from baseline to endpoint. Prior to the study, children were either medication naive or taken off medication for at least two months. Square root of the mean squared difference of successive normal-to-normal intervals (RMSSD) and high frequency (HF) were calculated as indicators of parasympathetic vagal tone. Both of these measures were significantly decreased after introduction of methylphenidate treatment from baseline to endpoint. Average heart rate significantly increased from baseline to endpoint. These results may indicate that the children with ADHD may exhibit decreased parasympathetic activity as indicated by increased HRV following pharmacological intervention [13]. Another study by Rukmani et al. exhibited similar results, finding that medication-naive children with ADHD had reduced overall heart rate variability compared to age and gender-matched controls. They hypothesized that these results indicate catecholamine dysregulation and parasympathetic dominance in ADHD [14]. However, this needs to be further studied due to the heterogeneity of ADHD, as catecholamine and the autonomic nervous system imbalance may be different in subgroups of individuals with ADHD. Mind–body therapies may offer an effect on functioning of the autonomic nervous system. Future research should investigate effects of mind–body therapy on measures of heart rate variability in order to compare its effects to that of pharmacological treatment.

2.2. Current Treatments

ADHD presents with a complex etiology and has multiple treatment options. Stimulant medication is the most often used medication for the disorder in younger children, and more recently, non-stimulant medications are used for children and adolescent populations. Other treatments include behavior modification, which includes therapy from clinicians, family or parent training and therapy, and school-based interventions in the classroom [15].

A recent study of 152 children with ADHD revealed that initial treatment behavior modification was less costly than initial treatment with a low dose of stimulant medication. This experimental study found that, on average, children who underwent successful behavior modification training had a cost of $392 versus $1448 for pharmacological treatment over a 10-month school year [16]. In addition, the Multimodal Treatment Study demonstrated that medication did have any long-term benefits in reducing ADHD symptom severity [17]. Adverse effects that are most common of stimulant medications are appetite loss, abdominal pain, headaches, and sleep disturbance [15]. Common effects of non-stimulant medications, such as atomoxetine, include initial somnolence, gastrointestinal disturbances, and decreased appetite. Other non-stimulant medications, such as clonidine or guanfacine, may cause somnolence and dry mouth [15].

Behavioral interventions and pharmaceutical regimens have been shown to be effective at reducing ADHD symptoms significantly, especially when used in combination [18]. It deserves to be explored if the integration of mind–body therapy, with these already accepted treatments would further decrease ADHD symptoms and improve functioning. Mind–body therapies offer a wide range of effects on psychosocial, emotional, and neurobiological functioning, making it a promising addition to current therapy regimens.

3. Mind–Body Therapies

3.1. Current Treatments

Integrative medicine offers an alternative or addition to pharmacological or cognitive-behavioral therapies for treatment of ADHD. There are limited well-designed studies of integrative therapies, making it difficult to generalize results. Current therapies to improve ADHD symptoms identified through evidence-based medicine include diet, nutrient supplementation, gut health, environmental health, and neurofeedback [19].

Mind–body therapy includes but is not limited to mindfulness, biofeedback, deep breathing, guided imagery, progressive relaxation, hypnotherapy, and yoga [20]. A reason for incorporating more integrative therapies is motivated by consumer interest and the need to improve treatment outcomes. Mind–body medicine encompasses various therapies that are non-invasive techniques with the aim of "harnessing positive thought and emotion for the purpose of enhancing health" (p. 102) [20]. The practice of mindfulness and meditation is a conscious exercise that builds attention control and inhibitory skills [21].

3.2. Yoga

One field of mind–body medicine is the practice of yoga. Yoga is an ancient physical practice, derived from Sanskrit word "yuj" meaning "to yoke," and refers to uniting the body, mind and spirit. Yoga teaches individuals to master certain poses and breathing techniques which may promote self-control, attention, awareness and adaptive skills. Yoga has been used as a form of exercise and meditation. It has been currently studied as therapy for the treatment of stress, chronic pain, asthma, irritable bowel syndrome, and ADHD [20].

Yoga has various components to unite the body, mind and spirit. It is comprised of the asanas (physical postures), pranayamas (breathing techniques), and dharana/dhyana (meditation practices) [22]. The goal of these components is to connect the breathing, thoughts, emotions, and body into awareness of the present moment. The conditions affected by yoga explored by Rosen et al. included emotional, mental and behavioral health. The studies reviewed showed significant decreases among children practicing yoga in a variety of measures such as: negative stress response behaviors, total mood disturbance, negative affect, anger, resilience, and fatigue/inertia [22]. There are few studies that may suggest that yoga influences HRV and autonomic function, but more rigorous studies are needed to report any firm conclusions [23].

One study by Hariprasad et al. investigated the effects of yoga as a complementary therapy for children with ADHD who were admitted in a child psychiatry unit [24]. The sample was made of nine children, ages 5–16 years. Eight of the nine children were on medications. The children underwent eight yoga sessions over the course of their inpatient stay. The children were rated on Conners' abbreviated rating scale (CARS), ADHD-rating scale IV (ADHD-RS IV), and clinical global impression (CGI)-Severity. They were rated at the beginning of the study, discharge, and at one month, two months and three months following the study. It was found that CARS, and ADHD-RS IV, and CGI-S were significantly improved among the patients upon discharge. Confounding variables are that this study lacked a control group and the group represents a more severely impaired population of ADHD individuals as evidenced by their need for inpatient treatment. Additionally, the children were taking medication and influenced by other inpatient interventions besides yoga. While yoga may offer some benefit as a complementary therapy in an inpatient setting, this study lacks controls and a large enough sample needed to recommend yoga as an add-on intervention [24].

Sahaja yoga practice as family therapy may have a positive effect on ADHD symptoms and could possibly reduce dosage of medication in some cases. Another study investigated effects of Sahaja yoga meditation as a family treatment for children with ADHD [25]. There were 48 participants in the study, 31 receiving medication, 14 not on medication, and 3 unknown. The participants went through a six-week program of 90-minute clinic sessions twice a week and regular meditation at home.

Effects of the yoga were measured by pre- and post-assessment of child self-ratings and parent's rating of ADHD symptoms, self-esteem and child–parent relationship quality. The results of the study indicated that parents reported significant improvements in ADHD symptoms, with an average decrease calculated at 35%. The researchers also compared scores of the six non-medicated versus the medicated children and found that there were no significant differences in symptoms, indicating that the changes were likely not due to pharmacologic treatment. In addition, 11 of the 20 children who were medicated could reduce their dose of medication throughout the yoga program. In addition to improvement in symptoms, parents also reported improved self-esteem and relationships, feeling less stressed and had a better ability to handle their children's behavior. Children self-reported better sleep patterns, less anxiety, more ability to focus at school, and less conflicts. However, this study relies on unblended ratings of parents and lacked a control group, which makes it difficult to infer that Sahaja yoga may be an effective adjunctive therapy for ADHD. Sahaja yoga has also been reported to increase gray volume matter associated with sustained attention, self-control, compassion, and interoceptive perception in older adults [26]. Additionally, the yoga as a form of stress reduction for parents of children with ADHD is a valid topic to be explored by future research.

Yoga may also help increase time on task for students with ADHD in the educational setting. One study investigated the effect of a yoga practice intervention on children's time on task in school [27]. The participants were 10 children, ages 6–10, with attention problems. The children completed three weeks of two sessions per week for 30 min in each session. The time to task was measured by observation during morning class work in school. The observers used the Behavioral Observation Form where time on task was defined as the percentage of intervals when students had eye contact with the teacher or assigned task and performed assignments. Cohen's effect size was calculated, with small effect being 0.20 or greater, moderate 0.50 or greater and, large effect 0.80 or greater. Effect size for each grade was calculated by taking the difference between the mean of the baseline and intervention phases divided by the standard deviation of the baseline phase. The effect sizes regarding behavioral observation scores were found to be from 1.51 to 2.72 for the three grade groups, showing a large effect. At follow-up, the effect sizes were decreased, but still showing a moderate to great effect at 0.77 and 1.95. Observation as a measurement of student behavior has both strengths and limitations. A limitation is that observation may include rater bias, especially when the observer is not blinded to the purpose of the study as was the case in the present study. On the other hand, teacher-ratings are often used in ADHD research such as the Conner's parent/teacher rating scale. Another positive result of this study was that children reported enjoying the yoga videos and that video format is an inexpensive and easy method of presenting the therapy. Yoga may have the potential to increase time on task in class and be an enjoyable and cost-effective treatment for children with attention problems [27].

There are few experimental studies exploring the effects yoga on attention mechanisms. One study investigated how 20 yoga sessions for boys with ADHD would help attention versus a control of cooperative game activities [28]. The experimental group consisted of 11 participants and control of eight boys. The two groups were assessed pre-and post-intervention using the Conners' Parent and Teacher Rating scale and scores were compared by one-way ANOVA. Qualitative data was also taken from parents. The scores in five subscales of the measurement were improved for the yoga group post-intervention. Parents also reported that the relaxation and breathing techniques were beneficial when their children were restless, needed sleep, and affected their behavior in the immediate period after class. The participants in both groups were receiving medication throughout the study. This experiment shows that yoga can be an effective complementary therapy for children with ADHD that are receiving medication [28]. The breathing and relaxation techniques that are learned through yoga practice may be used by children to focus attention and decrease hyperactivity.

In reference to the theory of executive dysfunction being the hallmark of ADHD, yoga practice must be evaluated in regards of its effect on these functions. Chou and Huang found that an eight-week yoga program significantly improved sustained attention and discrimination function in children with

ADHD compared with a control group [29]. The researchers created two groups of children 8–12 years old from the same suburban area: yoga (*n* = 24) and control (*n* = 25). The two groups were matched, so there were no significant differences in extraneous variables. They measured children at baseline and after intervention on the Visual Pursuit Test and Determination Test. These types of measurements may limit the application of this study because these two tests have not been used among ADHD populations. However, the Visual Pursuit Test is used in psychological diagnostics for selective and sustained attention and was used because attention deficits are symptoms of ADHD. Additionally, the Determination Test assesses for reaction speed, attention deficits, and reactive stress tolerance in the presence of external sensory stimuli. Findings revealed that the group who underwent yoga intervention had significantly better reaction time and response accuracy at the two measurements [29].

Another recent study investigated yoga and physical activity on measures of executive functioning [30]. They examined 30 female undergraduate students' scores on the Flanker task, a measure relating to inhibitory control, and the N-back task, a measure relating to working memory, under three different conditions: baseline, aerobic exercise and yoga. It was found that response accuracy to the Flanker task was significantly increased under the yoga condition compared to aerobic exercise. The researchers believe that the positive effects exhibited under the yoga condition on the two measures may be due to improvements in mood and its focus on body awareness and breathing. By these mechanisms, it is hypothesized that yoga would have positive effects on attentional ability [30].

3.3. Tai Chi

Tai Chi is an ancient Chinese martial art consisting of slow movements coordinated with balancing body weight and breathing deeply. There may be potential benefit for improving ADHD symptoms of anxiety and hyperactivity with regular Tai Chi practice. A sample of 13 adolescents with ADHD was studied to find the effect of a five-week Tai Chi intervention on symptoms according to the Conners' Scale rated by teachers. The participants were rated at baseline, at the end of the five weeks and two weeks after intervention. During the five weeks, participants completed two 30-minute sessions per week. It was found that the adolescents exhibited significantly decreased anxiety, decreased daydreaming, decreased inappropriate emotions, decreased hyperactivity, and increased conduct after the Tai Chi intervention. The scores persisted to be significantly affected even at the two-week post-intervention post-test [31]. Researchers hypothesized that these effects may be due to lower levels of stress and cortisol release, which has been shown as an effect of Tai Chi in previous research studies [32]. According to the theory that executive functions are impaired in ADHD, Tai Chi may help improve executive functioning because it requires a combination of focused attention on movement and breath as guided by the teacher. This study shows that Tai Chi may have some beneficial effects on adolescents with ADHD as an adjunctive therapy [31].

3.4. Physical Activity

In human studies, physical activity and fitness has shown to affect brain structure and increase brain activity that is associated with conflict and attentional control. Though ADHD is a disorder with a complex etiology, there are a few factors contributing to the likelihood of ADHD that may be affected by physical activity. Exercise has also been shown to improve dopamine function, known to be dysregulated in ADHD [33]. Brain derived neurotrophic factor (BDNF) has also been found to play a role in ADHD symptoms through recent research [34]. This factor helps development of neurons in the dopaminergic pathways in the brain, which may be of importance to impulse control and attention. According to animal studies, BDNF expression is increased with stimulant medications [35]. The prefrontal and frontal regions contribute to regulation of catecholaminergic pathways involved in ADHD. According to Madras et al., there may be a decreased ability for people with ADHD to reload these catecholamines effectively [36]. Physical activity may affect these same neurological factors and brain regions. It has been shown that physical activity increases cerebral blood flow, thereby potentially helping where ADHD exhibits a deficit in blood flow to the prefrontal and frontal regions. Hunter et al.

demonstrated that physical activity may increase the amount of dopamine and norepinephrine in synaptic clefts which activate catecholaminergic pathways [37]. High impact running significantly increased measurements of dopamine, epinephrine and BDNF activity. Additionally, these increases were correlated with significant improvements in memory and learning ability tasks among the study participants [37].

A recent meta-analysis demonstrated that physical activity increases executive function and cognitive functioning with an effect size of 0.535 [38]. In another meta-analysis, pre-adolescent children were found to have increased executive function after one aerobic exercise session (effect size 0.540) [39]. One study investigating karate and its impact on motor and cognitive development showed that this particular martial arts form resulted in improved attention through the Tower of London test (effect size 0.88, $p < 0.05$) [40]. Martial arts teach children to practice self-control, concentration and meditation that may ultimately result in improvements of executive function. A study by Medina et al. showed that boys with ADHD had significantly improved attention after high-intensity treadmill exercise lasting for 30 min with or without medication [33]. The impact on cognitive function and academic performance needs to be further studied, as a recent systematic review found that the evidence for the effect of exercise on ADHD is equivocal and limited in quantity and quality [41]. While the preliminary evidence supports physical activity as an adjunctive treatment for ADHD, the data is insufficient to support it as a stand-alone treatment. A literature review by Gapin et al. suggests that future research should investigate physical activity as a stand-alone therapy for individuals that prefer alternative treatments as this topic has not been extensively tested in research [42].

4. Mindfulness-Based Therapies

Mindfulness and meditation have been found to "change brain activation patterns, contribute to enhanced mood, reduce anxiety, improve stress management, reduce pain and enhance immune function" [43] (p. 510). These effects imply that mind–body therapies could be well-suited for symptoms of ADHD in children. Mindfulness is "defined as a process of bringing one's complete attention to the present experience on a moment-to-moment basis" (p. 64) [44]. In other descriptions, it has been known as bringing awareness to the present experience without a judgmental attitude, but rather attentive and curious [45]. Mindfulness was developed from ancient cultural meditation practices and has now been adopted by Western psychology and medicine as treatment for stress reduction therapy [44]. Additionally, mindfulness therapy has been found to be satisfying and without unwanted side effects for persons with ADHD [45,46]. Meditation has been defined as a mental training technique that can enhance an altered state of consciousness, resembling its similarity to mindfulness [47]. Mindfulness and meditation have also been found to increase connectivity amongst brain regions associated with executive function [48].

Meditation/Mindfulness

The effect of an eight-week mindfulness training program for adults and adolescents with ADHD was considered [46]. The group consisted of 24 adults and eight adolescents who completed the intervention of eight weeks with 2.5 hours of training per day and additional "homework" meditation of 5 to 15 min. Measurements for pre- and post-intervention included the ADHD Rating Scale IV and SNAP-IV scale (for ADHD symptoms), the Attention Network Test (ANT) (for alerting, orienting and conflict attention), and the Stroop task (for attentional conflict), the Trail Making Test (for set-shifting and inhibition), the Digit Span (for working memory) in addition to other measurements. Substantial effects of the meditation were exhibited. In addition, 78% of participants reported a significant reduction in their ADHD symptoms with 30% reporting at least a 30% reduction. Significant improvement in attentional conflict and set-shifting was also found from pre- to post-intervention. Participant satisfaction was rated at a 9/10 on the visual analog scale and no adverse side effects were reported from the therapy. This study supports the hypothesis that mindfulness training may reduce self-reported ADHD symptoms and improved performance on certain attentional and cognitive tests [46].

This study by Crescentini et al. examined the effects of mindfulness training on 16 healthy primary school children ages seven to eight years old. The training consisted of three sessions per week for eight weeks [45]. A pre-test and post-test were taken by the main teacher of the students measuring behavior, social, emotion, and attention regulation skills. The children also self-reported mood and depression symptoms. There was a positive effect of the intervention on reduction of attention and internalizing issues. Children did not report any change in depressive symptoms after the intervention. This study shows support that mindfulness training has beneficial effects on attention and ADHD symptoms [45]. Mindfulness training can be incorporated into classroom activities or at home easily. Unlike medications, there are no harmful side effects and the training can be virtually at no cost to parents or teachers if they are educated on how to carry out the sessions for children

The effects of meditation on attention were studied by Jha et al. [44]. Two experimental conditions were created to study mindfulness and its effect on attention. Three realms of attention were studied: alerting, orienting and conflict-monitoring. These areas of attention were measured by scores on the Attention Network Test (ANS) at Time 1 before treatment and Time 2 after treatment. Group 1 underwent an eight-week long, three-hour daily course. Group 2 underwent an intensive retreat for one month where they completed 10–12 h of mindfulness practice. Group 3 was a control group of persons with no previous mindfulness experience. Group 1 also had no previous mindfulness experience, while Group 2 had previous mindfulness practice and therefore could be compared as "experienced" in mindfulness. Results showed that participants in Group 1 had significantly improved scores of orienting-type attention and endogenous orient attention in comparison with the other two groups. Group 2 exhibited improved scores in exogenous stimulus detection when compared to the other two groups [44].

Another study by Van de Weijer-Bergsma et al. incorporated parents and tutors into the mindfulness intervention [49]. Ten adolescents, 19 parents and seven academic tutors underwent mindfulness training for eight weeks for 1.5 h sessions. The training consisted of sitting meditation, body scan, and breathing space exercises along with interventions to improve awareness of one's distractability, impulsivity, and hyperactivity. Measurements were completed before the training as a pretest, at the end of the eight-week training and then again after 16 weeks. Measures consisted of scales measuring behavior problems, executive functioning, mindful awareness, parenting stress, parenting style, fatigue, happiness, and a computerized test of attention. Statistical analysis was carried out from pre-test to post-test to follow-up by paired t-tests with significant effects at $p < 0.10$ in a two-tailed t-test. At eight weeks, it was found that the adolescents had improvements in attention problems, executive functioning and performance on the computerized attention test [49]. The significance of their findings should be interpreted with caution, as the significance level is more liberal at $p < 0.10$. Further study should explore effects on mindfulness, perhaps with the same measurements but with larger sample sizes and interpreted with more strict significance scoring.

Studies show that meditative practice causes measurable changes within brain-wave activity. One experiment by Lagopoulos et al. investigated the effects of nondirective meditation on theta and alpha activity in the brain as recorded by EEG [50]. Eighteen participants who engaged in regular meditation for many years were recruited for the study. The experiment compared the theta and alpha activity between 20 minutes of non-directed meditation to non-meditative relaxation among the participants. There was a significant increase in alpha and theta activity among all three brain regions during meditation when compared to the relaxation session. Delta activity was significantly greater in the temporal central region during meditation as compared to relaxation. There was significantly greater alpha activity in the posterior region when compared to the frontal region, whereas theta activity was greater in the frontal and temporal-central regions compared to the posterior [50]. Meditation's effects on brainwaves may be an important area of study to determine what brainwave changes occur in children with ADHD practicing mind–body therapies, such as meditation.

An important factor to consider in the discussion of mindfulness or meditation for ADHD treatment is the type of meditation being used. Certain forms of mindfulness lead participants to greater awareness or attention on breathing or emotions, while others encourage free, relaxed mental states of "inattention." For example, one form of meditation, known as Yoga Nidra, is characterized by leading participants to "lose executive control" and has been shown to cause decreased blood flow to areas of the brain that regulate executive functions [51]. This study showed increased theta activity, which supports other meditation studies on brain wave activity. Because persons with ADHD already exhibit increased theta activity, it is counterintuitive that meditation could exhibit a beneficial effect on symptoms by causing a potential further increase. One potential mechanism by which meditation might affect ADHD symptoms is through the regulation of dopamine. Kjaer et al. found that dopamine release was significantly increased in the ventral striatum during Yoga Nidra meditation practice [51]. Through a C-raclopride Positron Emission Tomography (PET) scan, they found that there was as great as a 65% increase in dopamine among their participants [51]. Since medications for ADHD primarily target dopamine and norepinephrine transporters to increase synaptic levels, there may be a possibility that meditation could exhibit similar effects to these medications by the same means [7,51].

5. Conclusions

Potential benefits and mechanism of action of mind–body therapies have been evidenced through research and continue to be explored. Compared to pharmacological treatment, mind–body therapies have little to no unwanted side effects. There is little cost compared to clinical therapy since the only cost is for training or sessions that are typically conducted in groups. Activities such as yoga or Tai Chi can be practiced at home or school. Families and teachers can access videos online or purchase videos from reliable sources as resources to guide the therapy.

Mindfulness and meditation can be done anywhere and at any time. Furthermore, mindfulness is a learned skill. It is counterintuitive that meditation has positive effects on ADHD symptoms because theta to beta ratios are typically increased in ADHD, and meditation further increases theta wave activity [48]. Meditation and mindfulness may improve symptoms not because of the quantity of brainwave activity, but because of the learned skill to control attention and focus to a specific purpose or action (i.e., the breath). Further study of whether persons with ADHD can perform meditation and mindfulness more effectively because of their naturally increased theta activity is worth exploration. How mind–body therapies affect neuroanatomical and neurotransmitter function may also support its therapeutic use.

Mind–body training for parents has an added benefit to children's ADHD symptoms. Parents who practice mindfulness with parenting techniques report better outcomes in ADHD symptoms of their children [48]. It is probable that the effects of the studies involving children and parents could be not only due to the intervention itself, but the lasting actions of the child–parent interaction at home following the mind–body sessions. A parent who learns mindfulness through yoga or meditation may have improved methods of disciplining and responding to a child's behavior, and, in turn, the child may learn from the parent how to change their behavior in a positive way. Furthermore, having parents involved in the same treatment as their children helps continuation of mindful practice at home rather than limiting training to individual sessions.

Limitations of current research are primarily due to small sample sizes and lack of control groups. More research needs to be done with larger sample sizes and more controlled settings. Many of the studies reviewed also gathered data from subjective self-report or parent/teacher surveys. More objective data should be measured alongside subjective data in future research.

Acknowledgments: No grants or funds were received for this review article. The authors wish to thank their division of KU Integrative Medicine and Department of Internal Medicine for their continued support and encouragement in the advancement of the field, integrative medicine.

Author Contributions: Anne Herbert contributed to the writing and editing of the manuscript. Anna Esparham contributed to the writing and editing of the manuscript.

Conflicts of Interest: The authors declare no conflict of interest.

References

1. Barry, R.J.; Clarke, A.R.; Johnstone, S.J. A review electrophysiology in attention-deficit/hyperactivity disorder: I. Qualitative and quantitative electroencephalopathy. *Clin. Neurophysiol.* **2003**, *114*, 172–183. [CrossRef]
2. Spencer, T.J.; Biederman, J.; Mick, E. Attention-deficit/hyperactivity disorder: Diagnosis, lifespan, comorbidities, and neurobiology. *Ambul. Pediatr.* **2007**, *7*, 73–81. [CrossRef] [PubMed]
3. Centers for Disease Control and Prevention. Attention-Deficit/Hyperactivity Disorder. 2013. Available online: http:www.cdc.gov/ncbddd/adhd/data.html (accessed on 18 November 2016).
4. Barkley, R.A. Behavioral inhibition, sustained attention, and executive function: Constructing a unified theory of ADHD. *Psychol. Bull.* **1997**, *121*, 65–94. [CrossRef] [PubMed]
5. Purper-Ouakil, D.; Ramoz, N.; Lepagnol-Bestel, A.M.; Gorwood, P.; Simonneau, M. Neurobiology of attention deficit/hyperactivity disorder. *Pediatr. Res.* **2011**, *69*, 69R–76R. [CrossRef] [PubMed]
6. Gizer, I.R.; Ficks, C.; Waldman, I.D. Candidate gene studies of ADHD: A meta-analytic review. *Hum. Genet.* **2009**, *126*, 51–90. [CrossRef] [PubMed]
7. Hohmann, S.; Hohm, E.; Treutlein, J.; Blomeyer, D.; Jennen-Steinmetz, C.; Schmidt, M.H.; Esser, G.; Banaschewski, T.; Brandeis, D.; Laucht, M. Association of norepinephrine transporter (*NET*, *SLC6A2*) genotype with ADHD-related phenotypes: Findings of a longitudinal study from birth to adolescence. *Psychiatry Res.* **2015**, *226*, 425–433. [CrossRef] [PubMed]
8. Sigurdardottir, H.L.; Kranz, G.S.; Rami-Mark, C.; James, G.M.; Vanicek, T.; Gryglewski, G.; Kautzky, A.; Hienert, M.; Traub-Weidinger, T.; Mitterhauser, M.; et al. Effects of norepinephrine transporter gene variants on NET binding in ADHD and healthy controls investigated by PET. *Hum. Brain Mapp.* **2016**, *37*, 884–895. [CrossRef] [PubMed]
9. Monastra, V.J. Quantitative electroencephalography and attention-deficit/hyperactivity disorder: Implications for clinical practice. *Curr. Psychiatry Rep.* **2008**, *10*, 432–438. [CrossRef] [PubMed]
10. Mohammadi, M.R.; Malmir, N.; Khaleghi, A.; Aminiorani, M. Comparison of sensorimotor rhythm (SMR) and beta training on selective attention and symptoms in children with attention deficit/hyperactivity disorder (ADHD): A trend report. *Iran. J. Psychiatry* **2015**, *10*, 165–174. [PubMed]
11. Ter Huurne, N.; Lozano-Soldevilla, D.; Onnink, M.; Kan, C.; Buitelaar, J.; Jensen, O. Diminished modulation of preparatory sensorimotor mu rhythm predicts attention-deficit/hyperactivity disorder severity. *Psychol. Med.* **2017**, 1–10. [CrossRef] [PubMed]
12. Lazzaro, I.; Gordon, E.; Li, W.; Lim, C.L.; Plahn, M.; Whitmont, S.; Clarke, S.; Barry, R.J.; Dosen, A.; Meares, R. Simultaneous EEG and EDA measures in adolescent attention deficit hyperactivity disorder. *Int. J. Psychophysiol.* **1999**, *34*, 123–134. [CrossRef]
13. Kim, J.H.; Yan, J.; Lee, M. Changes of heart rate variability during methylphenidate treatment in attention-deficit hyperactivity disorder children: A 12-week prospective study. *Yonsei Med. J.* **2014**, *56*, 1365–1371. [CrossRef] [PubMed]
14. Rukmani, M.R.; Sephardi, S.P.; Thennarasu, K.; Raju, T.R.; Sathyaprabha, T.N. Heart rate variability in children with Attention Deficit/Hyperactivity Disorder: A pilot study. *Ann. Neurosciences* **2016**, *23*, 81–88. [CrossRef] [PubMed]
15. Wolraich, M.; Brown, L.; Brown, R.T.; DuPaul, G.; Earls, M.; Feldman, H.M.; Ganiats, T.G.; Kaplanek, B.; Meyer, B.; Perrin, J.; et al. ADHD: Clinical practice guideline for the diagnosis, evaluation, and treatment of attention-deficit/hyperactivity disorder in children and adolescents. *Pediatrics* **2011**, *128*, 1007–1022. [PubMed]
16. Page, T.F.; Pelham, W.E., III; Fabiano, G.A.; Greiner, A.R.; Gnagy, E.M.; Hart, K.C.; Coxe, S.; Waxmonsky, J.G.; Foster, E.M.; Pelham, W.E. Comparative cost analysis of sequential, adaptive, behavioral, pharmacological, and combined treatments for childhood ADHD. *J. Clin. Child Adolesc. Psychol.* **2016**, *45*, 416–427. [CrossRef] [PubMed]

17. Swanson, J.M.; Arnold, L.E.; Molina, B.S.G.; Sibley, M.H.; Hechtman, L.T.; Hinshaw, S.P.; Abikoff, H.B.; Stehli, A.; Owens, E.B.; Mitchell, J.T.; et al. Young adult outcomes in the follow-up of the multimodal treatment study of attention-deficit/hyperactivity disorder: Symptom persistence, source discrepancy, and height suppression. *J. Child Psychol. Psychiatry.* **2017**. [CrossRef] [PubMed]
18. Pelham, W.E.; Fabiano, G.A.; Waxmonsky, J.G.; Greiner, A.R.; Gnagy, E.M.; Pelhamm, W.E., III; Coxe, S.; Verley, J.; Bhatia, I.; Hart, K.; Karch, K.; et al. Treatment sequencing for childhood ADHD: A multiple-randomization study of adaptive medication and behavioral interventions. *J. Clin. Child Adolesc. Psychol.* **2016**, *45*, 396–415. [CrossRef] [PubMed]
19. Esparham, A.; Evans, R.G.; Wagner, L.E.; Drisko, J.A. Pediatric integrative medicine approaches to attention deficit hyperactivity disorder (ADHD). *Children* **2014**, *1*, 186–207. [CrossRef] [PubMed]
20. McClafferty, H. Complementary, holistic and integrative medicine. *Pediatrics Rev.* **2011**, *32*, 201–203. [CrossRef] [PubMed]
21. Kaunhoven, R.J.; Dorjee, D. How does mindfulness modulate self-regulation in pre-adolescent children? An integrative neurocognitive review. *Neurosci. Biobehav. Rev.* **2017**, *74*, 163–184. [CrossRef] [PubMed]
22. Rosen, L.; French, A.; Sullivan, G. Complementary, holistic, and integrative medicine: Yoga. *Pediatrics Rev.* **2015**, *36*, 468–474. [CrossRef] [PubMed]
23. Tyagi, A.; Cohen, M. Yoga and heart rate variability: A comprehensive review of the literature. *Int. J. Yoga* **2016**, *9*, 97–113. [PubMed]
24. Hariprasad, V.R.; Arasappa, R.; Varambally, S.; Srinath, S.; Gangadhar, B.N. Feasibility and efficacy of yoga as an add-on intervention in attention deficit-hyperactivity disorder: An exploratory study. *Indian J. Psychiatry* **2013**, *55*, S379–S384. [PubMed]
25. Harrison, L.J.; Manocha, R.; Rubia, K. Sahaja yoga meditation as a family treatment programme for children with attention deficits-hyperactivity disorder. *Clin. Child Psychol. Psychiatry* **2004**, *9*, 479–497. [CrossRef]
26. Hernández, S.E.; Suero, J.; Barros, A.; González-Mora, J.L.; Rubia, K. Increased grey matter associated with long-term Sahaja yoga meditation: A voxel-based morphometry study. *PLoS ONE* **2016**, *11*, 1–16. [CrossRef] [PubMed]
27. Peck, H.L.; Kehle, T.J.; Bray, M.A.; Theodore, L.A. Yoga as an intervention for children with attention problems. *Sch. Psychol. Rev.* **2005**, *34*, 415–424.
28. Jensen, P.S.; Kenny, D.T. The effects of yoga on the attention and behavior of boys with attention-deficit/hyperactivity disorder (ADHD). *J. Atten. Disorders* **2004**, *7*, 205–216. [CrossRef] [PubMed]
29. Chou, C.; Huang, C. Effects of an 8-week yoga program on sustained attention and discrimination in children with attention deficit hyperactivity disorder. *PeerJ* **2017**. [CrossRef] [PubMed]
30. Gothe, N.; Potifex, M.B.; Hillman, C.; McAuley, E. The acute effects of yoga on executive function. *J. Phys. Act. Health* **2013**, *10*, 488–495. [CrossRef] [PubMed]
31. Hernandez-Reid, M.; Field, T.M.; Thimas, E. Attention deficit hyperactivity disorder: Benefits from Tai Chi. *J. Bodyw. Mov. Ther.* **2000**, *5*, 120–123. [CrossRef]
32. Converse, A.K.; Ahlers, E.O.; Travers, B.G.; Davidson, R.J. Tai chi training reduces self-report of inattention in healthy young adults. *Front. Hum. Neurosci.* **2014**, *8*, 1–7. [CrossRef] [PubMed]
33. Medina, J.A.; Netto, T.L.; Muszkat, M.; Medina, A.C.; Botter, D.; Orbetelli, R.; Scaramuzza, L.F.; Sinnes, E.G.; Vilela, M.; Miranda, M.C. Exercise impact on sustained attention of ADHD children, methylphenidate effects. *Atten. Defic. Hyperact. Disord.* **2010**, *2*, 49–58. [CrossRef] [PubMed]
34. Chen, C.; Nakagawa, S.; An, Y.; Ito, K.; Kitaichi, Y.; Kusumi, I. The exercise-glucocorticoid paradox: How exercise is beneficial to cognition, mood, and the brain while increasing glucocorticoid levels. *Front. Neuroendocrinol.* **2017**, *44*, 83–102. [CrossRef] [PubMed]
35. Fumagalli, F.; Cattaneo, A.; Caffino, L.; Ibba, M.; Racagni, G.; Carboni, E.; Gennarelli, M.; Riva, M.A. Sub-chronic exposure to atomoxetine up-regulates BDNF expression and signalling in the brain of adolescent spontaneously hypertensive rats: Comparison with methylphenidate. *Pharmacol. Res.* **2010**, *62*, 523–529. [CrossRef] [PubMed]
36. Madras, B.K.; Miller, G.M.; Fischman, A.J. The dopamine transporter and attention-deficit/hyperactivity disorder. *Biol. Psychiatry* **2005**, *57*, 1397–1409. [CrossRef] [PubMed]
37. Winter, B.; Breitenstein, C.; Mooren, F.C.; Voelker, K.; Fobker, M.; Lechtermann, A.; Krueger, K.; Fromme, A.; Korsukewitz, C.; Floel, A.; et al. High impact running improves learning. *Neurobiol. Learn. Mem.* **2007**, *87*, 597–609. [CrossRef] [PubMed]

38. Vyniauske, R.; Verburgh, L.; Oosterlaan, J.; Molendijk, M.L. The effects of physical exercise on functional outcomes in the treatment of ADHD: A meta-analysis. *J. Atten. Disord.* **2016**. [CrossRef]

39. Ludyga, S.; Gerber, M.; Brand, S.; Holsboer-Trachsler, E.; Pühse, U. Acute effects of moderate aerobic exercise on specific aspects of executive function in different age and fitness groups: A meta-analysis. *Psychophysiology* **2016**, *53*, 1611–1626. [CrossRef] [PubMed]

40. Alesi, M.; Bianco, A.; Padulo, J.; Vella, F.P.; Petrucci, M.; Paoli, A.; Palma, A.; Pepi1, A. Motor and cognitive development: the role of karate. *Muscle Ligaments Tendons J.* **2014**, *4*, 114–120.

41. Li, J.W.; O'Connor, H.; O'Dwyer, N.; Orr, R. The effect of acute and chronic exercise on cognitive function and academic performance in adolescents: A systematic review. *J. Sci. Med. Sport* **2017**. [CrossRef] [PubMed]

42. Gapin, J.I.; Laban, J.D.; Etnier, J.L. The effects of physical activity on attention deficit hyperactivity disorder symptoms: The evidence. *Prev. Med.* **2011**, *52*, 570–574. [CrossRef] [PubMed]

43. Edwards, E.; Mischoulon, D.; Rapaport, M.; Stussman, B.; Weber, W. Building an evidence base in complementary and integrative healthcare for child and adolescent psychiatry. *Child Adolesc. Psychiatr. Clin. N. Am.* **2013**, *22*, 509–522. [CrossRef] [PubMed]

44. Jha, A.P.; Krompinger, J.; Baime, M.J. Mindfulness training modifies subsystems of attention. *Cogn. Affect. Behav. Neurosci.* **2007**, *7*, 109–119. [CrossRef] [PubMed]

45. Crescentini, C.; Capurso, V.; Furlan, S.; Fabbro, F. Mindfulness-oriented meditation for primary school children: Effects on attention and psychological well-being. *Front. Psychol.* **2016**, *7*. [CrossRef] [PubMed]

46. Zylowska, L.; Ackerman, D.L.; Yang, M.H.; Futrell, J.L.; Horton, N.L.; Hale, T.S.; Pataki, C.; Smalley, S.L. Mindfulness meditation training in adults and adolescents with ADHD. *J. Atten. Disord.* **2008**, *11*, 737–746. [CrossRef] [PubMed]

47. Nash, J.D.; Newberg, A. Toward a unifying taxonomy and definition for meditation. *Front. Psychol.* **2013**, *4*. [CrossRef] [PubMed]

48. Taren, A.A.; Gianaros, P.J.; Greco, C.M.; Lindsay, E.K.; Fairgrieve, A.; Brown, K.W.; Rosen, R.K.; Ferris, J.L.; Julson, E.; Marsland, A.L.; et al. Mindfulness meditation training and executive control network resting state functional connectivity: A randomized controlled trial. *Psychosom. Med.* **2017**. [CrossRef] [PubMed]

49. Van de Weijer-Bergsma, E.; Formsma, A.R.; de Bruin, E.I.; Bögels, S.M. The effectiveness of mindfulness training on behavioral problems and attentional functioning in adolescents with ADHD. *J. Child Fam. Stud.* **2012**, *21*, 775–787. [CrossRef] [PubMed]

50. Lagopoulos, J.; Xu, J.; Rasmussen, I.; Vik, A.; Malhi, G.S.; Eliassen, C.S.; Arnsten, I.E.; Sæther, J.G.; Hollup, S.; Holen, A.; et al. Increased theta and alpha EEG activity during nondirective meditation. *J. Altern. Complement. Med.* **2009**, *15*, 1187–1192. [CrossRef] [PubMed]

51. Kjaer, T.W.; Bertelsen, C.; Piccini, P.; Brooks, D.; Alving, J.; Lou, H.C. Increased dopamine tone during meditation-induced change of consciousness. *Cogn. Brain Res.* **2002**, *13*, 255–259. [CrossRef]

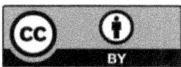

children

MDPI

Review

Immersive Virtual Reality for Pediatric Pain

Andrea Stevenson Won [1], Jakki Bailey [2], Jeremy Bailenson [2], Christine Tataru [2], Isabel A. Yoon [2] and Brenda Golianu [2,*]

1   Department of Communication, Cornell University, 417 Mann Library Building, Ithaca, NY 14853, USA; a.s.won@cornell.edu
2   Department of Anesthesiology and Perioperative Medicine, Stanford University, 300 Pasteur Dr. H3580A, Stanford, CA 94305, USA; jakki7@stanford.edu (J.B.); bailenso@stanford.edu (J.B.); ctataru5@stanford.edu (C.T.); iayoon@stanford.edu (I.A.Y.)
*   Correspondence: bgolianu@stanford.edu; Tel.: +1-650-723-5728

Academic Editor: Hilary McClafferty
Received: 12 March 2017; Accepted: 16 June 2017; Published: 23 June 2017

Abstract: Children must often endure painful procedures as part of their treatment for various medical conditions. Those with chronic pain endure frequent or constant discomfort in their daily lives, sometimes severely limiting their physical capacities. With the advent of affordable consumer-grade equipment, clinicians have access to a promising and engaging intervention for pediatric pain, both acute and chronic. In addition to providing relief from acute and procedural pain, virtual reality (VR) may also help to provide a corrective psychological and physiological environment to facilitate rehabilitation for pediatric patients suffering from chronic pain. The special qualities of VR such as presence, interactivity, customization, social interaction, and embodiment allow it to be accepted by children and adolescents and incorporated successfully into their existing medical therapies. However, the powerful and transformative nature of many VR experiences may also pose some risks and should be utilized with caution. In this paper, we review recent literature in pediatric virtual reality for procedural pain and anxiety, acute and chronic pain, and some rehabilitation applications. We also discuss the practical considerations of using VR in pediatric care, and offer specific suggestions and information for clinicians wishing to adopt these engaging therapies into their daily clinical practice.

Keywords: Virtual reality; pediatric pain; procedural pain; nonpharmacological; rehabilitation

1. Introduction

Children have always enjoyed games of "pretend." While immersed in a game, they often become deeply absorbed and able to ignore aversive stimuli. Immersive virtual reality (VR) is a promising and engaging intervention that may help to decrease pain and anxiety for children undergoing painful procedures and suffering from acute pain. In the context of their medical care, children may also endure chronic pain and discomfort. Because VR makes it possible to transform how patients perceive their bodies, it allows other, novel interventions that are possible in no other medium. Beyond providing distraction and enjoyment, virtual reality may provide a corrective psychological and physiological environment, and can facilitate rehabilitation for pediatric patients suffering from chronic pain, as well as neurorehabilitation for children suffering from stroke and cerebral palsy. With the advent of inexpensive consumer VR systems, the opportunities to research and deploy VR in the clinic have expanded. However, the powerful and transformative nature of many VR experiences may also pose some risks and should be utilized with caution in developing therapeutic VR interventions [1].

In this paper, we will review recent literature in pediatric virtual reality for procedural pain and anxiety, acute and chronic pain, and some rehabilitation applications. We will also discuss clinically relevant characteristics of VR experiences, such as the aspects of presence, interactivity, customization, social interaction, and embodiment. We will review how each of these requires special consideration, and in some cases adaptation of the hardware or software, for a child population. Finally, we will discuss the practical considerations of some currently available consumer VR systems, and offer specific suggestions and information for clinicians wishing to adopt these engaging therapies.

2. Review of Virtual Reality in Pediatrics

We conducted a review evaluating articles that describe the use of VR in pediatric procedural, acute and chronic pain. (see Table 1) We included articles detailing case studies or randomized trials of the use of VR. Where such studies were not available, we referred to adult studies that may offer insights into the potential use in pediatric populations, which are specifically described as pertaining to adult populations. We will discuss the selected articles and themes as they are relevant to the improved care of pediatric patients through VR. These articles can be roughly divided into two main areas of clinical relevance: acute and procedural pain and anxiety, and chronic pain and neurorehabilitation.

Table 1. The following terms were searched on PubMed (www.ncbi.nlm.nih.gov/pubmed/) between 2000 and 2017.

Key Word Search	Number of Articles Obtained	Number of Articles Deemed Relevant and Utilized in Review
Virtual Reality and Pediatric Procedures	94	13
Virtual Reality and Pediatric Anxiety	14	7
Virtual Reality and Procedural Anxiety	13	8
Virtual Reality and Pediatric Procedural Anxiety	5	5
Virtual Reality and Pediatric Chronic Pain	4	4
Virtual Reality and Pediatric Acute Pain	5	5
Virtual Reality and Pain	312	31
Virtual Reality and Acute pain	35	16
Virtual Reality and Chronic Pain	63	27

2.1. Acute and Procedural Pain

Acute pain is pain directly related to a temporary injury and typically lasts a short period of time (<6 weeks). Procedural pain and anxiety refers to distress derived from medical procedures, including intravenous (IV) injections, vaccinations, anesthesia administration, and other needle-related procedures, as well as other procedures required as part of routine care, such as burn wound dressing changes.

Virtual reality was first used to manage acute pain during painful repetitive dressing changes in patients with burn wounds [2]. Schmitt et al. demonstrated a reduction in pain of 27–44% in pediatric patients who participated in the virtual environment featuring a wintery scenario, called "SnowWorld", while undergoing dressing changes [3,4]. Jeffs et al. corroborated the efficacy of VR in burn wound pain management in adolescents [5]. In a randomized three-armed trial, 30 adolescents were assigned to standard care, watching a movie, and VR engagement with the "SnowWorld" virtual environment. The VR treatment group reported a decrease in pain compared to the passive distraction (movie) group, (difference 23.7 points decrease in pain score out of 100 total), 95% confidence interval (CI): 2.4–45.0, $p = 0.029$). In comparison to standard care, the VR group showed decreased pain as well, though the difference was not statistically significant. Of note, the VR group was the only one in which the patients' pain during the actual dressing change procedure was reported to be less than the pre-procedure pain [5].

Brown et al. performed a randomized controlled trial of an interactive VR intervention entitled "Ditto" and showed not only a decrease in self-reported pain and anxiety in pediatric patients undergoing dressing changes, but also an increased rate of epithelialization and faster wound healing in those patients undergoing VR intervention for their procedures (−2.14 days (wounds healed 2.14 days faster), CI: −4.38 to 0.1, $p = 0.061$), which was significantly faster when adjusted for mean burn depth (−2.26 days, CI −4.48 to −0.04, $p = 0.046$) [6]. Lastly, Miller et al. showed that not only was pain reduced during dressing changes, but when a multimodal intervention was utilized, the procedure required less time to complete ($p < 0.05$) [7]. Additional notable studies investigating the efficacy of VR distraction on pain and anxiety in children and adults undergoing severe burn wound care are referenced below [8,9].

Virtual reality has also proven successful at lessening procedural pain and distress related to IV placement and other needle-related procedures. In a 2006 study, Gold et al. performed a randomized control trial on 20 pediatric patients requiring IV placement [10]. The VR group received a multisensory VR experience including visual stimulation from a HMD device, tactile feedback, and music, for 5 min prior to IV placement until 5 min after placement. The control group received local anesthetic spray, but no VR intervention for the procedure. They were permitted to utilize the VR equipment for 3 min following IV placement. While children in the control group experienced a four-fold increase in pain as measured by the Wong-Baker FACES scale [11], the VR group showed no increase in affective pain following IV placement [10]. Nilsson et al. performed a similar study ($N = 42$) using a screen-based three-dimensional (3D) program [12]. Pediatric and adolescent patients undergoing venous punctures or subcutaneous venous port device insertion were randomized either to this non-immersive VR and standard care, or standard care alone. Patients did not report a significant decrease in self-reported pain for either condition; however, they did report that the VR distraction was a pleasant experience that succeeded at distraction. (We note that this intervention was not immersive).

Beyond VR's use in acute pain, it can potentially be used to make patients more familiar and comfortable with procedures. Most hospital procedures are accompanied by some stress or anxiety on the part of pediatric patients. He et al. looked at the effect of therapeutic play on perioperative anxiety, negative emotional manifestation, and postoperative pain [13]. Ninety-five children were assigned randomly to receive one hour of face-to-face therapeutic play involving objects to be used in the operation, or no intervention. Those children that participated in therapeutic play exhibited significantly lower levels of anxiety and negative emotion manifestation associated with their upcoming operation, and even showed lower levels of post-operative pain [13]. Virtual reality has the potential to familiarize children with the operation environment in a safe, controlled and playful way, and potentially decrease their pain and anxiety.

2.2. Chronic Pain

Unlike procedural or acute pain, chronic pain is persistent for a period greater than six weeks, often for months or years. It may include chronic headache, abdominal, limb, joint or back pain, neuropathic or sympathetically maintained pain such as complex regional pain syndrome (CRPS), and pain related to other medical conditions. In addition to symptom control, interventions often strive to maintain or improve function and minimize disability. While there is little research on using VR for the treatment of chronic pain in children [14], promising results in adults indicate that further research in this area is advisable. Below, we describe the use of virtual reality in neuromodulation, in physical therapy, and in biofeedback. We describe the limited research in children, and attempt to extend relevant research in adults to pediatric patients.

Virtual reality may have the potential to amplify the neuromodulatory effects of traditional mirror visual feedback (MVF), which can modify patients' pathological cortical representations in the group of chronic pain syndromes that includes phantom limb pain, complex regional pain syndrome and fibromyalgia. Mirror visual feedback was first applied to adult patients suffering from phantom limb pain (PLP) by Ramachandran and Rogers-Ramachandran [15]. This technique may exert some of its benefits by encouraging the remapping of motor and somatosensory cortices, allowing a return to a homeostatic processing mechanism and facilitating the improvement or resolution of the painful experience. Mirror visual feedback was also found to be of benefit for CRPS in a randomized controlled trial with adult patients [16]. Virtual reality has also been used in an open-label case study of five adults with CRPS, four of whom reported reduced pain intensity over five to eight sessions [17].

Besides providing a new medium for mirror therapy, VR also allows other avatar configurations to be altered. For example, patients can also experience augmented motion such that a small motion in the physical world maps to a large motion in the virtual one, or vice versa. Thus, a small movement of the arm made in real life could be rewarded by a larger, more apparent arm movement in VR. Conversely, for patients prone to guarding, movements made by patients in real life could be depicted as more restrained in the virtual world [18], which might encourage such patients to move more freely. Two studies demonstrated that adult patients with neck pain moved further and reported less pain as a result of movement when VR was used to reduce their apparent movement [18,19]. In the pediatric population, there is currently one feasibility study exploring the neuromodulatory effects of VR. Won et al. showed that a VR experience with MVF and movement augmentation properties was well tolerated by pediatric patients with CRPS during physical therapy sessions [20].

The hypothesis supporting the efficacy of neuromodulatory chronic pain therapies is founded in the association between brain connectivity changes and improvement in chronic pain symptoms. A study conducted by Lebel and colleagues found significant changes in the somatosensory processing of symptomatic pediatric CRPS when compared to post-treatment CRPS patients and control patients [21]. Because this processing resumes normality after months of traditional physical therapy, it is possible that directly altering somatosensory processing (i.e., via mirror therapy), might itself be helpful in resolving pain. Becerra et al. and Simons et al. [22,23] both showed changes in connectivity in various intrinsic brain networks after therapies that reduced pain and improved function. It is still under debate whether the association of successful recovery from CRPS symptoms is directly related to changes in brain connectivity or brain plasticity, and further research is required to determine what other factors may be involved in remapping somatosensory processing [24]. However, another piece of evidence supporting this hypothesis comes from graded motor imagery, a therapy that involves the imaginary mental rotation of one's limbs. Adult studies have shown that this therapy is associated with both changes in connectivity in the central nervous system as well as reduction in pain [25], and pediatric patients may also benefit from such therapy.

As discussed above, VR offers an engaging opportunity for children to practice motions that would be impossible or unsafe in the real world [26]. Especially in diseases like cerebral palsy, where motion is difficult, the opportunity to engage in active/repetitive motor and sensory practice can increase neuroplasticity and allow for learning to overcome some limitations of the disease [27]. In a study by Biffi et al., 12 children with Acquired Brain Injury (ABI) participated in 10 sessions using an interactive VR system called GRAIL (Gait Real-time Analysis Interactive Lab); treatment sessions led to improvement in walking abilities and enhanced engagement during training, suggesting that VR may play a role in the field of rehabilitation [28]. Although not discussing efficacy, Meyns et al. demonstrated the feasibility of using VR training to improve balance in children with cerebral palsy after lower limb surgery [29]. For a more in-depth review on neurorehabilitation applications of VR, please refer to the following excellent review by Wang et al. [26].

In addition to alterations in neuronal representation, patients with chronic pain often exhibit a debilitating fear of inducing more pain through movement. This fear not only seriously affects patients' ability to function; it can also inhibit physical therapy efforts. Trost et al. discusses the use of VR interventions to provide graded exposure treatment for pain-related fear and disability in adults with chronic low back pain [30]. Collado-Mateo et al. also found that a combined program of physical exercise and non-immersive VR improved adult patients' mobility, balance, and fear of falling in adult fibromyalgia patients [31]. Senkowski et al. cite significant promise in the use of VR-assisted therapy to aid in the decrease of fear-avoidance behavior and improvement in distorted body images [32]. Fear-avoidance is noted to be an issue in the pediatric population with chronic pain [33]; however, no VR interventions have yet been specifically designed to address this phenomenon.

2.3. Other Applications

Another possible application is the use of a virtual pain coach. A VR experience could reinforce therapeutic movements and exercises in an out-of-clinic environment. This is especially useful for long-distance patients or patients who are unable to be physically present for other reasons [34]. The variety of VR therapy options makes it an effective intervention to integrate into existing interdisciplinary programs, combining medical treatment, physical therapy and psychological interventions [35].

Finally, the effects of VR may potentially be augmented by other techniques such as biofeedback or hypnosis. Biofeedback is the process of providing the patient with information on his or her own neurological data such as heart rate variability, temperature, or muscle tension. In a recent pilot study, non-immersive VR mirror visual feedback was used successfully in combination with biofeedback to treat pediatric patients with chronic headaches [36]. Virtual reality was also used in conjunction with hypnosis in an adult case report [37].

3. Qualities of Virtual Reality

In the next section, we will discuss five qualities of VR that are of interest in considering clinical applications for children: presence, interactivity, social interactions, customization, and embodiment. We will then summarize current research on how these qualities may be useful for treating children, and note some potential areas of caution (see Table 2).

Table 2. Possible benefits and side effects of VR.

Benefits	<ul><li>Provides distraction from pain</li><li>Promotes movement</li><li>Promotes imagination</li><li>Fosters sense of internal health locus of control</li><li>Promotes cortical repatterning (potentially)</li></ul>
Side Effects	<ul><li>Visually-induced motion sickness (dizziness, nausea)</li><li>Collisions with nearby objects</li><li>As with other media, risks social isolation</li><li>In younger children, possible potential for "false memories"</li></ul>

3.1. Presence

Presence is the subjective feeling that the user is experiencing the environment and interactions in the virtual world are [38]. It is often measured by self-report, has been linked to physiological processes such as changes in hear rate and skin resistance [39] and behavioral measures such as not responding to stimuli in the real world [40]. Feelings of presence can be evoked by even a simple VR system, such as a 360° video viewed through a smartphone in a cardboard housing. However, a recent meta-analysis indicates that features such as improved tracking, stereoscopy, and wide field of view can make VR experiences feel more real [1]. VR is particularly promising as a distractor for procedural and acute pain because of the deep sense of presence created by virtual worlds. The immersive features of virtual reality technology immerse the patient with rich sensory stimuli, creating a realistic experience and effectively directing attention away from adverse stimuli [41,42].

Age may influence how virtual environments are experienced. For example, during burn wound care treatment with VR, pediatric patients reported higher levels of presence compared to adults receiving the same treatment [43]. Experiencing virtual environments as extremely real has important implications for how children behave and understand the world after the VR treatment. Baumgartner et al. showed that children's brains process virtual experiences differently than adults and young children may require different types of immersive experiences [44]. During early childhood (e.g., three to five-years-old) children's sense of fantasy and reality is rapidly developing [45,46]. Virtual reality can create realistic environments that may seem extremely real, particularly to young children.

Given that children may be more vulnerable to believing virtual experiences as real, virtual environments may need to be carefully selected and contextualized so that children are able to interpret their memories of the experience as derived from media rather than real life. In addition, for some age groups, debriefing post-VR experience may be necessary.

3.2. Interactivity

Virtual reality therapies incorporating tracked body movements allow for greater interactivity. In a study examining cold pressor-induced pain in 40 children of age 5–13, greater interactivity led to greater pain tolerance [47]. Children with disorders requiring intensive physical therapy, such as those with CRPS [20] or cerebral palsy [48], may benefit especially from interactive VR scenarios. Such scenarios can encourage them to engage in physical therapy while simultaneously increasing their pain tolerance.

High levels of interactivity, while effective in reducing pain, can be accompanied by a sense of nausea and increased potential for collisions with objects in the real world. Clinicians using VR as therapy should be aware of these minor risks and take appropriate precautions for pediatric patients. The more immersed users are in a virtual environment, the more the sensory input from the real world is occluded, and active users risk painful collisions.

Even adults can be at risk of falling or colliding with objects; during set-up, consumer VR systems require users to define a safe "play space", and displays are equipped with safety warnings and reminders to be careful when users approach the edge of this area. As children move around a virtual space, they may come dangerously close to objects in the real world. Even if children are seated, they should be monitored. Careful spotting is necessary to prevent them from injuring themselves or bystanders by accidentally colliding with real-world objects.

In addition, although both children and adults can be prone to "cybersickness" or feeling nausea or dizziness, children may be less able to anticipate and articulate their discomfort. Caretakers and clinicians will need to be aware of the possible signs of sickness and develop ways to measure children's discomfort in non-verbal and unobtrusive ways such as how children are moving their bodies. Another alternative is to set pre-determined timers to take short breaks.

3.3. Social Interactions in Virtual Reality

Many factors affect children's and adolescents' attraction to video games, one being their ability to share the experience with friends [49]. The use of social interactions may be particularly effective during adolescence, a time in which children are particularly sensitive to social environments [50]. Children as young as five years old respond to digital others in social ways, such as using information from a virtual character and a live person at equal rates to solve a decision-making task [51].

Children with chronic pain may have particular deficiencies in their abilities to develop and maintain peer relationships due to increased school absences, decreased physical ability to engage in sports or social activities, and decreased mood and motivation [52]. Virtual environments may offer an alternative platform for children to build these relationships by giving them access to near-real experiences that they can share with others. Children with high medical acuity, such as those in post-transplant oncology, who may be confined to a single room or unit, may benefit from access to virtual interactions if they are not able to engage with peers due to their ongoing medical condition. Since older children are already actively involved in virtual environments [53], the presence of virtual others offers new opportunities. For example, physical therapists might incorporate their own behavior into the environment via an avatar, which could help patients visualize or mimic the correct movements.

However, as in real life, children need age-appropriate environments. Social virtual environments where children can interact with others such as High Fidelity (highfidelity.io) or AltspaceVR (altVR.com) may require additional permissions so that outsiders cannot interact with patients. In addition, the risks and benefits of social media are also applicable when social media platforms provide opportunities for patients to engage virtually. While Facebook's current beta application, Spaces (oculus.com/experiences/rift/), and other environments linked with social media platforms may make it easy for children to engage with Facebook friends in immersive virtual reality, such interactions should not allow children to isolate themselves from face-to-face interactions.

3.4. Customization

Clinicians or patients themselves can select different virtual scenarios, and as commercial VR experiences become more common, there will be more entertainment options from which to choose. Allowing children to contribute towards selecting their virtual experience allows them agency and the ability to tailor content to their interests, as in a study by Ni et al. [54] in which pediatric patients and therapists evaluated games for degree of engagement and therapeutic usefulness together. For example, children undergoing chemotherapy who selected from a variety of virtual scenarios demonstrated reduced symptom distress [55].

Another area in which customization can be advantageous is in avatar representation. Children can select and customize their own avatar, providing them with a sense of control in a clinical setting that can significantly reduce patient stress [56]. When embodying stock avatars, children may need guidance in selecting age-appropriate material, as research suggests that users may conform their behavior to their preconceptions about the avatars they embody [57,58].

3.5. Embodiment

When body trackers, such as hand trackers, are used in virtual reality, participants can move their tracked limbs in real life and see their movements represented by the movements of their avatars in virtual reality. Thus, when patients are embodied in an avatar, they gain the sense that their avatar body has replaced their real body. This allows interventions that are possible in no other medium.

The tracking capabilities inherent in embodied VR experiences also offer clinicians the ability to monitor their patients' physical movements and quantify rehabilitative effort without relying on self-report data. As wearable monitors for tracking physiological data such as gait and posture become increasingly used, clinicians may observe their patients on multiple levels and tailor their treatment accordingly. As with all patient data, movement data in children must be carefully protected.

Movement is not the only aspect of patient activity that can be visualized. Biofeedback is one arena that would lend itself well to the flexibility of virtual reality, allowing the visualization of pain-linked physiological signals. This could be particularly useful for children who may not be as adept as adults at verbally describing sensory information, or translating verbal instruction into action. An example is described in a recent pilot study mentioned above, where non-immersive VR mirror visual feedback was used in combination with biofeedback to treat pediatric patients with chronic headaches [56].

In VR, patients can also be embodied in novel avatars, or avatars that do not conform to the limitations of their physical bodies [57,58]. As discussed above, Jäncke et al. propose that children may be more susceptible than adults to developing a feeling of presence in virtual environments, even in novel avatar bodies [59]. Thus, as with virtual environments, the experience of embodiment in an avatar, especially an avatar that is dissimilar to a child's real body must be contextualized. Debriefing post-VR may be necessary.

4. Practical Aspects of Virtual Reality: Hardware and Software

Clinicians looking to integrate virtual reality into their practice may benefit from the following information about the strengths and limitations of current consumer VR set-ups.

At a minimum, virtual reality requires a display in which the user sees the virtual environment. In the most common consumer systems, this is done through a head-mounted display (HMD). An HMD is a type of VR headset that displays digital images on two screens in front of the user's eyes. In phone-based VR systems such as Gear VR, Google Cardboard or Google Daydream, the HMD consists of a smartphone wrapped in an inexpensive case with lenses, such that the phone provides both the computing power and display. In more powerful VR systems, such as the Oculus Rift or HTC Vive, the content displayed on the headset is generated by a desktop or laptop computer certified as "VR ready" by the manufacturer, or, in the case of PlayStation, by a video game console. In all of these systems, the user's movements are tracked, and the system updates the content that is displayed to the user based on these tracked movements. Thus, as a child turns her head when looking around a virtual environment through an HMD, the content updates on the screens in front of her eyes, just as it would in the physical world if she turned her head to look at a different part of the room. Brief descriptions of some currently available consumer systems are found in Table 3.

4.1. Tracking Movement

Tracking users' movements while they experience VR is a key factor in creating realistic and compelling scenarios [1]. Two kinds of tracking are used in VR: orientation and position. Orientation, shown in Figure 1, tracks the user's head movements and allows her to gaze around her virtual environment.

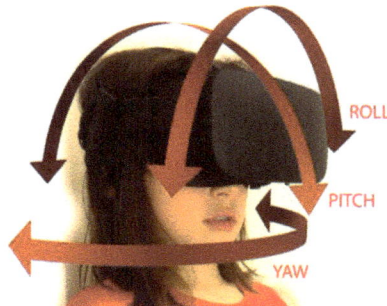

Figure 1. The child may move her head in pitch orientation, as in nodding her head, in yaw orientation, as in moving her head from side to side to look around the environment, or in roll orientation, as in touching her ear to her shoulder.

In VR systems that only have orientation, users are unable to move through scenes using their own body movement (i.e., walking). Instead, users might navigate through virtual environments using gaze, touchpad input or other less-embodied navigation techniques. Currently, smartphone-based devices tend to track only head orientation. While these systems are more limited in some respects, they are generally portable and self-contained, and require very little set-up time or space to use. They are also lighter, cheaper and potentially easier to clean and/or have disposable components, all of which may provide significant advantages when using them for pediatric patients.

In addition to orientation tracking, systems can also have positional tracking (e.g., moving forwards or backwards in VR). Position, shown in Figure 2, tracks the user's body and allows him to relocate within his environment. If the user holds hand trackers, his or her hands will also be tracked. This allows the user to interact with objects in the environment using his or her hands, and optionally see his or her hands represented by an avatar's hands. Positional tracking typically uses external sensors placed around a room that capture the position of the headset and/or additional tracked objects. Such systems allow users to walk around in the virtual space.

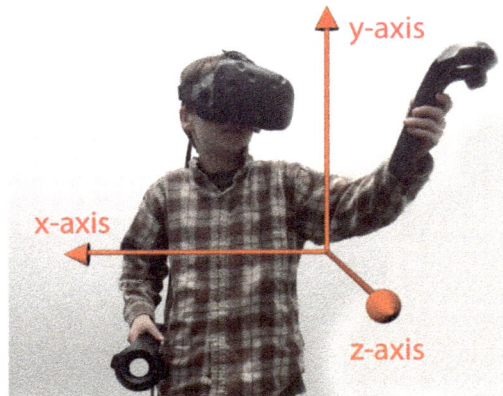

Figure 2. Virtual Reality (VR) coordinate system. In this picture, movement in the *y*-axis corresponds to moving up and down, movement in the *x*-axis corresponds to moving left and right, and movement in the *z*-axis corresponds to moving forward and backward. While global positional coordinates may vary according to set up, *y* is the up–down direction and the *z*-axis will often reflect movement towards the monitor of the desktop computer.

While they increase the level of interaction available, systems with sophisticated tracking capabilities that include hand trackers tend to be more expensive than those that only capture orientation. While still portable to an extent, more complex systems also require sufficient space for patients to safely move around, and the headsets may be heavier. They will also require more set-up time.

4.2. Hardware Issues to Consider for Children

Although consumer headsets are designed to be adjustable, they can be too heavy or too large to be easily used by smaller children, as Dahlquist, et al. speculate in their 2009 study [41]. An additional issue for hospital use is that headsets, along with hand-tracking devices, which come into close contact with users' bodies, will need to be cleaned.

These issues and more can be easily addressed through modular additions and adaptations to the basic VR unit, which would allow the technology to be effective in a wide range of clinical situations. Some consumer systems have washable covers to protect the parts of the headset that come into contact with patients' skin. Cleansing wipes can also be used on both trackers and sensors. In a 2014 study on a patient who had burn wounds on his head, a consumer HMD was mounted to an articulated arm so that the patient did not actually need to wear the device [9]. Very young children may also need the unfamiliar equipment to be decorated or disguised to be more appealing. As one of the authors has found, by introducing an HMD as a mask with a soft cover designed with a friendly face, children were more open to wearing the virtual reality equipment [60]. If trends in lightness, portability, and decreased price continue, VR systems are likely to become increasingly better adapted for pediatric patients.

Table 3. Virtual Reality (VR) head-mounted display (HMD) hardware. This table provides a non-exhaustive list of hardware

Product Name	Pricing for Headset at Time of Publication	Product Information	Description	Appropriate Ages	Limitations	Tracking
Head and Hand Tracking						
HTC Vive	$799	https://www.vive.com/us/	HMD & hand trackers, whole-room VR	(minimum 7+)	Requires "VR ready" personal computer (PC)	Positional and rotational
Oculus Rift &Touch Controllers	$599.98	https://www.oculus.com/rift/	HMD & hand trackers, can be set up on a desktop	13+	Requires "VR ready" PC	Positional and rotational
PlayStation VR	$499	https://www.playstation.com/en-us/explore/playstation-vr/	Video game console HMD and hand trackers	12+	Requires Sony PS4, compatible only with PlayStation games	Positional and rotational
Head Tracking						
Google Cardboard	$5 and up	https://vr.google.com/cardboard/	Phone-based	Unspecified; with adult supervision (single use <5–10 min)	No hand tracking; limited interactivity; requires VR-compatible phone	Rotational
Google Daydream	$79	https://vr.google.com/daydream/	Phone-based; lightweight; includes controller	13+	Currently limited software library; requires VR-compatible phone	Rotational with one controller
Gear VR	$129.99	https://www.oculus.com/gear-vr/	Phone-based, adjustable headset with hand controller	13+	Limited features compared to PC-based VR; requires VR-compatible phone	Rotational

4.3. Virtual Content

Researchers seeking virtual content have three options. They may use existing free or inexpensive consumer content. They may develop their own content. Finally, they may work with industry partners focused on the clinical use of virtual reality. The following section lists some resources available at press time.

Free or pre-existing games designed for virtual reality are becoming increasingly available and may be an appropriate option, particularly for procedural pain. Such games can be purchased and downloaded; for example, through the Steam and Oculus libraries. Another type of frequently free virtual content is 360° videos, which can be downloaded directly to the device. Some main content libraries are currently YouTube360, Within, Jaunt, NYTVR, Condition One, WSJ, and LifeVR [61]. Most content in these libraries consists of 360° videos, which allow for orientation tracking without much interaction. Finally, social interactions in a virtual space can be facilitated using social platforms such as Facebook Spaces, High Fidelity, AltSpaceVR, etc.

Virtual content can be also created for specific clinical purposes using development platforms such as Unity3D (unity3d.com), Unreal (unreal.com) and Vizard (vizard.com). Researchers seeking to create customized content, which might include those investigating rehabilitation or neurorehabilitation, may require specialized tracking and rendering or customization. Such researchers might consider collaborating with university departments, for example computer science, information science, or communication departments, or work with existing software companies. Recording one's own immersive video is also an option. Cameras ranging in complexity and price from the hundreds to thousands of dollars allow researchers to record their own video content and prepare it for viewing through a phone-based HMD.

Finally, there is increasing commercial interest in supplying clinicians with virtual reality applications. While it is outside the scope of this paper to recommend specific companies, searching for "virtual reality therapy" online will provide a list of suppliers. In addition, it is possible to make some recommendations for clinicians to take into consideration when working with a supplier. If patient data is collected as part of treatment, it may raise confidentiality issues. Developers should have experience working in a clinical setting. Compatibility with hardware should also be considered, as some application developers use proprietary hardware, while others allow the use of consumer systems. A brief list of currently available free games can be found in Table 4, below.

Table 4. Suggestions for VR games and their applications.

Game Title	Hardware Compatibility	Where to Find It	Potential Applications	Qualities
Google Earth VR	-HTC Vive -Oculus Rift	https://vr.google.com/earth/	-Anxiety -Distraction therapy -Procedural pain	-Hands-free -Cinematic -Engaging
Minecraft	-HTC Vive -Oculus Rift -Samsung -GearVR -Google -Cardboard	1. Install PC version of Minecraft 2. Install Vivecraft (http://www.vivecraft.org/) for VR compatibility	-Anxiety -Distraction therapy	-Controller required -Well-known by kids -Engaging
Guided Meditation VR	-HTC Vive -Oculus Rift -Samsung -GearVR	https://guidedmeditationvr.com/download/	-Anxiety -Distraction therapy -Procedural pain	-Hands Free -Calming
The Lab	-HTC Vive -Oculus Rift	http://store.steampowered.com/app/450390/The_Lab/	-Anxiety -Distraction therapy	-Exploration -Specific movements (archery + slingshot) -Scenic
The Blu	-HTC Vive -Oculus Rift	http://store.steampowered.com/app/451520/theBlu/	-Anxiety -Distraction therapy	-Hands-free -Cinematic -Exploration

While more research is necessary to determine the more complex aspects of VR in pediatric care, VR can be used immediately to improve the quality of life for pediatric patients. A clinician may order one of the above-mentioned devices to be kept in the clinic and made available to patients who require one of the procedures described earlier in this review. For example, a child might be given a headset and immersed in a relaxing forest scene while they are receiving an immunization or IV placement. Alternatively, a child requiring frequent dressing changes, or other painful procedures may choose to purchase a unit for home use to assist with pain management. A patient with chronic pain may find it beneficial to use VR interventions to temporarily alleviate symptoms, or to assist in performing challenging tasks while in physical or occupational therapy. The number of applications is unlimited, and can be adapted to the individual child's interests and the clinical therapeutic need.

5. Conclusions

In summary, VR is a promising new technology that offers unique opportunities to modulate the experience of pain. These opportunities include the management of acute and procedural pain and familiarizing children with future procedures via simulation. In addition, extrapolating from current evidence in adults, we propose that virtual reality may assist in the treatment of pediatric chronic pain via neuromodulation, as well as physical therapy.

Given the reduction in cost and increased ease of access, we hope that clinicians will be encouraged to explore the potential of this new modality. While the immediate adoption of VR can already engage and entertain children in a clinical setting with potential therapeutic benefits, continued study of the applications and efficacy of virtual reality in the treatment of pediatric pain is needed to better understand the impact upon quality of life for pediatric patients.

Acknowledgments: Andrea Stevenson Won's research was supported by a gift from the MAYDAY Fund through Program Officer Christina M. Spellman. Jakki O. Bailey was funded by the Sesame Workshop Dissertation Award.

Conflicts of Interest: The authors declare no conflict of interest.

References

1. Cummings, J.J.; Bailenson, J.N. How immersive is enough? A meta-analysis of the effect of immersive technology on user presence. *Media Psychol.* **2016**, *19*, 272–309. [CrossRef]
2. Hoffman, H.G.; Doctor, J.N.; Patterson, D.R.; Carrougher, G.J.; Furness, T.A., III. Virtual reality as an adjunctive pain control during burn wound care in adolescent patients. *Pain* **2000**, *85*, 305–309. [CrossRef]
3. Human Photonics Laboratory. Available online: www.Vrpain.com (accessed on 7 March 2017).
4. Schmitt, Y.S.; Hoffman, H.G.; Blough, D.K.; Patterson, D.R.; Jensen, M.P.; Soltani, M.; Carrougher, G.J.; Nakamura, D.; Sharar, S.R. A randomized, controlled trial of immersive virtual reality analgesia, during physical therapy for pediatric burns. *Burns* **2011**, *37*, 61–68. [CrossRef] [PubMed]
5. Jeffs, D.; Dorman, D.; Brown, S.; Files, A.; Graves, T.; Kirk, E.; Meredith-Neve, S.; Sanders, J.; White, B.; Swearingen, C.J. Effect of virtual reality on adolescent pain during burn wound care. *J. Burn Care Res.* **2014**, *35*, 395–408. [CrossRef] [PubMed]
6. Brown, N.J.; Kimble, R.M.; Rodger, S.; Ware, R.S.; Cuttle, L. Play and heal: Randomized controlled trial of Ditto™ intervention efficacy on improving re-epithelialization in pediatric burns. *Burns* **2014**, *40*, 204–213. [CrossRef] [PubMed]
7. Miller, K.; Rodger, S.; Bucolo, S.; Greer, R.; Kimble, R.M. Multi-modal distraction. Using technology to combat pain in young children with burn injuries. *Burns* **2010**, *36*, 647–658. [CrossRef] [PubMed]
8. Pardesi, O.; Fuzaylov, G. Pain management in pediatric burn patients: Review of recent literature and future directions. *J. Burn Care Res.* **2017**. [CrossRef] [PubMed]
9. Hoffman, H.G.; Meyer, W.J., III; Ramirez, M.; Roberts, L.; Seibel, E.J.; Atzori, B.; Sharar, S.R.; Patterson, D.R. Feasibility of articulated arm mounted Oculus Rift Virtual Reality goggles for adjunctive pain control during occupational therapy in pediatric burn patients. *Cyberpsychol. Behav. Soc. Netw.* **2014**, *17*, 397–401. [CrossRef] [PubMed]
10. Gold, J.I.; Kim, S.H.; Kant, A.J.; Joseph, M.H.; Rizzo, A.S. Effectiveness of virtual reality for pediatric pain distraction during IV placement. *CyberPsychol. Behav.* **2006**, *9*, 207–212. [CrossRef] [PubMed]
11. Wong, D.L.; Baker, C.M. Pain in children: comparison of assessment scales. *Pediatr. Nurs.* **1988**, *14*, 9–17. [PubMed]

12. Nilsson, S.; Finnström, B.; Kokinsky, E.; Enskär, K. The use of virtual reality for needle-related procedural pain and distress in children and adolescents in a paediatric oncology unit. *Eur. J. Oncol. Nurs.* **2009**, *13*, 102–109. [CrossRef] [PubMed]

13. He, H.G.; Zhu, L.; Chan, S.W.C.; Liam, J.L.W.; Li, H.C.W.; Ko, S.S.; Klainin-Yobas, P.; Wang, W. Therapeutic play intervention on children's perioperative anxiety, negative emotional manifestation and postoperative pain: A randomized controlled trial. *J. Adv. Nurs.* **2015**, *71*, 1032–1043. [CrossRef] [PubMed]

14. Shahrbanian, S.; Ma, X.; Aghaei, N.; Korner-Bitensky, N.; Moshiri, K.; Simmonds, M.J. Use of virtual reality (immersive vs. non immersive) for pain management in children and adults: A systematic review of evidence from randomized controlled trials. *Eur. J. Exp. Biol.* **2012**, *2*, 1408–1422.

15. Ramachandran, V.S.; Rogers-Ramachandran, D. Synaesthesia in phantom limbs induced with mirrors. *Proc. Biol. Sci.* **1996**, *263*, 377–386. [CrossRef] [PubMed]

16. McCabe, C.; Haigh, R.; Ring, E.; Halligan, P.; Wall, P.; Blake, D. A controlled pilot study of the utility of mirror visual feedback in the treatment of complex regional pain syndrome (type 1). *Rheumatology* **2003**, *42*, 97–101. [CrossRef] [PubMed]

17. Sato, K.; Fukumori, S.; Matsusaki, T.; Maruo, T.; Ishikawa, S.; Nishie, H.; Takata, K.; Mizuhara, H.; Mizobuchi, S.; Nakatsuka, H. Nonimmersive virtual reality mirror visual feedback therapy and its application for the treatment of complex regional pain syndrome: An open-label pilot study. *Pain Med.* **2010**, *11*, 622–629. [CrossRef] [PubMed]

18. Harvie, D.S.; Broecker, M.; Smith, R.T.; Meulders, A.; Madden, V.J.; Moseley, G.L. Bogus visual feedback alters onset of movement-evoked pain in people with neck pain. *Psychol. Sci.* **2015**, *26*, 385–392. [CrossRef] [PubMed]

19. Chen, K.B.; Sesto, M.E.; Ponto, K.; Leonard, J.; Mason, A.; Vanderheiden, G.; Williams, J.; Radwin, R.G. Use of virtual reality feedback for patients with chronic neck pain and kinesiophobia. *IEEE Trans. Neural Syst. Rehabil. Eng.* **2016**. [CrossRef] [PubMed]

20. Won, A.S.; Tataru, C.A.; Cojocaru, C.M.; Krane, E.J.; Bailenson, J.N.; Niswonger, S.; Golianu, B. Two virtual reality pilot studies for the treatment of pediatric CRPS. *Pain Med.* **2015**, *16*, 1644–1647. [CrossRef] [PubMed]

21. Lebel, A.; Becerra, L.; Wallin, D.; Moulton, E.; Morris, S.; Pendse, G.; Jasciewicz, J.; Stein, M.; Aiello-Lammens, M.; Grant, E. fMRI reveals distinct CNS processing during symptomatic and recovered complex regional pain syndrome in children. *Brain* **2008**, *131*, 1854–1879. [CrossRef] [PubMed]

22. Becerra, L.; Sava, S.; Simons, L.E.; Drosos, A.M.; Sethna, N.; Berde, C.; Lebel, A.A.; Borsook, D. Intrinsic brain networks normalize with treatment in pediatric complex regional pain syndrome. *NeuroImage Clin.* **2014**, *6*, 347–369. [CrossRef] [PubMed]

23. Simons, L.; Pielech, M.; Erpelding, N.; Linnman, C.; Moulton, E.; Sava, S.; Lebel, A.; Serrano, P.; Sethna, N.; Berde, C. The responsive amygdala: Treatment-induced alterations in functional connectivity in pediatric complex regional pain syndrome. *Pain* **2014**, *155*, 1727–1742. [CrossRef] [PubMed]

24. Makin, T.R.; Scholz, J.; Henderson Slater, D.; Johansen-Berg, H.; Tracey, I. Reassessing cortical reorganization in the primary sensorimotor cortex following arm amputation. *Brain* **2015**, *138*, 2140–2146. [CrossRef] [PubMed]

25. Walz, A.D.; Usichenko, T.; Moseley, G.L.; Lotze, M. Graded motor imagery and the impact on pain processing in a case of CRPS. *Clin. J. Pain* **2013**, *29*, 276–279. [CrossRef] [PubMed]

26. Wang, M.; Reid, D. Virtual reality in pediatric neurorehabilitation: Attention deficit hyperactivity disorder, autism and cerebral palsy. *Neuroepidemiology* **2011**, *36*, 2–18. [CrossRef] [PubMed]

27. Weiss, P.L.; Tirosh, E.; Fehlings, D. Role of virtual reality for cerebral palsy management. *J. Child Neurol.* **2014**, *29*, 1119–1124. [CrossRef] [PubMed]

28. Biffi, E.; Beretta, E.; Cesareo, A.; Maghini, C.; Turconi, A.C.; Reni, G.; Strazzer, S. An immersive virtual reality platform to enhance walking ability of children with acquired brain injuries. *Methods Inf. Med.* **2017**, *56*, 119–126. [CrossRef] [PubMed]

29. Meyns, P.; Pans, L.; Plasmans, K.; Heyrman, L.; Desloovere, K.; Molenaers, G. The Effect of additional virtual reality training on balance in children with cerebral palsy after lower limb surgery: A feasibility study. *Games Health J.* **2017**, *6*, 39–48. [CrossRef] [PubMed]

30. Trost, Z.; Zielke, M.; Guck, A.; Nowlin, L.; Zakhidov, D.; France, C.R.; Keefe, F. The promise and challenge of virtual gaming technologies for chronic pain: The case of graded exposure for low back pain. *Pain Manag.* **2015**, *5*, 197–206. [CrossRef] [PubMed]

31. Collado-Mateo, D.; Dominguez-Muñoz, F.J.; Adsuar, J.C.; Merellano-Navarro, E.; Gusi, N. Exergames for women with fibromyalgia: A randomised controlled trial to evaluate the effects on mobility skills, balance and fear of falling. *PeerJ* **2017**, *5*, e3211. [CrossRef] [PubMed]

32. Senkowski, D.; Heinz, A. Chronic pain and distorted body image: Implications for multisensory feedback interventions. *Neurosci. Biobehav. Rev.* **2016**, *69*, 252–259. [CrossRef] [PubMed]

33. Simons, L.E.; Kaczynski, K.J. The Fear Avoidance model of chronic pain: Examination for pediatric application. *J. Pain* **2012**, *13*, 827–835. [CrossRef] [PubMed]

34. Pekyavas, N.O.; Ergun, N. Comparison of virtual reality exergaming and home exercise programs in patients with subacromial impingement syndrome and scapular dyskinesis: Short term effect. *Acta Orthop. Traumatol. Turc.* **2017**, in press. [CrossRef] [PubMed]

35. Odell, S.; Logan, D.E. Pediatric pain management: The multidisciplinary approach. *J. Pain Res.* **2013**, *6*, 785–790. [CrossRef] [PubMed]

36. Shiri, S.; Feintuch, U.; Weiss, N.; Pustilnik, A.; Geffen, T.; Kay, B.; Meiner, Z.; Berger, I. A virtual reality system combined with biofeedback for treating pediatric chronic headache—A pilot study. *Pain Med.* **2013**, *14*, 621–627. [CrossRef] [PubMed]

37. Soltani, M.; Teeley, A.M.; Wiechman, S.A.; JENSEN, M.P.; SHARAR, S.R.; Patterson, D.R. Virtual reality hypnosis for pain control in a patient with gluteal hidradenitis: A case report. *Contemp. Hypn. Integr. Ther.* **2011**, *28*, 142–147.

38. Lombard, M.; Ditton, T. At the heart of it all: The concept of presence. *J. Comput. Med. Commun.* **1997**, *3*. [CrossRef]

39. Wiederhold, B.K.; Jang, D.; Kaneda, M.; Cabral, I.; Lurie, Y.; May, T.; Kim, I.; Wiederhold, M.D.; Kim, S. An investigation into physiological responses in virtual environments: an objective measurement of presence. In *Towards Cyberpsychology: Mind, Cognitions and Society in the Internet Age*; Riva, G., Galimberti, C., Eds.; IOS Press: Amsterdam, 2001; pp. 176–182.

40. Sanchez-Vives, M.V.; Slater, M. From presence to consciousness through virtual reality. *Nat. Rev. Neurosci.* **2005**, *6*, 332–339. [CrossRef] [PubMed]

41. Dahlquist, L.M.; Weiss, K.E.; Clendaniel, L.D.; Law, E.F.; Ackerman, C.S.; McKenna, K.D. Effects of videogame distraction using a virtual reality type head-mounted display helmet on cold pressor pain in children. *J. Pediatr. Psychol.* **2009**, *34*, 574–584. [CrossRef] [PubMed]

42. Law, E.F.; Dahlquist, L.M.; Sil, S.; Weiss, K.E.; Herbert, L.J.; Wohlheiter, K.; Horn, S.B. Videogame distraction using virtual reality technology for children experiencing cold pressor pain: The role of cognitive processing. *J. Pediatr. Psychol.* **2011**, *36*, 84–94. [CrossRef] [PubMed]

43. Sharar, S.R.; Carrougher, G.J.; Nakamura, D.; Hoffman, H.G.; Blough, D.K.; Patterson, D.R. Factors influencing the efficacy of virtual reality distraction analgesia during postburn physical therapy: Preliminary results from 3 ongoing studies. *Arch. Phys. Med. Rehabil.* **2007**, *88*, S43–S49. [CrossRef] [PubMed]

44. Baumgartner, T.; Speck, D.; Wettstein, D.; Masnari, O.; Beeli, G.; Jäncke, L. Feeling present in arousing virtual reality worlds: Prefrontal brain regions differentially orchestrate presence experience in adults and children. *Front. Hum. Neurosci.* **2008**, *2*, 8. [CrossRef] [PubMed]

45. Flavell, J.H.; Flavell, E.R.; Green, F.L.; Korfmacher, J.E. Do young children think of television images as pictures or real objects? *J. Broadcast. Electron. Media* **1990**, *34*, 399–419. [CrossRef]

46. Richert, R.A.; Robb, M.B.; Smith, E.I. Media as social partners: The social nature of young children's learning from screen media. *Child Dev.* **2011**, *82*, 82–95. [CrossRef] [PubMed]

47. Dahlquist, L.M.; McKenna, K.D.; Jones, K.K.; Dillinger, L.; Weiss, K.E.; Ackerman, C.S. Active and passive distraction using a head-mounted display helmet: Effects on cold pressor pain in children. *Health Psychol.* **2007**, *26*, 794–801. [CrossRef] [PubMed]

48. Bryanton, C.; Bosse, J.; Brien, M.; Mclean, J.; McCormick, A.; Sveistrup, H. Feasibility, motivation, and selective motor control: Virtual reality compared to conventional home exercise in children with cerebral palsy. *Cyberpsychol. Behav.* **2006**, *9*, 123–128. [CrossRef] [PubMed]

49. Olson, C.K. Children's motivations for video game play in the context of normal development. *Rev. Gener. Psychol.* **2010**, *14*, 180. [CrossRef]

50. Blakemore, S.-J.; Mills, K.L. Is adolescence a sensitive period for sociocultural processing? *Annu. Rev. Psychol.* **2014**, *65*, 187–207. [CrossRef] [PubMed]

51. Claxton, L.J.; Ponto, K.C. Understanding the properties of interactive televised characters. *J. Appl. Dev. Psychol.* **2013**, *34*, 57–62. [CrossRef]
52. Forgeron, P.A.; King, S.; Stinson, J.N.; McGrath, P.J.; MacDonald, A.J.; Chambers, C.T. Social functioning and peer relationships in children and adolescents with chronic pain: A systematic review. *Pain Res. Manag.* **2010**, *15*, 27–41. [CrossRef] [PubMed]
53. Beals, L.; Bers, M.U. A developmental lens for designing virtual worlds for children and youth. *Int. J. Learn. Media* **2009**, 51–65. [CrossRef]
54. Ni, L.T.; Fehlings, D.; Biddiss, E. Design and evaluation of virtual reality-based therapy games with dual focus on therapeutic relevance and user experience for children with cerebral palsy. *Games Health J.* **2014**, *3*, 162–171. [CrossRef] [PubMed]
55. Schneider, S.M.; Workman, M. Effects of virtual reality on symptom distress in children receiving chemotherapy. *CyberPsychol. Behav.* **1999**, *2*, 125–134. [CrossRef] [PubMed]
56. Li, H.C.W.; Lopez, V.; Lee, T.L.I. Effects of preoperative therapeutic play on outcomes of school-age children undergoing day surgery. *Res. Nurs. Health* **2007**, *30*, 320–332.
57. Fox, J.; Bailenson, J.N.; Tricase, L. The embodiment of sexualized virtual selves: The Proteus effect and experiences of self-objectification via avatars. *Comput. Hum. Behav.* **2013**, *29*, 930–938. [CrossRef]
58. Yee, N.; Bailenson, J. The Proteus effect: The effect of transformed self-representation on behavior. *Hum. Commun. Res.* **2007**, *33*, 271–290. [CrossRef]
59. Jäncke, L.; Cheetham, M.; Baumgartner, T. Virtual reality and the role of the prefrontal cortex in adults and children. *Front. Neurosci.* **2009**, *3*, 6. [CrossRef] [PubMed]
60. Bailey, J.O.; Bailenson, J.N.; Obradović, J.; Aguiar, N.R. The influence of Immersive virtual reality on children's inhibitory control and social behavior. Presented at the International Communication's 67th Annual Conference, San Diego, CA, USA, 25–29 May 2017.
61. Rasmussen, N.B. Top 10 Most Viewed 360° Videos of 2016. *Time*, 26 July 2016.

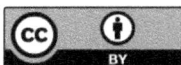

© 2017 by the authors. Licensee MDPI, Basel, Switzerland. This article is an open access article distributed under the terms and conditions of the Creative Commons Attribution (CC BY) license (http://creativecommons.org/licenses/by/4.0/).

MDPI AG

St. Alban-Anlage 66

4052 Basel, Switzerland

Tel. +41 61 683 77 34

Fax +41 61 302 89 18

http://www.mdpi.com

Children Editorial Office

E-mail: children@mdpi.com

http://www.mdpi.com/journal/children

www.ingramcontent.com/pod-product-compliance
Lightning Source LLC
Chambersburg PA
CBHW051855210326
41597CB00033B/5912